American Cancer Society's

COMPLETE GUIDE TO
COLORECTAL
CANCER

Books published by the American Cancer Society

A Breast Cancer Journey: Your Personal Guidebook, Second Edition

American Cancer Society Consumers Guide to Cancer Drugs, Second Edition, Wilkes and Ades

American Cancer Society's Complementary and Alternative Cancer Methods Handbook

American Cancer Society's Complete Guide to Prostate Cancer, Bostwick et al.

American Cancer Society's Guide to Pain Control: Understanding and Managing Cancer Pain, Revised Edition

Angels & Monsters: A child's eye view of cancer, Murray and Howard

Because...Someone I Love Has Cancer: Kids' Activity Book

Cancer in the Family: Helping Children Cope with a Parent's Illness, Heiney et al.

Cancer: What Causes It, What Doesn't

Caregiving: A Step-By-Step Resource for Caring for the Person with Cancer at Home, Revised Edition, Houts and Bucher

Coming to Terms with Cancer: A Glossary of Cancer-Related Terms, Laughlin

Couples Confronting Cancer: Keeping Your Relationship Strong, Fincannon and Bruss

Crossing Divides: A Couple's Story of Cancer, Hope, and Hiking Montana's Continental Divide, Bischke

Eating Well, Staying Well During and After Cancer, Bloch et al.

Good for You! Reducing Your Risk of Developing Cancer

Healthy Me: A Read-along Coloring & Activity Book, Hawthorne (illustrated by Blyth)

Informed Decisions: The Complete Book of Cancer Diagnosis, Treatment, and Recovery, Second Edition, Eyre, Lange, and Morris

Kicking Butts: Quit Smoking and Take Charge of Your Health

Lymphedema: Understanding and Managing Lymphedema After Cancer Treatment

Our Mom Has Cancer, Ackermann and Ackermann

When the Focus Is on Care: Palliative Care and Cancer, Foley et al.

Also by the American Cancer Society

American Cancer Society's Healthy Eating Cookbook: A celebration of food, friends, and healthy living, Third Edition

Celebrate! Healthy Entertaining for Any Occasion

Kids' First Cookbook: Delicious-Nutritious Treats to Make Yourself!

American Cancer Society's

COMPLETE GUIDE TO
COLORECTAL
CANCER

FOREWORD BY
KATIE COURIC

Edited by

Bernard Levin, MD
Terri Ades, MS, APRN, AOCN
Durado Brooks, MD, MPH
Christopher H. Crane, MD
Paulo M. Hoff, MD, FACP
Paul J. Limburg, MD, MPH
David A. Rothenberger, MD

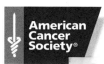

Published by
American Cancer Society
Health Promotions
1599 Clifton Road NE
Atlanta, Georgia 30329, USA

Printed in the United States of America
Designed by Shock Design Inc, Atlanta, GA and Jill Dible Design, Atlanta, GA
Cover designed by Shock Design, Inc. Atlanta, Georgia

5 4 3 2 1   05 06 07 08 09

Library of Congress Cataloging-in-Publication Data

Levin, Bernard, 1924-
     [Complete guide to colorectal cancer]
     American Cancer Society's complete guide to colorectal cancer / by
Bernard Levin, Terri B. Ades, Durado Brooks. -- Rev. ed.
        p. cm.
     Includes bibliographical references and index.
     ISBN 0-944235-55-7
     1. Colon (Anatomy)--Cancer.   2. Rectum--Cancer.   I. Ades, Terri
B. II. Brooks, Durado.   III. American Cancer Society.   IV. Title.
     RC280.C6L46 2006
     616.99'4347--dc22

                                                            2005024711

A Note to the Reader

The information contained in this book is not intended as medical advice and should not be relied upon as a substitute for talking with your doctor. This information may not address all possible actions, treatments, medications, precautions, side effects, or interactions. All matters regarding your health require the supervision of a medical doctor or appropriate health care professional who is familiar with your medical needs. For more information, contact your

American Cancer Society's

COMPLETE GUIDE TO
COLORECTAL
CANCER

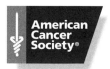

Advisory Panel and Medical Review

Terri Ades, MS, APRN, AOCN
Director of Cancer Information, American Cancer Society, Atlanta, GA

Durado Brooks, MD, MPH
Director, Prostate and Colorectal Cancer, American Cancer Society, Atlanta, GA

John M. Dorso
Volunteer, American Cancer Society, *Member,* United Ostomy Association,
and *Colorectal Cancer Survivor*, Marietta, GA

Ted Gansler, MD
Director of Medical Strategy, American Cancer Society, Atlanta, GA

Amy E. Kelly
Co-founder and *Director,* Colon Cancer Alliance, New York, NY

John S. Macdonald, MD
Professor of Medicine, Medical Director, and *Chief,* Gastrointestinal Oncology Service,
St. Vincent's Comprehensive Cancer Center, New York, NY

Bruce D. Minsky, MD
Professor and *Vice Chairman,* Department of Radiation Oncology,
Memorial Sloan-Kettering Cancer Center, New York, NY

Joel E. Tepper, MD
Professor and *Chair,* Clinical Research, Radiation Oncology, University of North Carolina
Chapel Hill School of Medicine and Lineberger Comprehensive Cancer Center, Chapel Hill, NC

Copyeditor
Rodney Atkins

Editor
Amy Brittain

Managing Editor
Gianna Marsella, MA

Book Publishing Manager
Candace Magee

Book Publishing Director
Len Boswell

Strategic Director, Content
Chuck Westbrook

*We would like to thank the many people who generously shared their
personal experiences with colorectal cancer with us.*

Brief Contents

CONTENTS

CHAPTER 6
Understanding Your Prognosis

CHAPTER 7
Coping With Your Diagnosis

CHAPTER 8
Making the Medical System Work for You

CHAPTER 13
Clinical Trials and Emerging Therapies 209

CHAPTER 14
Complementary and Alternative Medicine 221

CHAPTER 15
Strategies for Coping With Symptoms and Side Effects 237

FOREWORD

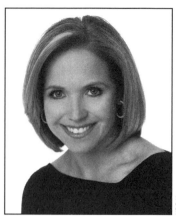

Katie Couric

WHEN I FIRST STARTED AS CO-ANCHOR of the TODAY show 15 years ago, I was concentrating on my family and my career, which were both exceeding my wildest expectations. At the center of that happy little world were my husband, Jay Monahan, and our two beautiful daughters, Ellie and Carrie.

How Colorectal Cancer Changed My Life

In 1997, Jay was 41 years old and seemed to be in perfect health. He was tired, but after all, we had two little girls and he was traveling a lot for his work as a lawyer and legal commentator on TV. He had lost some weight, but who isn't happy to shed a few pounds? He had a sour stomach and always had a roll of antacids in his pocket…but really, nothing seemed out of the ordinary.

Then one morning I got a call at my office: Jay was doubled over with severe abdominal pain. We went quickly to my internist; like so many men his age, Jay didn't really have a doctor he went to on a regular basis. Within a few hours our lives were turned upside down. We learned that Jay had a tumor the size of an orange that was almost completely blocking his colon. Even worse, the cancer had spread.

Jay underwent chemotherapy, radiation, and surgery, enduring cancer's terrible toll with courage, grace, and even a sense of humor. He lost his valiant battle with the disease nine months later.

Raising Awareness to Increase Screening and Early Detection

After Jay's death, I was determined to spare other families of the same terrible experience. If only we could have detected the cancer earlier, Jay's life might have been saved. I didn't want others to die of lack of knowledge or embarrassment. I was desperate to bring colorectal cancer out of the closet—to get people talking and get people screened. Public awareness and education is vital to prevention when it comes to this disease.

My NBC colleagues were enormously supportive, and we began a regular, annual multi-part series designed to demystify the disease. I had a colonoscopy that was broadcast on the TODAY show. After the segment aired, the number of colonoscopies nationwide jumped twenty percent—a development medical researchers have dubbed the "Couric Effect." I'm so proud of that increase which, I'm happy to report, has been sustained over time.

So we've made some real headway on the awareness front, but more than half of the people for whom testing is recommended still aren't getting checked. If you are reading this and have not yet been screened, please talk to your doctor to find out more and to arrange appropriate testing. If you're living with a diagnosis of colorectal cancer, please talk to your friends and loved ones about getting screened. Heck, talk to your coworkers and neighbors and the teller at the bank and the cashier at the grocery store and everyone else you can think of about getting screened. You may very well save their lives.

How This Book Can Help

When we first found out about Jay's diagnosis, we quickly realized how much we had to learn about colorectal cancer and the many decisions we would have to make—finding a doctor, undergoing tests, choosing the right treatment, telling our family (including our young children) about Jay's cancer, and getting the physicians and other health care professionals to work together as a team. The process of gathering all the necessary information and running around New York City from one doctor's office to another was exhausting and overwhelming. We needed a place to go for reliable, unbiased information. We longed to feel comforted and supported. We wanted to feel confident that we were making the best decisions for Jay and our family.

These days, I often find myself wishing that I had known then what I know now. Not only about screening and early detection, but about the resources that are available to help people facing colorectal cancer.

The American Cancer Society provides a wealth of information and services to educate, comfort, and support people with colorectal cancer and their families. This book is one example of the many ways they can help.

Whether you've been diagnosed with colorectal cancer or simply want to learn more about the disease, *American Cancer Society's Complete Guide to Colorectal Cancer* is a wonderful resource. Written in plain language with clear explanations, this book will help you understand and cope with the disease, find quality care, and make the best treatment decisions for your situation. Think of it as a helpful conversation with a doctor you trust—a doctor with a comforting bedside manner who really "knows his stuff."

The information in this book represents the latest research and state-of-the-art treatments for colorectal cancer, gathered together in one place and distilled by the leading experts in the field. The support and resources it provides are invaluable. I hope this book can help you as you face colorectal cancer. Good health and good wishes.

PREFACE

Bernard Levin, MD

Advancements in Colorectal Cancer

SO MUCH HAS CHANGED IN THE FIELD OF COLORECTAL CANCER in the past few years, making it a particularly appropriate time for the American Cancer Society to publish this book. Much new knowledge has emerged recently from basic science laboratories about how colorectal cancer develops. New information about genetics has given us a better understanding of how colorectal cancer is inherited, and has also provided more opportunities for early detection. Similarly, many exciting advances have occurred in prevention, screening, and treatment. The medical community has also come to realize the value and importance of informing and educating our patients and their family members about this disease. Increased awareness has led to a wider network of support and resources for people with colorectal cancer and their families

All of these factors have led to an encouraging decline in the incidence and mortality of colorectal cancer over the last decade. And each of these critical advances directly affects the day-to-day care we provide our patients at every stage of their colorectal cancer experience:

- *Prevention*: supporting positive lifestyle changes like improved diet, increased physical activity, and avoidance of tobacco, as well as the need for genetic counseling and testing in those with a family history of the disease.
- *Early detection*: following the American Cancer Society's recommended screening guidelines.
- *Treatment*: helping patients to better understand their treatment options, providing state-of-the-art care, and following up through recovery or advanced disease.
- *Quality of life*: effectively managing side effects and controlling pain, acknowledging the emotional and psychological impact of the disease, and supporting patients, their loved ones, and caregivers.

Why We Wrote This Book

We know that the nearly 150,000 people newly diagnosed with colorectal cancer each year in the United States want and need reliable, trustworthy information from the experts on a broad range of colorectal cancer topics. We also know that for this information to be helpful, it has to be understandable. *American Cancer Society's Complete Guide to Colorectal Cancer* was designed to be comprehensive and useful, but not overwhelming. This book provides up-to-date, essential information about the disease, its prevention and treatment, and the many resources that are available for people with colorectal cancer as well as their loved ones and caregivers.

If you are reading this book to learn more about colorectal cancer in general, we hope that it will convince you of the need to be regularly screened for colorectal polyps and cancer after the age of 50–earlier if you have a family history of the disease. If you or a loved one have been diagnosed with colorectal cancer, we hope this book will educate you about the disease and help you face the many challenges that cancer can pose.

Acknowledgements

I have many to thank who have contributed to this book. Gianna Marsella, Managing Editor for Books at the American Cancer Society, has been extraordinarily conscientious and effective in nurturing and leading this project from its inception.

My coeditors Terri B. Ades, Durado Brooks, Christopher H. Crane, Paulo M. Hoff, Paul J. Limburg, and David A. Rothenberger deserve special praise—without their hard work, patience, and wisdom this book would not have appeared.

I am also very grateful to the many chapter authors and colorectal cancer survivors who enthusiastically joined in this effort.

On behalf of the American Cancer Society and the many participants in this book project, I am appreciative of Katie Couric for her willingness to write the Foreword. Her unswerving personal commitment to increasing public knowledge about colorectal cancer, enhancing wider acceptance of screening, and supporting innovative research through the National Colorectal Cancer Research Alliance is admirable and unequalled.

INTRODUCTION

COLORECTAL CANCER IS THE THIRD MOST COMMON CANCER found in men and women in this country. Yet many people are embarrassed to talk to their doctor or family members about their risk of colorectal cancer, or don't know what to ask once they've been diagnosed. This book can help start the dialogue.

Who This Book Is For

You may be reading this book as a person interested in learning how you can reduce your risk of developing colorectal cancer, or you may be facing the challenges that accompany a colorectal cancer diagnosis. This book is a step-by-step guide through the physical and emotional aspects of the colorectal cancer experience, from testing for colorectal cancer to diagnosis to thinking about the future. It explores the experiences and challenges you're likely to face, provides important information and practical advice, and offers emotional support so that you can make the best decisions possible *for your unique situation.*

There is no "right way" to make decisions about cancer, and this book doesn't assume a single solution is best. Each person faces a diagnosis of colon or rectal cancer in an individual way. Each person's cancer is different, and the way cancer affects a person's body is unique. Some people with colorectal cancer choose to play an active role in their treatment decisions; others rely more heavily on their cancer care team to guide them through the decision-making process. Whatever choices you make, *American Cancer Society's Complete Guide to Colorectal Cancer* will help you through your experience with colorectal cancer.

What This Book Is About

American Cancer Society's Complete Guide to Colorectal Cancer takes a helpful, matter-of-fact approach to risk factors and prevention, diagnosis, treatment options, and coping with the disease. Written by experts in cancer screening, oncology, nursing, research, and patient care and services, this up-to-date, evidence-based text explores every aspect of colorectal cancer, including:

- what colorectal cancer is, who gets it, and why
- screening tests and how colorectal cancer is diagnosed
- treatment options for different types and stages of colorectal cancer
- managing side effects, including caring for a colostomy
- coping with emotional issues and practical matters such as work, insurance, and money
- the role of family, relationships, and support groups during and after cancer

It also includes insights from real people with colorectal cancer, lists of suggested questions to ask your health care team, and valuable resources to help you cope and move forward with your treatment, recovery, and life after colorectal cancer. There's even a chapter written especially for loved ones and caregivers of someone with colorectal cancer.

How This Book Is Organized

American Cancer Society's Complete Guide to Colorectal Cancer will walk you through the issues and details most important to you at different times during your colorectal cancer experience. You may find it most helpful to read the chapters in consecutive order, considering each phase from beginning to end and anticipating future issues. Or you may want to read only the chapter (or chapters) most applicable to your current experience.

The chapters in Section I explore the nature of colorectal cancer, the terminology and concepts used by medical professionals, who is at risk for the disease, and what people can do to prevent colorectal cancer.

In Section II, we'll look at diagnostic tests and the initial colorectal cancer evaluation, with a special focus on helping you understand what the test results and pathology reports mean for your particular situation.

Section III guides you through coping with your diagnosis, building your health care team, and navigating the sometimes complicated medical system to ensure you get the best care possible.

Section VI is all about treatment options: which ones are available and how to make an informed decision about what course of treatment to pursue. In addition to discussing surgery, radiation therapy, and chemotherapy, we also cover emerging therapies, clinical trials, and complementary and alternative methods to ensure that you'll be aware of all your options before deciding on a treatment plan.

The chapters in Section V guide you through the treatment process, with a focus on coping with symptoms and side effects. A chapter on living with a colostomy provides practical tips and is also a good introduction to the topic for those whose surgery may involve an ostomy. Other practical issues, such as balancing work and managing insurance and finances, are also discussed.

Life after treatment is discussed in Section VI, including maintaining your health and pursuing follow-up care as well as facing the possibility of recurrence. Ideas for making the most of life after cancer are also provided.

Finally, Section VII is devoted to helping family members, friends, and caregivers know what to do and how to cope when a loved one has colorectal cancer. You may want to share this chapter with those people most closely involved in your care.

The Resources section in the back of the book lists resources that may be helpful to people with colorectal cancer and their loved ones. It includes a directory of American Cancer Society resources, colorectal cancer organizations, cancer information sources, patient and family services, Internet sources and information. The Glossary offers definitions of terms you are likely to encounter as you learn about colorectal cancer. Cross-references within the book will refer you to additional sections where a topic is addressed.

A Note About Colon Cancer and Rectal Cancer

Colon and rectal cancer are sometimes discussed separately because they have somewhat different prognoses, diagnostic approaches, and treatment regimens. However, they both arise from the same type of cell, they have the same screening tests, and they have an overlapping set of symptoms that lead to their diagnosis. Therefore, they will often be referred to as the same disease, and termed colorectal cancer in this book, unless otherwise noted.

About the American Cancer Society

Represented in more than 3400 communities throughout the United States, Guam, and Puerto Rico, the American Cancer Society is a nonprofit health organization dedicated to eliminating cancer as a major health problem. Its mission is to save lives and diminish suffering from cancer through research, education, advocacy, and service.

The American Cancer Society is the largest private source of cancer research dollars in the United States. Founded in 1913 by ten physicians and five concerned members of the community, the organization now has over two million volunteers.

The Society's Efforts in the Fight Against Colorectal Cancer

In the past 90 years, there have been a handful of significant opportunities for the American Cancer Society to save lives and reduce the impact cancer has on human lives. For example, in the 1960s, the Society undertook an aggressive campaign to encourage the use of the Pap test among women and healthcare providers, and since then, cervical cancer death rates have decreased by 70 percent. Today, the Society is taking the lead in efforts to reduce the number of Americans who get and die from colorectal cancer. The opportunity to save lives from colorectal cancer is so great that the American Cancer Society has identified colorectal cancer as its top priority for the immediate future.

This book is one example of the American Cancer Society's broad commitment to helping those concerned about or diagnosed with colorectal cancer. *American Cancer Society's Complete Guide to Colorectal Cancer* will help you explore the issues ahead and educate you about your options. Being informed and empowered to make knowledgeable decisions about your care will help you better understand and meet the challenge of colorectal cancer.

For additional information, support, or referrals to resources in your community, please call the American Cancer Society at 800-ACS-2345/800-227-2345 to find out what we can do for you.

How Much Do You Know About Colorectal Cancer?

How many of these common colorectal cancer myths have you heard or believed? Take a look at the truth behind the myths, below.

1. **Colorectal cancer only affects older people.**

   FALSE. *Although more than 90 percent of cases are diagnosed in people older than 50 years, colorectal cancer can develop in younger people too—even those with no known risk factors and no family history of the disease.*

2. **The rate of new diagnoses of colorectal cancer is increasing at an alarming rate.**

   FALSE. *The rate of new colorectal cancer diagnoses has actually decreased in the last 20 years in the general population.*

3. **Men get colorectal cancer much more often than women.**

   FALSE. *Colorectal cancer affects men and women nearly equally, and it is the second leading cause of cancer death for both men and women in the United States.*

4. **People cannot control their risk of getting colorectal cancer.**

   FALSE. *Colorectal cancer is one of the most preventable types of cancer. Physical inactivity, poor diet, obesity, smoking, and alcohol use are all colorectal cancer risk factors that people can change and control. In addition, colorectal cancer screening tests often find precancerous growths (called polyps); removing these can help prevent cancer.*

5. **If you don't have symptoms, you don't have colorectal cancer.**

   FALSE. *In its early stages, colorectal cancer often causes no symptoms. Symptoms often don't appear until the disease has become more advanced. Common symptoms that may develop include rectal bleeding, a change in bowel habits, a feeling of needing to have a bowel movement that is not relieved by doing so, abdominal pain, weight loss or loss of appetite, or weakness and fatigue.*

6. **Hispanics/Latinos are more likely than other ethnic groups to develop colorectal cancer.**

   FALSE. *Hispanics/Latinos have some of the lowest colorectal cancer incidence rates. However, despite these lower rates of diagnosis, colorectal cancer is the second leading cause of cancer death among Hispanic/Latino men and women. African Americans and Ashkenazi Jews appear to have the highest rates of colorectal cancer.*

7. **A diagnosis of colorectal cancer is like a death sentence.**

   FALSE. *When colorectal cancer is detected early, it has a 90 percent survival rate. And because colorectal cancer often progresses slowly, people have time to treat the disease before it advances.*

8. **Because colorectal cancer is a common disease, most people are already screened by their doctors.**

   FALSE. *Despite recommendations, many Americans are not currently screened for colorectal cancer. In fact, only about half of the population at risk for colorectal cancer is regularly screened for the disease.*

9. **Most colorectal cancers are due to inherited or genetic factors.**

   FALSE. *Fewer than 10 percent of colorectal cancers are caused by inherited gene mutations. Having benign colon polyps or a family history of colorectal cancer is linked to increased risk, but most cases occur in people whose primary risk factor is being over the age of 50.*

CHAPTER ONE

OVERVIEW OF COLORECTAL CANCER

Dennis Ahnen, MD
Aaron C. Baltz, MD

How much do you know about colorectal cancer? Take this quick true-or-false quiz (on facing page) to test your colorectal cancer IQ.

The fact is that many Americans don't know much about colorectal cancer, even though it is the third most common cancer and second leading cause of cancer death in both men and women in the United States. For example, only one in three adults age 50 and older knows that he or she is at risk for the disease.

This lack of awareness may exist because many people feel embarrassed or uncomfortable talking about the disease, especially because of the body parts it involves. An American Cancer Society survey

> *"Part of our fear with colorectal cancer is the fear of embarrassment. Our society doesn't talk about bladder and colon problems—like these are dirty words and not part of our normal body constitution."*
>
> —KRIS

found that colorectal cancer actually tops politics and religion as a topic Americans are most uncomfortable talking about with someone they just met.

1

The Profile of Colorectal Cancer in the United States

Cancer is the leading cause of death in Americans younger than age 85. Colorectal cancer accounts for approximately 10 percent of all new cancer diagnoses and deaths each year. This year alone, more than 140,000 Americans are expected to be diagnosed with colorectal cancer, and an estimated 56,000 will die.

An average American man has an approximate 1 in 17 chance of developing colorectal cancer at some time in his life, and an average American woman has an approximate 1 in 18 chance (an approximate 5 to 6 percent chance). Overall, men and women have an approximate 1 in 45 (2.25 percent) chance of dying from the disease. But not everyone is at the same risk of developing colorectal cancer. (The risk factors for colorectal cancer are discussed in greater detail in chapter 2.) If colorectal cancer is found and treated at an early stage, the five-year survival rate exceeds 90 percent, yet fewer than four of every ten colorectal cancers are detected at this early stage.

The good news is that the death rate from colorectal cancer is declining in the United States. Overall death rates have been decreasing in women since the 1950s and in men since the 1980s. This progress is thought to be due in part to earlier detection (see chapter 3), advancements in therapy (see chapters 10 through 14), and people taking preventive steps such as eating healthier diets (see chapter 2), leading to an improved survival rate for patients diagnosed with colorectal cancer.

The rate of new colorectal cancer diagnoses has also decreased in the general population over the last 20 years. It is likely that screening for and removing colon polyps before they can develop into cancer has contributed to this decline. These encouraging trends suggest that with a better informed public, increased use of screening tests by primary care physicians, and wider availability of state-of-the-art treatment approaches, we will continue to see a decline in the toll that colorectal cancer can take.

Now that you know a little bit about who colorectal cancer affects and how often it strikes, let's talk about the disease itself: what it is and how it develops.

About the Digestive System

The human body is made of different systems that perform unique and critical functions to keep it in a state of balance. To understand colorectal cancer, it is

Figure 1.1 The Digestive System

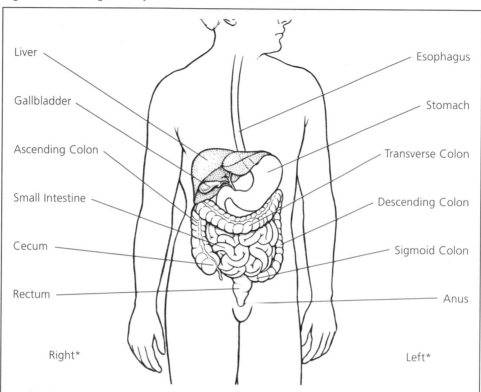

Liver

Gallbladder

Ascending Colon

Small Intestine

Cecum

Rectum

Right*

Esophagus

Stomach

Transverse Colon

Descending Colon

Sigmoid Colon

Anus

Left*

* When doctors talk about the right and left colon, these directions refer to the sides of the patient's body as the patient would identify them, not the right and left side a doctor sees when facing the patient or that you see when looking at a picture of the human body.

important to know a little bit about the digestive system, which includes the colon and rectum.

The digestive system (also called the gastrointestinal, or GI, system) carries out the important tasks of digesting food, absorbing nutrients and water, and eliminating solid waste.

The first part of the digestive system is often referred to as the upper GI tract. Digestion of food begins in the mouth, where chewing breaks food down into smaller pieces. Pieces of food are then swallowed and travel down the esophagus into the stomach, where food is mixed with acid and stored until its release into the small intestine. (The small intestine is called "small" because of its diameter, not its length. At about 20 feet long, it is the longest segment of the digestive system.)

The contents of the stomach are gradually emptied into the first part of the small intestine (duodenum). In the duodenum, digestive juices from the pancreas and bile from the liver and gall bladder are added to the intestinal contents. By the time the contents have passed through the small intestine, the body has absorbed almost all of the fat, protein, and carbohydrates. The remaining contents are mostly liquid.

About one and a half quarts of liquid empty from the small intestine into the large intestine each day. The large intestine absorbs water and electrolytes (minerals such as sodium, potassium, calcium, and magnesium) and converts the liquid intestinal contents into formed stool. The large intestine is about six feet long and is composed of two major parts: the colon and the rectum.

The colon is divided into multiple segments (see Figure 1.1 on page 3). The first part of the large intestine is called the cecum. The cecum is located in the lower right part of the abdomen and is attached to the appendix. The next sections of the colon are named for their position in the abdomen: the ascending colon extends upward from the cecum, the transverse colon crosses the upper abdomen from right to left, and the descending colon extends down to the left lower abdomen and connects to the sigmoid colon, which typically has an "S"-shaped turn. The final part of the large intestine is called the rectum. Stool is stored in the rectum until it is evacuated through the anus during a bowel movement.

When doctors talk about the "proximal" portion of the colon, they mean the area where it *begins* near the stomach, whereas the "distal" portion is the junction with the anus, or the *end*.

What Is Cancer?

Cancer is not the same disease in every part of the body. Each type of cancer has its own unique characteristics. Although there are many kinds of cancer, they all start when cells begin to grow in an uncontrolled manner.

Normally, cells grow, divide, and die in an orderly fashion. But cancer cells continue to grow and divide, forming new abnormal cells.

What Is Colorectal Cancer and How Does It Develop?

Colorectal cancer is cancer that develops in the colon or the rectum. The wall of the colon and rectum is made up of several layers of tissue (see Figure 1.2).

Figure 1.2 Cross Section of the Digestive Tract

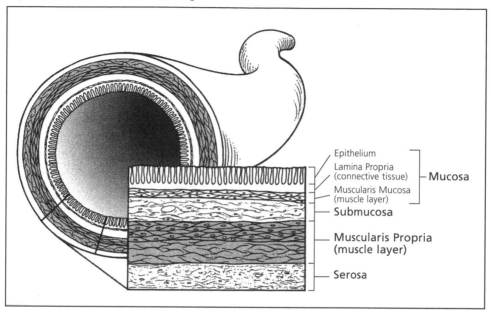

Colorectal cancer starts in the innermost layer and can extend through some or all of the other layers.

The walls of the digestive tract have four layers of tissue: mucosa, submucosa, muscularis propria, and serosa. The innermost layer is the mucosa, a tissue layer that forms a continuous lining of the gastrointestinal tract from the mouth to the anus. In the large bowel, this tissue layer contains cells that produce mucus to lubricate and protect the smooth inner surface of the bowel wall. Connective tissue and muscle separate the mucosa from the second layer, the submucosa, which contains vessels and nerves. Next to the submucosa is the muscularis propria, consisting of two layers of muscle fibers—one that runs lengthwise and one that encircles the bowel. The fourth layer, the serosa, is a thin membrane that produces fluid to lubricate the outer surface of the colon so that it can slide against the organs and structures that surround it. (In the rectum, the muscular layer is surrounded mostly by fat.)

The layer of cells that lines the inner surface of the colon and rectum is a part of the mucosa and is called the epithelium. Almost all cancers of the colon and rectum arise from the epithelial cell layer. Epithelial cells are continuously exposed to substances that pass through or are produced by the digestive system.

These substances include a broad variety of ingested foods and chemicals, as well as abundant bacteria, viruses, bile acids, and enzymes. Scientists believe that these colonic contents contain carcinogens (substances that can lead to an increased risk of cancer development) and also contain chemopreventive agents (substances that may protect against cancer).

> "It surprises me the ignorance there is about cancer. A gentleman that I know is a college graduate—very articulate, very intelligent— and when I was telling him that I had colon cancer, his comment to me, with just a totally puzzled look on his face, was, 'How did you catch cancer?' I was speechless. I just looked at him and said, 'You can't CATCH cancer.'"
>
> —JACY

Colorectal cancer usually begins as a non-cancerous (or benign) polyp. A polyp is simply a growth that develops on the lining of the colon or rectum. When cancer forms within a polyp, it can eventually grow through the lining and into the wall of the colon or rectum. Once there, the cancer cells may extend into the circulatory system, which can then carry cancer cells to more distant parts of the body. The process of cancer spreading to other body sites is called metastasis.

The Role of Polyps

Some polyps are precancerous and will grow into malignancies if not removed. Others pose less risk; they will remain benign even if left alone. Some examples of colon polyps are shown in Figure 1.3.

Figure 1.3 Colon Polyps

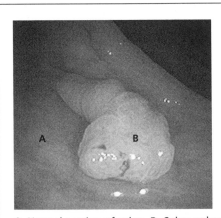 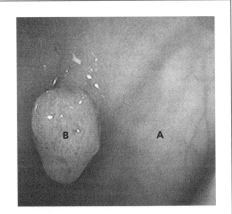

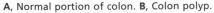
A, Normal portion of colon. **B,** Colon polyp.

Images courtesy of Dennis Ahnen, MD.

There are several types of polyps. Inflammatory polyps are not precancerous. For the most part, neither are hyperplastic polyps. (Recently, however, scientists have discovered that some hyperplastic polyps may be precancerous, particularly if they grow in the right side of the colon or are detected in multiple family members).

Adenomatous polyps, or adenomas, are the most likely to become cancers. Adenomas, growths formed from glandular tissue, are common. They are found in approximately one third of the general US population by age 50, and approximately half the population will develop one or more adenomas by age 70.

Adenomas start from a single cell and typically grow slowly, but over time they can grow to be larger than an inch. The risk of cancer within an adenoma increases as the size of the adenoma increases. Not all adenomas grow into cancer. In fact, fewer than 10 percent of adenomas become cancerous.

Adenocarcinomas are the cancerous counterpart of adenomas. They grow from the glandular cells that line the inside layer of the wall of the colon and rectum. The progression from normal epithelial cells in the colon or rectum to adenomas/ adenomatous polyps to adenocarcinoma (cancer) is illustrated in Figure 1.4. Because more than 95 percent of colorectal cancers are adenocarcinomas, we focus on this type of colorectal cancer in this book.

Figure 1.4 The Adenoma-Carcinoma Sequence

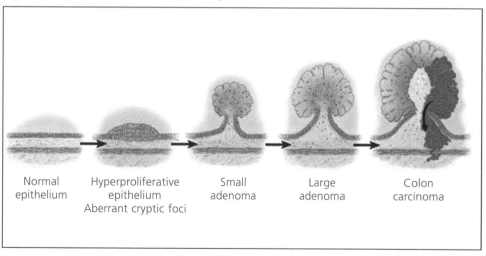

| Normal epithelium | Hyperproliferative epithelium Aberrant cryptic foci | Small adenoma | Large adenoma | Colon carcinoma |

Types of Adenomatous Polyps

There are two major types of adenomatous polyps:
- Tubular adenomas are the most common type found in the colon and rectum. They get their name from the round or tubular appearance of the glands in the polyp.
- Villous adenomas are so named because their glands have a villous, or frond-like, appearance under the microscope.

Some adenomas contain both tubular and villous features and are called tubulovillous adenomas. Villous and tubulovillous adenomas are less common than tubular adenomas, but they are more likely to give rise to cancer than tubular adenomas.

Where Do Colorectal Cancers Arise?

Cancer can arise in any part of the colon or rectum (see Figure 1.5). About 25 to 30 percent of all colorectal cancers are located in the rectum. Another 20 to 25 percent occur in the S-shaped sigmoid colon, 15 to 20 percent arise in the cecum (the beginning of the large intestine, where it attaches to the small intestine), and the remainder are relatively evenly distributed across the other segments of the colon.

Figure 1.5 Cancer Occurrence in Different Parts of the Colorectum

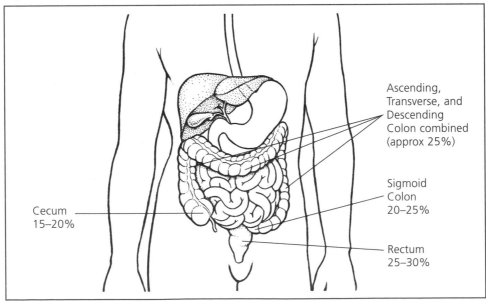

How Long Does It Take for Colorectal Cancer to Develop?

In most people, colorectal cancers develop slowly over a period of several years. It is thought that the progression from normal epithelial cells to cancer takes, on average, 10 to 20 years. Because it takes such a long time for a small adenoma to develop into an adenocarcinoma, colorectal cancer is a highly preventable disease.

The Importance of Screening and Early Detection

Once a benign adenoma is removed from the body, it will never have the chance to develop into a cancer. Scientists estimate that with regular screening and removal of colorectal polyps, a person's lifetime risk of dying from colorectal cancer can be reduced by up to 80 percent. In addition, when colorectal cancer is detected early, it is highly curable.

Finding and removing benign adenomas is important, and there are many different ways to effectively screen for colorectal polyps and cancers. These methods are discussed in detail in chapter 3.

Why Does Colorectal Cancer Develop?

Cancer cells are thought to develop because of damage to DNA, the genetic material in every cell that directs its activities. People can inherit damaged DNA, which accounts for hereditary cancers. Many times, though, a person's DNA becomes damaged by exposure to something in the environment, such as smoking or carcinogens in the diet. Cancer may also be caused by a combination of factors. We'll talk more about why people get colorectal cancer in the next chapter.

CHAPTER TWO

RISK FACTORS AND PREVENTION

Amy S. Oxentenko, MD, Esther K. Wei, ScD
Paul J. Limburg, MD, MPH, and Edward Giovannucci, MD, ScD

The complex way that cancer develops makes it difficult to predict exactly who will get colorectal cancer and who will not. Fortunately, colorectal cancer is one of the most widely studied cancers, and researchers have identified many risk factors for the disease. A risk factor is anything that increases your chance of getting a disease, such as cancer. (Some factors actually *reduce* the risk of colorectal cancer, and therefore *not having enough* of one of them is considered a risk factor). While having many risk factors puts you at increased risk, it does not guarantee that you will get colorectal cancer—just as having very few risk factors does not guarantee that you will avoid developing it.

Some risk factors can be affected by changes in lifestyle. For example, you can lower your risk of developing colorectal cancer (as well as the risk of other cancers) by improving your diet, increasing your physical activity, not smoking, and limiting your use of alcohol. Preventing a chronic disease from developing, whenever possible, is preferable to treating it once it has appeared.

Other risk factors, such as family history and age, are not controllable. Learning about their role in the development of colorectal cancer, however, can help ensure that you seek appropriate tests (sometimes called screening; see chapter 3), which can help detect the disease at an earlier, more treatable stage.

Sometimes, people mistakenly think certain factors put them at great risk or offer substantial protection, but these factors actually have relatively little effect on their likelihood of getting colorectal cancer. Gender is a good example of this. A general misconception about colorectal cancer is that it is a man's disease, that it affects men much more frequently than women. However, the lifetime risk of developing colorectal cancer is similar for both men and women in the United States: approximately 1 in 17 for men and 1 in 18 for women.

> "The life lesson I learned from being diagnosed with colon cancer is even if you have no family history of cancer, have always been healthy, are not overweight, ate a healthy diet, and don't smoke, you can still get cancer."
> —JENNIFER

Age

Colorectal cancer, like most cancers, is rare in people younger than 40. The occurrence of colorectal cancer starts to increase after age 40 and becomes increasingly common with advancing age. In fact, more than 90 percent of all colorectal cancer diagnoses happen after age 50, making age the primary risk factor for colorectal cancer. Table 2.1 shows the probability of developing colorectal cancer for men and women at various ages.

Race and Ethnicity

No racial or ethnic group is spared from colorectal cancer, although some groups seem to be at lower risk of developing the disease (incidence) and dying from it (mortality). For example, colorectal cancer rates are lowest for Hispanics, while African Americans—both men and women—have the highest incidence and mortality rate (see Table 2.2 on page 14). Jews of Eastern European descent (Ashkenazi Jews) also have unusually high rates of colorectal cancer.

Survival statistics also differ by race. For example, the five-year survival rate (the number of individuals who survive five years after a colorectal cancer diagnosis) is lower among African Americans than whites (see Table 2.3 on page 14). This is in part because African Americans tend to be diagnosed with colorectal cancer (and other cancers) at later stages than whites; however, even when diagnosed with the same stage of disease, African Americans tend to have lower five-year survival rates than whites. (See Table 2.4 on page 15, which classifies cancer by

Table 2.1 Probability of Developing Colorectal Cancer for United States Men and Women, 1999–2001

Men

Age (years)	Percent	Risk (approximate)
20–29	.01	1 in 8312
30–39	.06	1 in 1802
40–49	.21	1 in 474
50–59	.71	1 in 140
60–69	1.69	1 in 59
70–79	2.75	1 in 36
Lifetime	5.90	1 in 17

Women

Age (years)	Percent	Risk (approximate)
20–29	.01	1 in 8228
30–39	.05	1 in 1999
40–49	.19	1 in 535
50–59	.51	1 in 195
60–69	1.20	1 in 84
70–79	2.09	1 in 48
Lifetime	5.54	1 in 18

Data from: DEVCAN: Probability of Developing or Dying of Cancer Software, Version 5.3. Statistical Research and Applications Branch, National Cancer Institute, 2004. http://srab.cancer.gov/devcan
Source: American Cancer Society, Surveillance Research, 2005.

whether it is contained locally or if it has spread to nearby tissues or more distant areas of the body; see chapter 5 for a more detailed explanation of staging).

Among whites, both the occurrence of and death caused by colorectal cancer have steadily decreased since 1985; African Americans, however, have not experienced such a decline over time. The reasons for these racial and ethnic differences are unclear and need to be studied further to better establish the underlying causes.

Your Health History

Two aspects of a person's health history affect his or her risk of developing colorectal cancer: personal health history and family health history. First we'll explore the

Table 2.2 Colorectal Cancer Incidence and Mortality Rates* by Race/Ethnicity and Sex, 1997–2001

	Incidence		Mortality	
Race/Ethnicity	Male	Female	Male	Female
African Americans	72.9	56.5	34.3	24.5
Whites	63.1	45.9	24.8	17.1
Asian Americans/Pacific Islanders	56.3	38.6	15.8	10.8
Hispanics/Latinos	49.6	32.5	18.0	11.6
American Indians/Alaska Natives	38.3	32.7	17.1	11.7
All Races/Ethnicities	63.4	46.4	25.3	17.7

Per 100,000, age-adjusted to the 2000 US Standard Population

Data from: Surveillance, Epidemiology and End Results (SEER) program (www.seer.gov) SEER Stat Database: Incidence—SEER 9 Registries (1973–2001), SEER 11 Registries plus Alaska Public-Use, Nov 2003 Sub for Expanded Races (1992–2001), National Cancer Institute, DCCPS, Surveillance Research Program, Cancer Statistics Branch, Released April 2004, based on the November 2003 submission.

Source: American Cancer Society, Colorectal Cancer Facts and Figures, Special Ed., 2005. Atlanta, GA: American Cancer Society; 2005:3.

Table 2.3 Five-Year Colorectal Cancer-Specific Survival and Age-Adjusted Relative Risk of Colorectal Cancer Deaths by Race/Ethnicity and Sex, 1992–2000.

	Cause-Specific Survival*		Adjusted Relative Risk[†] (95% CI[‡]) of Deaths	
Race/Ethnicity	Male	Female	Male	Female
Non-Hispanic whites	64.0	63.4	1.00	1.00
Hispanics/Latino whites	60.9	61.3	1.05 (0.99–1.11)	1.05 (0.99–1.11)
African Americans	56.1	57.0	1.26 (1.20–1.32)	1.18 (1.13–1.23)
Asian Americans/Pacific Islanders	66.7	68.2	0.95 (0.90–1.00)	0.90 (0.85–0.96)
American Indians/Alaska Natives	62.3	58.2	1.14 (0.95–1.35)	1.38 (1.16–1.64)

Cause-specific survival rates are the probability of not dying of colorectal cancer within 5 years after the date of diagnosis. They do not account for stage and age at diagnosis.
[†]Relative risk estimates that controlled for age and tumor stage at diagnosis were calculated to compare probability of death from colorectal cancer within 5 years after diagnosis between racial/ethnic groups.
[‡]95% confidence intervals represent the range in which we are 95% confident that the true value falls. Wider confidence intervals generally reflect smaller sample sizes.

Data from: Jemal A, Clegg LX, Ward E, et al. Annual report to the nation on the status of cancer, 1975–2001, with a special feature regarding survival, Cancer. Jul 1 2004;101(1):3–27.

Source: American Cancer Society, Colorectal Cancer Facts and Figures, Special Ed., 2005. Atlanta, GA: American Cancer Society; 2005:6.

Table 2.4 Stage at Diagnosis of Colorectal Cancer, by Race and Ethnicity, 1996–2000

Race/Ethnicity	Stage Distribution			
	Local	Regional	Distant	Unstaged
Non-Hispanic whites	38.1	37.8	19.0	5.2
Hispanics/Latino whites	34.9	38.4	21.4	5.3
African Americans	34.5	34.7	23.8	7.0
American Indians/Alaska Natives	34.8	38.7	23.3	3.2
Asian Americans/Pacific Islanders	38.7	39.5	17.2	4.6

Data from: Surveillance, Epidemiology and End Results (SEER) program (www.seer.gov) SEER Stat Database: Incidence—SEER 9 Registries (1973–2001), SEER 11 Registries plus Alaska Public-Use, Nov 2003 Sub for Expanded Races (1992–2001), National Cancer Institute, DCCPS, Surveillance Research Program, Cancer Statistics Branch, Released April 2004, based on the November 2003 submission.

Source: American Cancer Society, Colorectal Cancer Facts and Figures, Special Ed., 2005. Atlanta, GA: American Cancer Society; 2005:5.

illnesses or diseases that might be linked to an increased risk for colorectal cancer. Then we'll look at family health history and the role of genetics in colorectal cancer.

Personal History of Cancer

People who have already been treated for colorectal cancer are at increased risk for developing another colorectal cancer in the future. In addition, some studies have found that people who have been diagnosed with other cancers (such as cancer of the breast or uterus in women) may also be at future increased risk for colorectal cancer.

Personal History of Polyps

Colorectal cancers usually grow slowly, taking many years to progress from normal colorectal cells to cancer. Cancer often starts with a single cell becoming abnormal. This abnormal cell can multiply and grow into polyps. Some of these polyps are benign; left alone, they will not have any serious consequences. However, one group of polyps known as adenomatous polyps contain abnormal cells that multiply and may eventually become cancerous. Polyps are usually diagnosed at a screening test; if a polyp is found during one of these tests, it can be removed during a test called a colonoscopy.

Cancer Disparities

In the past decade there has been increasing awareness of cancer disparities (the unequal burden of cancer on racially and ethnically diverse populations, the poor, and medically underserved populations). Economic, social, and cultural factors, often in combination, can influence individual and community health. (Of course, biological or inherited characteristics play a role, but research suggests that these factors are less important than socioeconomic factors in explaining differences among cancer incidence and mortality among the major racial and ethnic populations in the United States.) For example, low socioeconomic status is linked to lack of access to medical care as well as to increases in risk factors, such as tobacco use and obesity. Social inequities, such as the legacy of racial discrimination in the United States, can still influence the interactions between patients and their doctors. And cultural factors, including language, values, and traditions, can influence health behaviors, beliefs about illness, and approaches to medical care.

Poor, diverse, and medically underserved populations generally have higher risks of developing cancer and poorer chances of early diagnosis, optimal treatment, and survival. Moreover, these groups have not benefited equally from recent improvements in prevention, early detection, and treatment.

Many groups, including the American Cancer Society, are working hard to reduce these inequities. The National Institutes of Health (NIH), National Cancer Institute (NCI), Centers for Disease Control and Prevention (CDC), and other public, private, and nonprofit organizations have recognized the importance of reducing or eliminating disparities in the fight against cancer. See the section on cancer in diverse populations in the Resources section at the end of this book for more information.

If you have had a polyp removed from your colon before, you are no longer at risk of that particular polyp developing into cancer. However, having had an adenomatous polyp means you are more likely to have other polyps in the future. Therefore, people who have had a previous diagnosis of colorectal polyps should be screened carefully and tested more frequently in order to detect and remove any more polyps that may develop.

Personal History of Inflammatory Bowel Disease

Inflammatory bowel disease (IBD) includes ulcerative colitis and Crohn's disease (granulomatous colitis). Persons with either one of these conditions have a much higher risk of developing colorectal cancer compared with persons who do not have these conditions. However, because of the relative rarity of these conditions and the treatment for them (which can involve removing the colon entirely, or in part), only about 1 percent of people with colorectal cancer have a previous history of inflammatory bowel disease. The overall increased risk of colorectal cancer for someone with IBD has been estimated to be 4 to 20 times higher than normal. Having IBD increases one's risk of colorectal cancer. However, the amount of the increase depends on several factors, including how long a person has experienced symptoms and how inflamed the large intestine is.

About half of the people who have inflammatory bowel disease for 25 to 35 years will eventually develop colorectal cancer. People who have either ulcerative colitis or Crohn's disease often need to begin screening at an earlier age and should be screened frequently and carefully for colorectal cancer (see page 36 for more information on screening).

Personal History of Type 2 Diabetes

Type 2 diabetes is a condition characterized by high blood glucose levels caused either by a lack of insulin or the body's inability to use insulin efficiently. (Type 2 diabetes has also been called "adult-onset" diabetes because it generally affects people older than 40. However, type 2 diabetes is being seen in younger people in increasing numbers because of the steep rise in obesity in the United States in the last decade, making the term "adult-onset" less accurate.)

Researchers began to suspect a connection between the causes of colorectal cancer and type 2 diabetes when they studied the similarity in the geographical occurrence of the two diseases. Besides genetic influences, the main risk factors for diabetes include excess body fat (especially when it is concentrated in the abdomen), lack of physical activity, and high intake of calories. These diabetes risk factors are similar to the risk factors for colorectal cancer (see pages 20–25). Having diabetes is associated with an approximate 50 percent increase in risk for colorectal cancer and colorectal polyps. If you have been diagnosed with type 2 diabetes, you should be aware of this increased risk and discuss it with your doctor.

Family History and the Role of Genetics in Colorectal Cancer

People with one or more immediate family members (a parent, sibling, or child) who have been diagnosed with colorectal cancer are at higher risk of developing the disease themselves. The risk increases further if the relatives were diagnosed at an earlier age.

Having immediate family members with other types of cancer (such as uterine or stomach cancer) may also increase the risk of colorectal cancer.

You cannot rewrite your family health history. However, if you do have a family history of colorectal cancer, you can still make changes in your lifestyle to help reduce your risk. We'll discuss how to do this later in this chapter. People with a family history of colorectal cancer should also talk with their doctors about this history and follow special screening guidelines that have been developed specifically for persons with a family history. (Current guidelines state that colorectal cancer screening should generally begin at age 50. However, special guidelines apply to some people who have a family history of colorectal cancer or colorectal adenomas. See chapter 3 for more information on screening.)

> *"Both my parents had been treated for colorectal cancer, which probably put me at higher-than-average risk for the disease. Still, I felt blindsided by the diagnosis and was deeply stunned when told I had cancer in my 30s."*
> —DICK

About 20 percent of all people with colorectal cancer have family members who have also had the disease. Having a family history of colorectal cancer is linked to an increased risk of colorectal cancer because, in some cases, there may be a genetic component to the disease that is passed on and carried through the family.

About 5 percent of people with colorectal cancer have a specific genetic abnormality that causes the cancer. Two familial genetic syndromes that are linked to colorectal cancer are familial adenomatous polyposis (FAP) and hereditary non-polyposis colorectal cancer (HPNCC). Other people who have a family history of colorectal cancer but do not have FAP or HPNCC may have other specific genetic syndromes, but these seem to be less common than FAP or HNPCC.

Familial Adenomatous Polyposis Syndrome

Familial adenomatous polyposis (also called familial polyposis coli or adenomatous polyposis of the colon, but most commonly abbreviated as FAP) is a relatively rare genetic syndrome that accounts for approximately 1 percent of all colorectal cancers. It occurs in 1 of 10,000 births and appears in men and women equally.

FAP is characterized by hundreds to thousands of adenomatous (precancerous) polyps throughout the colon. People with FAP may experience symptoms such as bleeding, abdominal pain, or a change in bowel habits.

Almost all people with FAP will develop colorectal cancer if the condition is left untreated. Most people with FAP will be diagnosed with colorectal adenomas in their early teenage years, with more than 95 percent of people with FAP developing adenomas by their mid-30s. As a result, people with a family history of FAP should be routinely screened for colorectal adenomas starting in their teens. (See chapter 3 for more information on screening.) Genetic testing and counseling may also be helpful (see page 21).

Hereditary Nonpolyposis Colorectal Cancer Syndrome

Hereditary Nonpolyposis Colorectal Cancer (HNPCC), also known as Lynch syndrome, is another form of familial colorectal cancer. HNPCC accounts for approximately 3 to 5 percent of all colorectal cancers, making it the most common form of hereditary colorectal cancer.

For someone with HNPCC, the chance of developing colorectal cancer sometime in his or her lifetime is about 80 percent (as opposed to about 6 percent in the general population). People with HNPCC are also at increased risk for other cancers, such as cancer of the uterus, bile duct, stomach, and urinary tract. If HNPCC is suspected based on a family history of colorectal and other cancers, specific genetic tests can help confirm the diagnosis. (See the feature box on page 21 for more information on genetic testing).

Cancer in people with HNPCC usually develops when they are relatively young (mid-40s), and about two thirds of these cancers occur on the right side of the colon. HNPCC can be more difficult to diagnose than FAP because people with HNPCC typically have far fewer adenomas than those with FAP. However, if adenomas are present in someone with HPNCC, they tend to progress more rapidly. Interestingly, people with HNPCC-related colorectal cancer often have better survival compared with people with colorectal cancer in the general population.

Other Familial Colorectal Cancer Syndromes

Other colorectal cancer syndromes with genetic or inherited components exist, but they occur less often than HNPCC and FAP. These include the following syndromes:

- The hallmarks of Peutz-Jeghers syndrome are polyps in the gastrointestinal tract, dark freckled pigmentation that occurs in and around the mouth and face, and an increased risk of colorectal cancer. About half of the people who develop this syndrome have a family history of Peutz-Jeghers. Genetic testing can isolate the defective gene in about 70 percent of people with a family history of Peutz-Jeghers syndrome.
- Juvenile polyposis is another rare syndrome characterized by excessive growth of polyps throughout the gastrointestinal tract that appear similar to polyps occasionally seen in young children. People with juvenile polyposis have a 40 percent risk of developing colon cancer and a slightly lower risk for rectal cancer. Genetic testing is not currently available for this syndrome, so doctors diagnose the disease based on laboratory studies of the polyps and a thorough family history.
- Other familial colorectal cancer cases have been described in association with various breast cancer syndromes. Certain genes linked to higher rates of breast and ovarian cancers may also be linked to a higher risk of colorectal cancer.

Lifestyle Factors for Risk and Prevention

Lifestyle factors are risk factors that—unlike your genetic profile—you can change and control. They include being overweight, being physically inactive, using alcohol and tobacco, and eating a poor diet.

The evidence is quite strong that not smoking during adolescence and early adulthood, maintaining a healthy weight, and exercising regularly in adulthood can prevent a large number of colorectal cancers. Avoiding excessive alcohol

Table 2.5 Summary of Personal and Familial Health Factors Associated With an Increased Risk of Colorectal Cancer

Personal Health Factors Associated with an Increased (↑) Risk of Colorectal Cancer	Familial Factors Associated with an Increased (↓) Risk of Colorectal Cancer
Personal history of colorectal cancer (and some other cancers)	Family history of colorectal cancer (and some other cancers)
Personal history of adenomatous polyps	Family history of genetic syndromes linked to colorectal cancer (including FAP and HPNCC)
Personal history of IBD	
Personal history of type 2 diabetes	

Genetic Testing

Genetic testing is conducted to see if a person has a certain gene mutation known to increase the risk for a specific disease (such as colorectal cancer) or to confirm a suspected mutation in an individual or family.

If you are concerned about your family history of colorectal or other cancers, you may want to consider genetic testing. The benefits of genetic testing for those at high risk include more certain diagnoses, which can direct family members toward testing if appropriate, and being able to develop a management plan for people known to be predisposed to colorectal cancer before symptoms or cancer develop. The knowledge obtained can also affect family planning decisions.

But genetic testing is not for everyone, so if you decide to move forward, you should receive counseling before genetic testing. Genetic counselors have specialized training to help people understand how families inherit cancers and how genes are transmitted, as well as the types of cancer seen in the family, and a person's estimated risk. Counselors discuss benefits, risks, costs, and limitations of testing and help people decide who in the family should be tested. They also educate those considering genetic testing about the testing process and help people cope with fears about test results, the potential for discrimination, and the risk of disease for children.

A person considering genetic testing should carefully consider the following issues before being tested:

- **Limited answers.** Genetic tests can tell what *might* happen, but not what *will* happen. Tests may be flawed, or results misinterpreted. A positive test result does not necessarily mean a disease will occur. A negative result does not mean you have no risk.

- **Psychological impact.** Learning that you have or might develop a serious disease is frightening. Testing and waiting for results can produce stress and anxiety. Inconclusive results may cause depression or hopelessness. Family members who learn that they have a gene or have passed a gene on to their children may experience guilt and anger.

- **Privacy issues and discrimination.** People with a genetic disorder (or their family members) may be refused health insurance on the basis of their genetic profile. Employers might wrongfully use genetic information to discriminate when making hiring or promotion decisions. The law is not yet settled in this area.

consumption may also reduce the occurrence of some colorectal cancers. These factors influence many other major health-related conditions in addition to colorectal cancer.

Getting screened can also reduce your risk of developing colorectal cancer. See chapter 3 for more information on screening and early detection of colorectal cancer.

Body Weight and Fat Distribution

Energy balance occurs when the food you eat is equivalent to the amount required for you to do the activities of your daily life and maintain your weight. Over time, if you eat more than you require, you will store the excess energy as body fat and you will gain weight. If you eat less than you require, you will burn stored fat and lose weight. The number of calories that you require is determined by many factors, including your age, height, amount of muscle, and how many calories you burn through daily living and exercise. Having a positive energy balance for an extended period of time can lead to excess body weight.

Doctors define "overweight" and "obesity" using a scale called the body mass index (BMI). Your BMI is a ratio of your weight to your height (see Table 2.6). "Overweight" applies to those with a BMI between 25 and 29 and "obese" to those with a BMI of 30 or higher.

Many research studies in this area have found people who have a high BMI are at an increased risk of colorectal cancer. Any additional weight above the healthy range appears to increase your risk of colorectal cancer. Compared with people in the normal weight range, being very obese (having a BMI of 40 or greater) increases your risk of colorectal cancer by approximately 50 percent if you are a woman and by about 80 percent if you are a man. Being overweight also increases the risk for both men and women, but not as markedly.

Some evidence indicates that regardless of your BMI, a tendency to store fat in your abdominal area may increase your risk of colorectal cancer. In addition, adenoma growth over time has been found to be linked to higher levels of body fat and higher BMI.

Excess body weight seems to be a more significant colorectal cancer risk factor for men than for women, but further research is needed to confirm this finding.

Physical Activity

Exercise provides many health benefits, including lowering blood pressure, improving cholesterol measurements, and promoting cardiovascular well being. People who are physically active tend to have a lower risk of colorectal cancer as well.

Table 2.6 Body Mass Index (BMI)

To use the table, find the appropriate height in the left-hand column labeled Height. Move across to a given weight (in pounds). The number at the top of the column is the BMI at that height and weight. (Pounds have been rounded off.) "Overweight" applies to those with a BMI between 25 and 29; "obese" to those with a BMI of 30 and higher.

							Weight in pounds										
BMI	**19**	**20**	**21**	**22**	**23**	**24**	**25**	**26**	**27**	**28**	**29**	**30**	**31**	**32**	**33**	**34**	**35**
Height in inches (feet, inches)							**Overweight**					**Obese**					
58 (4'10")	91	96	100	105	110	115	119	124	129	134	138	143	148	153	158	162	167
59 (4'11")	94	99	104	109	114	119	124	128	133	138	143	148	153	158	163	168	173
60 (5')	97	102	107	112	118	123	128	133	138	143	148	153	158	163	168	174	179
61 (5'1")	100	106	111	116	122	127	132	137	143	148	153	158	164	169	174	180	185
62 (5'2")	104	109	115	120	126	131	136	142	147	153	158	164	169	175	180	186	191
63 (5'3")	107	113	118	124	130	135	141	146	152	158	163	169	175	180	186	191	197
64 (5'4")	110	116	122	128	134	140	145	151	157	163	169	174	180	186	192	197	204
65 (5'5")	114	120	126	132	138	144	150	156	162	168	174	180	186	192	198	204	210
66 (5'6")	118	124	130	136	142	148	155	161	167	173	179	186	192	198	204	210	216
67 (5'7")	121	127	134	140	146	153	159	166	172	178	185	191	198	204	211	217	233
68 (5'8")	125	131	138	144	151	158	164	171	177	184	190	197	203	210	216	223	230
69 (5'9")	128	135	142	149	155	162	169	176	182	189	196	203	209	216	223	230	236
70 (5'10")	132	139	146	153	160	167	174	181	188	195	202	209	216	222	229	236	243
71 (5'11")	136	143	150	157	165	172	179	186	193	200	208	215	222	229	236	243	250
72 (6')	140	147	154	162	169	177	184	191	199	206	213	221	228	235	242	250	258
73 (6'1")	144	151	159	166	174	182	189	197	204	212	219	227	235	242	250	257	265
74 (6'2")	148	155	163	171	179	186	194	202	210	218	225	233	241	249	256	264	272
75 (6'3")	152	160	168	176	184	192	200	208	216	224	232	240	248	256	264	272	279
76 (6'4")	156	164	172	180	189	197	205	213	221	230	238	246	254	263	271	279	287

Data from: the National Heart, Lung, and Blood Institute
Source: http://www.nhlbi.nih.gov/guidelines/obesity/bmi_tbl.htm

Excess Body Weight and Cancer

A frightening two thirds of the US population is considered overweight, and doctors are worried about rising numbers of obese children. In the United States alone, excess body weight contributes to more than 90,000 deaths from cancer each year—about 16 percent of the expected 563,700 deaths from cancer this year.

Maintaining a healthy weight is a good idea for many reasons. It is widely known that obesity increases a person's risk of heart disease, diabetes, arthritis, and high blood pressure, in addition to many different cancers, including cancer of the colon and rectum.

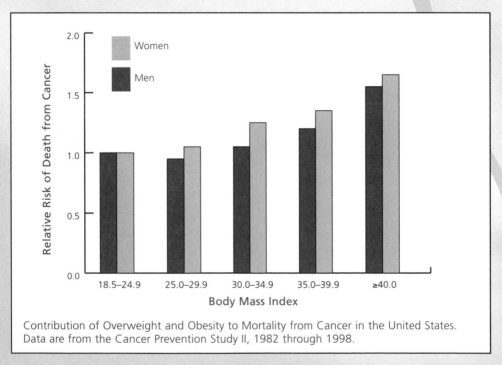

Contribution of Overweight and Obesity to Mortality from Cancer in the United States. Data are from the Cancer Prevention Study II, 1982 through 1998.

A convincing body of research has demonstrated that physical inactivity is a risk factor for colorectal cancer. In addition, people who are physically active appear to have a reduced risk of colorectal polyps, particularly the kind of polyps that are most likely to progress to cancer.

While physical activity may lower colorectal cancer risk, in part by reducing the occurrence of obesity, physical activity may also further lower risk beyond its benefit on BMI. The highest risk of colorectal cancer has been observed among persons who are both physically inactive and who have high BMI.

Overall, studies suggest that while greater risk reductions are possible with higher levels of activity, even moderate levels of physical activity (for example, brisk walking for three to four hours a week) are associated with substantial benefits.

Smoking

In the United States, about one in five colorectal cancer cases in men and about one in eight colorectal cancer cases in women may be due to smoking. Cigarette smokers have about a two- to three-fold increased risk of colorectal polyps. Smoking also increases a person's risk for colorectal cancer; the risk depends directly on the number of cigarettes smoked.

Smoking seems to influence the early stages of the process, when normal cells become cancerous. Therefore, exposure to cigarette smoking early in life can lead to colorectal cancer up to 30 years later. Burning tobacco generates a wide range of toxic compounds that can reach the lining of the colon—perhaps when chemicals in the smoke travel through the blood, when these chemicals become dissolved in saliva that is swallowed, or when smokers unintentionally swallow small quantities of tobacco.

People who quit smoking are still at a slightly increased risk compared with people who have never smoked. Because colorectal cancer can take many years to develop, and because of the increased risk even after quitting, former smokers should make a special effort to get screened. They should also make other lifestyle adjustments that will reduce their risk.

Colorectal cancer is only one of many conditions linked to smoking, including other cancers (including lung, mouth, throat, esophagus, pancreas, cervix, kidney, and bladder) as well as coronary heart disease, chronic lung disease, and stroke. Therefore, all smokers should be encouraged to quit, and children and teens should be strongly encouraged never to start.

Dietary Factors for Risk and Prevention

The complexity of most food substances makes recognizing specific cancer-causing and cancer-fighting dietary factors somewhat challenging. Nonetheless, scientists continue to study dietary factors to see if they might contribute to or help prevent colorectal cancer.

Avoiding red and processed meats and excessive alcohol consumption can probably help reduce your risk of colorectal cancer. Getting enough vitamins and minerals, such as calcium, folate, selenium, and vitamin D, also may be beneficial. Fiber in the diet may not play the important role in colorectal cancer prevention that scientists once thought it did.

While controversy exists regarding the exact role of these specific dietary factors, several studies show that dietary patterns composed of high intakes of red and processed meats, highly refined grains and starches, and sugars are related to a higher risk of colorectal cancer. Thus, replacing these foods with poultry, fish, and plant sources as primary protein sources, monounsaturated and polyunsaturated fats (such as those found in olive oil or canola oil) as primary fat sources, and whole grains, legumes, and fruits as primary carbohydrate sources is likely to lower risk of colorectal cancer.

The overall benefits of a healthful diet are clear, even though scientists are not always sure which specific food or nutrient is responsible, or how.

Dietary Factors Associated With Increased Risk for Colorectal Cancer

There is an important difference between asserting something is *known* to cause colorectal cancer and saying something is *linked to* or *associated with an increased risk* of colorectal cancer. Very few factors—dietary or otherwise—are scientifically proven to have an undeniable cause-effect relationship on cancer. But as our knowledge of diseases such as cancer grows, so does our understanding of which factors may play a role in its development and effects.

Alcohol Consumption

The relationship between alcohol use and colorectal cancer risk has been controversial, but the majority of evidence now indicates that consuming large amounts of alcohol increases a person's risk of colorectal cancer. For example, it appears that people who consume more than two alcoholic beverages a day over a long period of time are at a 24 percent increased risk for colorectal cancer. It is unclear whether drinking fewer than two drinks a day affects a person's risk for colorectal cancer.

Alcohol consumption is also linked to increased risk for cancers of the mouth, throat, esophagus, liver, and, for women, the breast.

Why consuming larger quantities of alcohol increases cancer risk is not entirely clear, but alcohol is known to reduce the positive effects of folate (discussed on page 29), and this may be one way alcohol increases risk for colorectal cancer.

Dietary Fat

High-fat diets have been thought to be associated with an increased risk of cancers of the colon, rectum, prostate, and uterus. It is not clear if this link is due to the total amount of fat, the type of fat, the high number of calories in fatty food, or some other factor. The relationship between dietary fat and cancer risk is being actively studied.

Scientists hypothesize that because dietary fats promote bile acid excretion from the liver, they may increase risk of colorectal cancer, since compounds in bile acids are thought to have cancer-causing effects. However, studies have not shown consistent results clearly linking dietary fat intake and colorectal cancer risk.

Red Meat, Charred Meat, and Processed Meat

Some studies have suggested a link between frequent consumption of red meat and an increase in colorectal cancer risk. The reason red meat, as opposed to other sources of protein, tends to be associated with increased risk of colorectal cancer remains unclear. One possibility is that red meat is a source of saturated fat (see previous section), protein, and iron, any of which may contribute to risk.

It is possible that the risk of colorectal cancer may be increased among meat-eaters who consume meat with a heavily browned or charred surface, but not among those who consume meat with a medium or lightly browned surface. (When meat undergoes prolonged frying, grilling, or broiling at high temperatures, cancer-causing substances may form.)

More evidence has recently shown that a high intake of processed meats such as bologna, luncheon meats, and hot dogs increases risk as well. Sources of protein other than red meat—including low-fat dairy products, legumes, fish, and chicken—have been associated with a lower risk of colorectal cancer and colorectal polyps.

Overall, reducing your intake of red meat and processed meat and consuming a diet rich in other sources of protein may help reduce your risk for colorectal cancer.

Dietary Factors Associated with Decreased Risk for Colorectal Cancer

To recap, dietary factors that are *linked to* or *associated with a decreased risk* of colorectal cancer will not necessarily prevent colorectal cancer or stop it from developing once it has started. But there is good scientific evidence that certain dietary factors may have strong health benefits, including preventive effects against colorectal cancer.

Calcium

Calcium is a mineral found in many of the things we eat and drink, such as dairy products (milk, yogurt, and cheese), leafy green vegetables (rhubarb, spinach, and turnips), and some fish (salmon and sardines). While calcium is essential for the development of strong bones and teeth in children, adults need calcium to maintain bone structure and prevent osteoporosis.

The amount of calcium a person needs depends on age, sex, and menopausal status. Adults generally need 1000 milligrams (mg) of calcium per day. In addition to its effects on bone health and metabolism, large, well-designed studies consistently show that calcium intake of 700 to 800 mg per day may be associated with a lower risk of colorectal cancer. It appears that getting adequate calcium minimizes the risk of the kind of polyps that are most likely to develop into cancer.

When digesting food, the lining of the intestine is directly exposed to bile acids, which may potentially be carcinogenic (cancer-causing). Calcium was originally hypothesized to reduce colorectal cancer risk by neutralizing some of the toxic effects of bile acids as they pass through the colon. However, some evidence now suggests that calcium may also have a direct effect on the cells of the colorectum.

Fiber

Fiber is a plant substance that remains relatively undigested and unabsorbed as it courses through the intestinal tract, which makes it beneficial as a stool-bulking agent. While fiber is found in many foods—including beans, whole-wheat products, and fruits and vegetables—most people in the United States do not meet the recommended daily allowance of 20 to 35 grams of fiber. Lack of sufficient dietary fiber can lead to bothersome complaints such as constipation, hemorrhoids, or diverticulosis (an intestinal disorder). Too much fiber can result in gas and bloating.

The concept that a diet high in fiber, especially from fruits and vegetables, lowers risk of colorectal cancer has been around for more than four decades, starting from the observation that certain groups of people in Africa who eat a high-fiber diet also have low rates of colorectal cancer. Since this original idea, the relationship between fiber, fruits and vegetables in general, and colorectal cancer risk has been evaluated, with somewhat conflicting results. Some studies suggest that fiber (or certain kinds of fiber) can reduce risk, while others have found no effect.

Doctors have several theories about how fiber might reduce colorectal cancer risk:

- Fiber stimulates the movement of materials through the intestine, so that any potentially harmful substances that enter the digestive system will have less contact time with the lining of the colon and rectum.
- Fiber helps eliminate bile acids that might have tumor-promoting capabilities. Enzymes that work to break down fiber products are thought to neutralize bile acids, again making them less toxic.
- Fiber may increase the levels of certain chemicals in the stool, which may provide a protective benefit.

While high intake of fiber may slightly reduce risk for colorectal cancer, the most recent data do not support increasing fiber intake specifically to prevent colorectal cancer. Diets high in fruits, vegetables, and fiber may have many health benefits, such as the prevention of several chronic diseases, including diabetes, but a substantial reduction in colorectal cancer risk may not be among the benefits.

Folate

Folate is a vitamin found in fruits and leafy green vegetables, as well as in fortified foods such as breakfast cereal and in supplements. The chemical form of folate used in supplements and fortified foods is called folic acid. (In 1996, the government issued a regulation requiring all enriched grain products to be fortified with folic acid because it has been shown to reduce the occurrence of birth defects.) Higher intakes of folate (or folic acid) are related to a 20 to 50 percent lower risk of colorectal polyps and colorectal cancer.

As mentioned in the section on alcohol consumption, alcohol is known to inhibit the positive effects of folate. So, although the effect of folate on risk for colorectal cancer is somewhat small, when combined with information on alcohol intake, the results are much more striking. In general, a two- to five-fold increased risk of colorectal cancer or polyp risk is seen among people who drink two or more alcoholic drinks a day and who also have low intakes of folate.

Regular multivitamin use and adequate intake of fruits, vegetables, and folate-fortified foods can ensure the proper folate intake for most people. Because of the fortification of grain products, outright folate deficiency is rare, and most people are probably already consuming enough folate without additional supplementation.

Selenium

Selenium is a trace element that exists in the soil and is absorbed by plant materials. Humans ingest selenium by eating grains, meat, poultry, and fish. Selenium-containing compounds activate tumor-suppressor genes and aid in the repair of genetic material.

Selenium gained support as a potential preventive agent for colorectal cancer after a study of people with skin cancer revealed that those who took selenium supplements had a reduced risk of colorectal and other cancers (but not skin cancer). Subsequent studies have found higher selenium levels may be associated with longer survival time after colorectal cancer diagnosis, and higher selenium levels may also decrease the risk of developing large colorectal adenomas. Additional research on the potential role of selenium in colorectal cancer prevention is under way. It is important to remember that there is a narrow margin between a safe dose and a toxic dose.

Vitamin D

Vitamin D may also play a role in reducing risk for colorectal cancer. Vitamin D is a unique nutrient because in addition to the vitamin D we obtain by eating foods containing or fortified with vitamin D (such as cod liver oil, fatty fish such as salmon, and fortified milk), we are able to produce vitamin D in our skin. When humans are exposed to the ultraviolet radiation in sunlight (UV-B), vitamin D is formed in our skin and circulated through our bodies. People who are exposed to sunlight more often have higher levels of vitamin D compared with those who have limited sun exposure.

Studies have found that people who have high levels of vitamin D (from supplement use, diet, exposure to ultraviolet light, or all of the above) have a lower risk of colorectal cancer. There also is some evidence that vitamin D can reduce risk for colorectal adenomas. The reduction in risk seen among those with high vitamin D levels may be due to vitamin D reducing abnormal rates of cell growth, which are sometimes involved in cancer.

Although some sun exposure may reduce risk of colorectal cancer via increased vitamin D levels, doctors do not recommend prolonged exposure to the sun because this has been linked to an increased risk of skin cancer.

Tumor-Blocking Medications

Cancer chemoprevention is the use of medicines or nutritional supplements to prevent or inhibit tumor growth. We've already discussed a variety of dietary factors and nutritional supplements that may potentially help reduce a person's risk of colorectal cancer. Next, we'll look at medications with potential tumor-blocking effects in the colon and rectum.

Hormone Replacement Therapy

Estrogen is a female sex hormone produced by the ovaries and adrenal glands. When women reach middle age and their hormone levels begin to drop, they may be prescribed estrogen replacement therapy (ERT) or hormone replacement therapy (HRT, a combination of estrogen plus a second hormone, progesterone, or its synthetic form, progestin), if indicated.

The use of ERT or HRT may slightly reduce the risk of colorectal cancer in postmenopausal women. However, the use of ERT and HRT may increase the risk of other serious diseases, such as coronary artery disease and breast cancer. Therefore, women should not begin using ERT and HRT as a colorectal cancer prevention strategy.

Nonsteroidal Anti-inflammatory Drugs

Nonsteroidal anti-inflammatory drugs (NSAIDs) reduce inflammation and are used to relieve pain from arthritis, headaches, joint pain, lower back strain, menstrual cramps, and certain injuries. Common NSAIDs include ibuprofen (Advil, Motrin), naproxen (Aleve), piroxicam (Feldene), and sulindac (Clinoril). Aspirin (Bayer, Ecotrin), the best-known NSAID, is also used for its blood-thinning qualities by many people who are at high risk for heart disease. Research has found daily aspirin use can reduce the occurrence of blood clots that trigger heart attacks and strokes.

NSAIDs have recently received a lot of press because of their possible chemo-preventive effects against colorectal cancer as well. Many studies have found that people who regularly use aspirin and other NSAIDs have a 20 to 50 percent lower risk of colorectal cancer and adenomatous polyps. Aspirin appears particularly effective in lowering risk when taken consistently for many years.

Studies in both animals and humans have suggested that regular NSAID use might play a role in preventing the development and recurrence of colorectal cancer. Aspirin and other NSAIDs may reduce risk of colorectal cancer by (1) reducing chronic inflammation and (2) interfering with the actions of certain proteins in the colorectum involved in the breakdown of specific types of unsaturated dietary fat. NSAIDs have also been found to decrease the growth and spread of abnormal tissue and to cause cell death, which are thought to help fight colorectal tumor growth.

ON THE HORIZON

Cholesterol-Lowering Statins May Protect Against Colorectal Cancer

Drugs taken by millions of Americans to reduce cholesterol levels may also reduce the risk of colorectal cancer. Early research suggests that statins—which block an enzyme that the body needs to make cholesterol—may also inhibit the growth of colon cancer cells in laboratory experiments. An unrelated clinical study showed that participants who had suffered from heart attacks and used statins benefited from a reduced risk of colorectal cancer. These findings are very preliminary, but plans are under way to launch a clinical study (see chapter 13) to determine whether statins reduce risk for colorectal cancer in people who have a family history of the disease.

Scientists are trying to learn more about how NSAIDs might help prevent colorectal cancer and what dosage would be most beneficial, especially because long-term use of NSAIDs for colorectal cancer prevention may irritate the lining of the stomach (causing indigestion, nausea, or even stomach bleeding or ulcers) or cause more serious problems, such as abnormal bleeding, liver or kidney damage, or stroke. Because of these potential side effects, the use of NSAIDs is not recommended as a cancer prevention strategy. Do not start using aspirin or any other medication without consulting your health care provider.

A special type of NSAID called a COX-2 inhibitor may also have chemopreventive effects—results of clinical studies are forthcoming. Celecoxib (Celebrex), a COX-2 inhibitor, has been approved by the FDA for reducing polyp formation in people with familial adenomatous polyposis (FAP). However, COX-2 inhibitors have come under great scrutiny because of the increased risk of heart attack, stroke, and other complications associated with their use in some but not all studies. Further studies to investigate the potential benefits as well as the risks of COX-2 inhibitors and other NSAIDs are ongoing.

You should not take celecoxib to prevent polyps without a careful discussion with your doctor about your personal risks and the potential benefits.

What Can You Do?

The goal of preventing most colorectal cancer is getting closer as scientists expand and refine their understanding of this disease and even begin to discover medications with possible chemopreventive or anticancer effects.

Fortunately, many important risk factors for colorectal cancer have already been identified (see Table 2.5 on page 20 and Table 2.7). Although some of these are not changeable, such as age, race and ethnicity, family history, or a previous diagnosis of colorectal polyps or cancer, the good news is that you can reduce your risk of colorectal cancers by making moderate changes in diet and lifestyle and by following the American Cancer Society guidelines for colorectal cancer screening.

Table 2.7 Summary of Controllable Factors Affecting Colorectal Cancer Risk

Note: Age, race and ethnicity and personal/family health history are considered fixed or uncontrollable risk factors.

Factors Associated With an Increased (↑) Risk of Colorectal Cancer	Factors Associated With a Decreased (↓) Risk of Colorectal Cancer
Lifestyle Factors	
Overweight or Obesity Tobacco	Physical Activity
Dietary Factors	
Alcohol Dietary Fat Red, Charred, or Processed Meat	Calcium Fiber Folate Selenium Vitamin D*
Medications	
	HRT* Non-steroidal anti-inflammatory drugs (NSAIDs)*

* Because of potentially dangerous risks associated with use, the use of NSAIDs and/or HRT is not recommended as colorectal cancer prevention strategies, and neither is Vitamin D when gained through sun exposure.

Therefore, making relatively small changes in the lifestyle and dietary factors discussed in this chapter—engaging in physical activity, achieving or maintaining a healthy body weight, following a healthful diet, and avoiding excessive alcohol use and smoking—are effective strategies people can use to reduce their risk of colorectal cancer. Although the epidemic of obesity suggests that maintaining a healthy body weight and getting adequate physical activity are not easy goals to achieve, all efforts to reach or maintain a healthy body weight and increase physical activity will lead to benefits, including lowering risk of colorectal cancer.

These changes are particularly important for those who may be at above-average risk (because of factors such as family history or medical conditions), but are useful for anyone who wants to reduce his or her risk of colorectal cancer.

In addition, it is very important to follow the guidelines for regular colorectal screening (see chapter 3), because finding and removing polyps in the colon can prevent colorectal cancer.

CHAPTER THREE

EARLY DETECTION

Kandice L. Knigge, MD

An estimated 56,000 people die from colorectal cancer each year, making colorectal cancer a leading cause of cancer death in the United States. But it doesn't have to be.

The most effective way to reduce your risk of colorectal cancer is to get screened for colorectal cancer routinely, starting at age 50 (earlier if you are at higher risk). That way, if you have polyps, they can be removed before they turn into cancer. And if colorectal cancer is found, it is often curable when it is detected in its early stages, before it has had a chance to metastasize, or spread.

Early Detection Makes a Difference

Early detection of colorectal cancer saves lives. As discussed in chapters 1 and 2, colorectal cancers can take many years to develop and are usually preceded by adenomatous polyps or adenomas. More than four in five colorectal cancers arise from these potentially precancerous polyps, but removal of polyps (a procedure referred to as "polypectomy") can prevent the disease from occurring. Early detection for colorectal cancer is the cornerstone of preventing this disease, since identifying and removing adenomatous polyps can decrease colorectal cancer risk by 60 to 90 percent.

The earlier colorectal cancer is discovered, the better the prognosis (or outcome) for the person with colorectal cancer (see chapter 6). Approximately 90 percent of people diagnosed with early stage colorectal cancer are alive five years after diagnosis and treatment. Unfortunately, only about a third of colorectal cancers are diagnosed at an early stage. Most colorectal cancers do not cause any symptoms until they have reached a late stage, at which point the chance for cure is significantly reduced. Once the cancer has spread, the likelihood of survival diminishes significantly. (We'll talk more about prognosis and interpreting survival statistics in chapter 6.)

To achieve early detection and prevent colorectal cancer, people should be tested, or screened, *before* the development of symptoms. (Screening is the term doctors use when they perform tests to diagnose or rule out diseases before the patient experiences any symptoms.) Anyone already experiencing symptoms such as abdominal pain, change in bowel habits, rectal bleeding, anemia, weakness, fatigue, or weight loss should visit a doctor immediately for an initial evaluation (see chapter 4).

> *"There definitely is not enough information for the public about colon cancer. It is not talked about openly, and I think it's because people just don't like to talk about colons and rectums and about their bodily functions. So, this cancer is simply not talked about, and most people are not aware of the symptoms. They're not aware that, beginning at age 50, or even younger if they have a family history, they need to have screening done to see if they have a colon cancer or a precancerous condition. This cancer, if it's detected early, or even before it becomes cancerous, has a very high survival rate."*
>
> —PAM

Who Should be Screened for Colorectal Cancer?

Everyone age 50 or older should be routinely screened for colorectal cancer (see Table 3.1 on page 41). People who are at higher risk of developing the disease because of personal health history or family health history should talk to their doctors about earlier or more frequent testing (see Table 3.2 on page 42).

Underuse of Screening for Colorectal Cancer

One of the primary reasons for the delay in diagnosis of colorectal cancer is that only about two in five Americans who are at risk for colorectal cancer undergo any type of screening for the early detection of colorectal cancer and adenomatous polyps.

Screening for colorectal cancer lags behind screening for other cancers. (For example, nearly four out of five at-risk women are screened for breast cancer.) Screening for colorectal cancer is particularly low among people who lack health insurance, those who don't visit the doctor annually, or those with no usual source of health care.

It is estimated that if everyone followed the American Cancer Society guidelines for colorectal cancer screening (see Table 3.1 on page 41 and Table 3.2 on page 42), it could reduce new cases by one fourth and cut the number of deaths from the disease in half.

Why Are Colorectal Cancer Screening Rates So Low?

Despite the availability of effective screening tests, colorectal cancer screening remains underused. There are many reasons for this unacceptably low rate of screening for colorectal cancer. Some of these reasons are:

1. *Some people may be embarrassed.* The colon and rectum are still considered by many to be "private" body parts, and many are embarrassed or unwilling to talk to their doctor about personal details such as a change in bowel habits or rectal bleeding.

2. *Some people prefer avoidance and denial to the possibility of "bad news."* People may fear that screening will lead to a diagnosis of colorectal cancer, which is news they don't want to hear.

3. *Many people still do not recognize the importance of screening for colorectal cancer.* Many at-risk people are unaware of their risk and do not understand the extreme difference in survival outcomes between early- and late-stage diagnoses.

4. *Doctors have not made screening for colorectal cancer a priority.* Physicians' time constraints often lead them to focus more on the treatment of active diseases than on prevention. This may mean that doctors may not recommend colorectal cancer screening to all of their at-risk patients and may also prevent them from spending large amounts of time and effort convincing reluctant people of the value of the tests.

5. *Many people are unaware of the variety of options available to screen for colorectal cancer.* They may not be informed about the advantages and disadvantages of each approach. People may therefore choose to undergo no screening at all.

6. *Until recently, the costs associated with certain colorectal cancer screening tests (such as colonoscopy) have been prohibitive for some people.* However, people age 50 and older with Medicare are eligible for colorectal cancer screening. All Medicare beneficiaries (no age limit) at average risk for colorectal cancer are now entitled to undergo colorectal cancer screening by any of the agreed-upon screening methods, including screening colonoscopy. (Call 800-MEDICARE/ 800-633-4227 or visit http://www. medicare.gov/Health/ColonCancer.asp for the most up-to-date information on Medicare coverage for colorectal cancer screening.) In addition, most private insurers are now paying for some form of colorectal cancer screening, often including screening colonoscopy.

At What Age Should Regular Screening Begin?

Less than 10 percent of all colorectal cancer cases occur among persons younger than 50 years of age. Colorectal cancer incidence rates begin to rise rapidly after 50 years of age and increase steadily thereafter. Colorectal polyps are also more common with advancing age and are present in about 30 percent of people aged 50, 40 to 50 percent of people aged 60, and 50 to 65 percent of people aged 70. Therefore, in the absence of known risk factors (see chapter 2), doctors recommend that regular colorectal cancer screening should begin for *most people* at age 50. (The American Cancer Society recommends earlier and more frequent screening for people at higher risk; see Table 3.2 on page 42.)

Types of Screening Tests

There are currently several effective options available for colorectal cancer screening for people at average risk for the disease. These options include fecal blood tests, endoscopy (a method of examining the interior of a body cavity or hollow organ, such as the colon, using an endoscope, a narrow, flexible, fiber optic instrument that conducts light), and the double-contrast barium enema (an X-ray procedure). Each screening test has unique advantages and limitations that may vary for individual people and settings, and no single screening test has been proven to be superior to all others.

Some new alternatives, fecal DNA tests and virtual colonoscopy (also known as CT colonography) are also being developed for colorectal cancer screening and may offer patient-friendly improvements over currently available screening tests (see the feature box on pages 48–49). However, the accuracy of these emerging options has not been fully determined, so doctors cannot confidently recommend their use.

Fecal Blood Tests: The Fecal Occult Blood Test and Fecal Immunochemical Test

The fecal occult blood test (FOBT) is a common method of colorectal cancer screening. The FOBT involves examining a small sample of stool to determine whether any occult (hidden) blood is present in the feces. Blood vessels at the surface of adenomatous polyps and cancers are often quite fragile. With the passage of feces, the blood vessels may become damaged and release a small amount of blood that is often too small to see with the naked eye or to color the stool red. The FOBT detects this blood through a chemical reaction.

If the FOBT is positive, a colonoscopy should always be performed to determine the source of the bleeding (the use of double-contrast barium enema to evaluate a positive FOBT is not recommended unless colonoscopy is unavailable). Despite this strong recommendation, only about half of those people with a positive FOBT currently undergo colonoscopy.

The test is noninvasive and does not require a bowel preparation (cleansing). It should be done at home using a special kit (tests done in a doctor's office at the time of a rectal exam are not adequate for detecting most polyps and colorectal cancers). The home test kits require specimens of stool from three separate bowel movements are smeared onto a small square of paper. Then the kit can be returned to a physician's office or medical lab to be evaluated. FOBT is the only colorectal cancer prevention test that has been conclusively linked in studies to a decreased number of deaths from colorectal cancer. By itself, FOBT only finds about one in four cases of colorectal cancer. But FOBT done annually, in combination with a flexible sigmoidoscopy every five years after age 50, may successfully detect as many as three in four colon tumors.

Fecal occult blood testing followed by colonoscopy for all positive tests results in up to 33 percent reduction in death from colorectal cancer when performed annually and a 21 percent reduction in mortality rates from colorectal cancer when performed every other year. This approach has also been shown to decrease the number of new cases of colorectal cancer among those who are screened.

Disadvantages of FOBT include the fact that the test is often negative in people who have adenomatous polyps and colorectal cancer. This is called a false negative (a result that shows there is no cancer when there really is). One-time testing with FOBT detects one sixth to one half of colorectal cancers. *To be an effective screening tool, FOBT must be repeated yearly.*

Even after an FOBT result comes back negative, if the patient experiences any rectal bleeding or significant change in bowel habits, he or she should be reevaluated with a colonoscopy.

A newer, less widely used form of fecal occult blood testing, called a fecal immunochemical test, can also be used to screen for colorectal cancer. Unlike conventional FOBT, which gives positive results for any type of blood present in the stool (including animal blood from ingested meat), the fecal immunochemical test detects a specific portion of a human blood protein. This test is done much the same way as a conventional FOBT, but is more specific and more accurate as a diagnostic tool. The fecal immunochemical test shares some of the same drawbacks of the conventional FOBT, including the inability to detect a tumor that is not bleeding.

Flexible Sigmoidoscopy

A sigmoidoscope is a thin, flexible, lighted tube that is inserted through the rectum into the lower part of the colon. The scope is about two feet long (60 cm) and about the thickness of a finger. The sigmoidoscope, which can be hooked up to video camera and display monitor, allows the doctor to directly view the lower third of the colon (see Figure 3.1).

Flexible sigmoidoscopy requires a bowel preparation (see page 43) to cleanse the colon for proper inspection. A typical sigmoidoscopy takes approximately 10 to 20 minutes to perform, and the procedure generally does not require the patient to be sedated. The procedure might be uncomfortable, but it should not be painful. The examination is inexpensive and can be completed by some primary care physicians in the office setting (see Figure 3.2 on page 42). Small polyps or other abnormalities may be treated or removed during this procedure. In this case, a colonoscopy should be performed to look for lesions in the upper part of the colon. If the results of the flexible sigmoidoscopy are normal, screening should be repeated in five years.

Studies have shown that sigmoidoscopy and removal of polyps (polypectomy) can reduce the risk of death from cancers within reach of the sigmoidoscope by 60 to 80 percent. However, as many as a third of people with adenomatous polyps or colorectal cancer have abnormalities only in the

> "My diagnosis was a complete surprise. I went in for my yearly gynecology checkup and had a wonderful physician whom I've gone to for over 30 years, who suggested to me that I was over 50 and I hadn't turned those [FOBT] envelopes in, and it was time for me to take that test and get those envelopes back in to his office. He made the point of telling me that he knew I probably wouldn't want to do it, but at my age, I'd better do it. So, I sent them in and they came back with an indication that more testing was necessary. I had a colonoscopy, a polyp was found, had surgery from that, and was diagnosed with stage III colorectal cancer with it already having entered my lymph nodes. So, I feel very blessed that I had a persistent doctor who knew the value of early screening and early detection and knew me well enough to know that he needed to lecture me to get the FOBT back in."
>
> —PATTI

Figure 3.1 Flexible Sigmoidoscopy

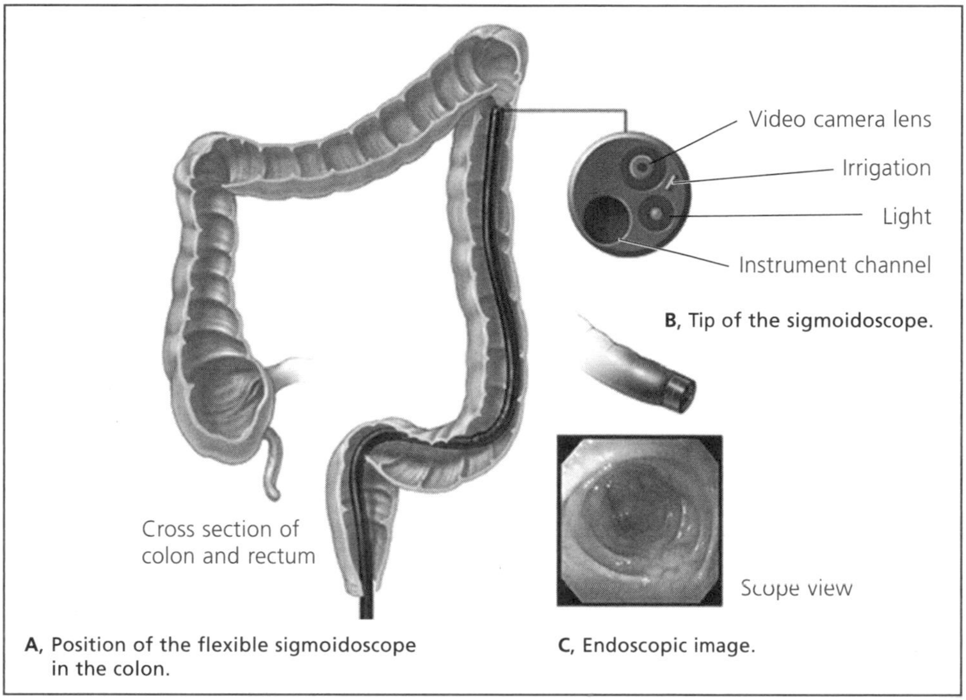
Video camera lens
Irrigation
Light
Instrument channel
B, Tip of the sigmoidoscope.
Cross section of colon and rectum
Scope view
A, Position of the flexible sigmoidoscope in the colon.
C, Endoscopic image.

Source: Copyright © 2005 The Johns Hopkins University. All Rights Reserved. Figure 12 from The Johns Hopkins Gastroenterology and Hepatology Resource Center, http://www.hopkins-gi.org, Digestive Disease Library, Colon & Rectum, Hereditary Colon Cancer.

upper part of the colon. (Some evidence suggests that precancerous polyps isolated to the upper right colon may occur more frequently in women than in men.) Since they have no abnormalities in the lower part of the colon, this portion of the population will have a normal flexible sigmoidoscopy. These people do not typically get a colonoscopy, and thus adenomatous polyps and colorectal cancer located in the upper part of the colon may go undetected.

When an experienced, trained health care professional performs a sigmoidoscopy, it is safe, well tolerated, and accurate. However, there are several disadvantages to sigmoidoscopy:

1. Patient discomfort may limit the depth of insertion of the sigmoidoscope and decrease accuracy.
2. There is small risk—about 1 in 10,000—of perforation (creating a hole in the bowel wall).

Figure 3.2 Patient Positioning for Sigmoidoscopy and Colonoscopy

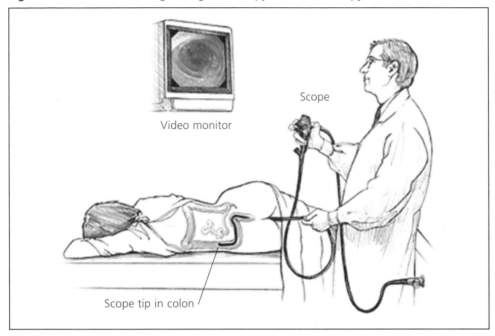

Video monitor

Scope

Scope tip in colon

3. Poor bowel preparation can limit the ability to adequately visualize the lining of the bowel.
4. Sigmoidoscopy only allows doctors to view the lower third of the colon. Therefore, polyps located in the upper part of the colon may go undetected.
5. If a polyp is found during sigmoidoscopy, the test needs to be followed by a colonoscopy.

Yearly fecal occult blood testing combined with flexible sigmoidoscopy every five years may increase the number of cases of colorectal cancer and adenomatous polyps detected over the use of either test alone. However, the additional benefits and potential drawbacks of combining the two tests are not known. As a rule, FOBT should precede flexible sigmoidoscopy because a positive FOBT should lead to a colonoscopy and will rule out the need for sigmoidoscopy.

It is important for people to understand that if they develop colorectal symptoms (such as rectal bleeding or significant change in bowel habits) after the flexible sigmoidoscopy, they should be evaluated with a colonoscopy.

What Is a Bowel Preparation?

Before a flexible sigmoidoscopy or colonscopy procedure, the colon must be thoroughly cleansed. This is called a bowel prep. If your colon is not completely clean, your doctor may not be able to get a good look at the inside of your colorectum, or he or she may mistake residual fecal matter for cancerous tissue.

There are a number of ways to prepare your colon for an endoscopic examination. These include the use of large volumes of fluids (PEG prep), small doses of liquid laxatives combined with large volumes of clear liquids, and a laxative in tablet form along with large volumes of clear liquids. (Clear liquids are liquids that you can see through such as water, apple juice, broth, and gelatin.) Both of the latter methods of bowel prep are generally more popular with patients than the PEG prep. You should discuss these options with your doctor so that you can find a method that works best for you.

Colonoscopy

A colonoscope is a longer version of a sigmoidoscope, and it allows for direct inspection of the entire lining of the colon (recall that a sigmoidoscope can only examine the lower third; compare Figure 3.1 on page 41 with Figure 3.3 on page 44). The colonoscopy requires a bowel preparation, is typically done in an outpatient endoscopy unit or in a clinic, and should be performed by a well-trained endoscopist with ample clinical experience.

Colonoscopy is usually done with "conscious sedation." This means that during the examination, medication is given through an intravenous (IV) line (a tube inserted through the skin into a vein). This helps you to remain calm and comfortable during the examination. Some patients sleep through their colonoscopy. Not all patients need sedation for their colon examination. Your doctor will evaluate a number of factors to determine what type of sedation, if any, would be best for you.

Figure 3.3 Colonoscopy

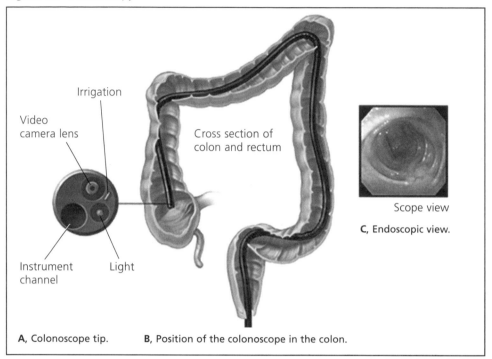

Irrigation

Video
camera lens

Cross section of
colon and rectum

Scope view

C, Endoscopic view.

Instrument
channel

Light

A, Colonoscope tip.   **B, Position of the colonoscope in the colon.**

Source: Copyright © 2005 The Johns Hopkins University. All Rights Reserved. Figure 14 from The Johns Hopkins Gastroenterology and Hepatology Resource Center, http://www.hopkins-gi.org, Digestive Disease Library, Colon & Rectum, Hereditary Colon Cancer.

Your heart rate, blood pressure, respiratory rate, and blood oxygen saturation are carefully monitored throughout the procedure. Patients are not allowed to drive home after the exam because the sedative medication can alter the ability to safely operate machinery for up to 24 hours.

Colonoscopy allows for diagnosis and treatment in a single session. The exam usually takes about 15 to 30 minutes to complete, but it may take longer if polyps are identified and need to be removed. In this process, called a polypectomy, polyps are removed by passing a wire loop (snare) through the scope to cut the polyp from the lining of the colon using an electrical current. Polyps are collected and sent to a laboratory for evaluation. At the lab, a pathologist (a doctor trained in the examination of tissue to detect disease) will use a microscope to identify the type of polyp and search for any evidence of cancer.

Figure 3.4 Polypectomy

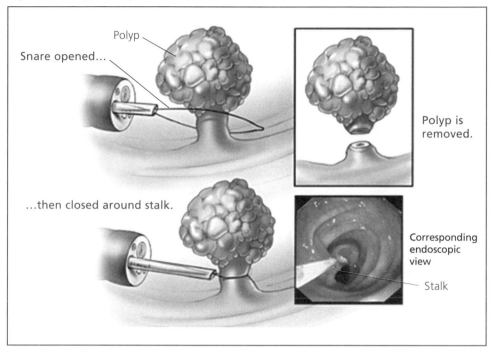

Endoscopic technique for snare resection of a polyp.

Source: Copyright © 2005 The Johns Hopkins University. All Rights Reserved. Figure 16 from The Johns Hopkins Gastroenterology and Hepatology Resource Center, http://www.hopkins-gi.org, Digestive Disease Library, Colon & Rectum, Sporadic Colon Cancer.

The accuracy of colonoscopy in detecting colorectal cancer exceeds 90 percent. Colonoscopy is not a perfect screening test and it can miss small polyps, although the accuracy for detecting large polyps is excellent. When comparing its ability to detect adenomas and cancers with that of other screening methods, colonoscopy is superior to FOBT, flexible sigmoidoscopy, and double-contrast barium enema (DCBE). In addition, if the results of colonoscopy are normal, additional screening is not needed for 10 years, unless new symptoms develop.

However, colonoscopy is associated with higher risks than other screening methods, both because it is a more invasive test and because it requires the patient to undergo conscious sedation. These risks are some of the disadvantages of the procedure:

1. The use of conscious sedation may cause complications, such as problems with low blood pressure, low respiratory rate, low blood oxygen saturation, and cardiac arrhythmias.

2. The risk for perforation of the bowel is significantly higher than other screening tests, particularly if polypectomy is performed. However, it is still less than 1 percent.

3. There is risk of serious bleeding (requiring blood transfusion or surgery) after polypectomy. Minor bleeding is more common.

4. Colonoscopy is initially more expensive than other screening methods. However, because a normal study requires no additional follow-up for 10 years, colonoscopy is a cost-effective screening strategy for colorectal cancer over time.

> *"I was awake through the whole procedure. The nurse kept telling me how glad she was that I had come in for the procedure. The visual monitor showed me why. There was a large soft polyp almost totally blocking the colon. It was found to be cancerous.... The only regret I have is that I didn't have the colonoscopy when I should have. If it weren't for [my wife], I'd be in bad shape because I would have waited for symptoms. I can do anything now that I did before. I just have this scar to remind me of my stubborn procrastination."*
>
> —KEVIN

It is not known whether the potential added benefits of colonoscopy outweigh the potential risks relative to other screening tests. When highly skilled examiners perform colonoscopy, it is a safe procedure. If a less experienced endoscopist performs the procedure, it may affect both the accuracy and safety of the test.

Double-Contrast Barium Enema

Double-contrast barium enema (DCBE), also known as a barium enema with air contrast, is a procedure that studies the colon using barium sulfate (a thick, chalky substance) that is administered by inserting a small tube into the patient's rectum. The barium spreads throughout the colon while the patient is positioned on an X-ray table. Air is introduced into the colon through the same tube to expand the colon and then X-rays are taken to produce images of the lining of the bowel (See Figure 3.5).

The test requires a complete bowel preparation (an oral laxative and one to two days of a clear liquid diet) and is administered without sedation. DCBE takes approximately 30 to 45 minutes to complete and is the least expensive test that examines the entire colon. The risk of perforation of the colon is low (about 1 in 25,000).

DCBE has not been studied as a screening tool to determine whether it decreases the incidence of or mortality rate from colorectal cancer in persons with

Figure 3.5 Patient Positioning for a Double-Contrast Barium Enema

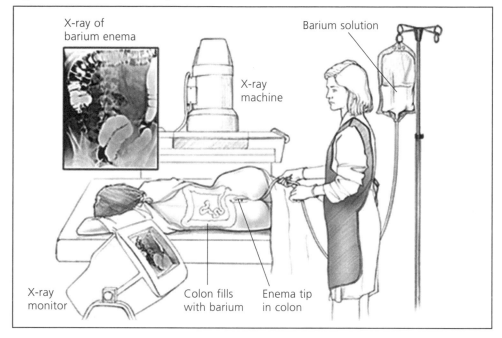

average risk. However, it is now apparent that DCBE is not as effective as endoscopy for detection of colon polyps or colorectal cancer. Studies have shown that DCBE detects only one half of adenomatous polyps greater than 1 cm in size (which are the adenomas that are most likely to progress to cancer), and less than a third of polyps smaller than 0.5 cm. In addition, DCBE may miss up to 15 percent of colorectal cancers.

In addition to potential false-negative results, DCBE has other disadvantages:

1. The procedure does not allow for removal of polyps. Therefore, if polyps are detected, the patient will have to undergo another complete bowel preparation and subsequent colonoscopy.
2. Certain findings, such as retained stool in the colon, may be misidentified as polyps. This could lead to further tests that may not be necessary.

The addition of flexible sigmoidoscopy to DCBE is generally not recommended for routine screening, because the increase in yield for detecting colorectal cancer with this combination approach is negligible.

ON THE HORIZON:

New Technologies for the Early Detection of Colorectal Cancer

Virtual Colonoscopy

First described in 1994, virtual colonoscopy is an imaging procedure that uses a CT scan (highly specialized X-ray) to create two- or three-dimensional images of the lining of the colon. Most commonly known as virtual colonoscopy, the exam is also known as CT colonography, which is actually the term many doctors prefer, because "virtual" colonoscopy suggests the examination is not a real endoscopic procedure.

The exam is performed without sedation, and a complete bowel preparation is required. A tube is inserted into the patient's rectum and the colon is distended with air, which can be uncomfortable. The patient lies flat on an X-ray table in the supine (on the back) position and the breath is held for several seconds while a CT scan of the abdomen and pelvis is performed. The patient then lies in the prone (on the stomach) position and a second CT scan is performed. The examination itself can usually be completed in 5 to 10 minutes, and then a radiologist reads and interprets the CT colonography findings

There is only limited information on the use of CT colonography in typical screening populations for colorectal cancer, and studies of CT colonography to date have shown a wide range of results. There are no data as to whether the test leads to pre-vention of colorectal cancer or death. On average, current information suggests that CT colonography is not as good as colonoscopy for the detection of colon polyps except in specialized centers where experts familiar with the technique are available.

CT colonography may offer some advantages over conventional colonoscopy, however. This risk of perforation of the bowel is very low with CT colonography. As the technology advances, CT colonography may prove to be a "roadmap" for endo-scopists to guide them to the correct location and number of polyps to be removed. In addition, some cancers that may not be detected by colonoscopy, such as those located near a large fold in the colon or above the level of an obstruction, may be detected by virtual colonoscopy.

A number of limitations of CT colonography have also been identified. False positive readings (readings that say cancer is present when there really isn't) can result in a follow-up colonoscopy that is unnecessary. Moreover, CT colonography is only a diagnostic procedure, and if polyps are detected (and they are in 30 to 50 percent of people), patients must have an additional procedure to have the polyps removed. Other questions about CT colonography have to do with comfort for those being examined, risk of radiation exposure, and high costs. Currently, CT colonography is considered experimental in most settings and is not covered by Medicare or private insurance companies.

At this time, CT colonography is not recommended for widespread use for colorectal cancer screening until further evidence for its accuracy is available. Large studies are now under way that may help determine whether CT colonography is as good as or better than current screening methods. Talk with your doctor about this option if you are interested, because the technology is rapidly advancing.

Altered DNA in Stool

Researchers have recently discovered DNA mutations that affect certain genes of colorectal cancer cells. These mutations can be distinguished from normal cells using highly specialized molecular techniques that detect abnormal DNA in the stool that is shed from colorectal cancers and adenomatous polyps. The test does not require a bowel preparation and can be performed at home. People send an entire bowel movement to a central laboratory in a prefabricated stool collection kit. The stool is then analyzed for the presence of abnormal DNA that is associated with colorectal cancer and premalignant polyps.

Early studies suggest that the fecal DNA test is only accurate about 60 percent of the time for detecting colorectal cancer and 20 percent of the time for detecting adenomatous polyps. False positives appear to be rare with this technique. False negative results remain a concern with available tests, and fecal DNA testing is currently much more expensive than FOBT.

The science of DNA stool testing is an emerging technology. If this technology evolves and proves to be accurate in large studies, it will probably supplement other screening tests rather than replace them. At the present time, fecal DNA testing is not ready for widespread application, but it represents an important step forward toward a more reliable, inexpensive, and noninvasive screening test for colorectal cancer.

Recommendations for Screening

The American Cancer Society currently recommends that men and women at average risk should be screened for colorectal cancer and adenomatous polyps beginning at age 50 years, using one of the following five options for screening:

- annual fecal occult blood test (FOBT)
- flexible sigmoidoscopy every 5 years
- annual FOBT plus flexible sigmoidoscopy every 5 years
- double-contrast barium enema (DCBE) every 5 years
- colonoscopy every 10 years

(For a brief review of these screening options, see Table 3.1.)

Other commonly performed methods of colorectal cancer screening and follow up *are not adequate*. These measures include:

- a digital rectal exam (DRE), in which the doctor inserts a gloved, lubricated finger into the patient's rectum
- the collection of a single-sample FOBT during a routine DRE
- a repeat FOBT after an initial positive test

A positive FOBT in a patient who has undergone screening should always be followed by a colonoscopy or by DCBE and flexible sigmoidoscopy in the rare instance where colonoscopy is not available. Speak to your doctor about the American Cancer Society guidelines if you think you or someone you love has not been adequately screened.

Recommendations for People at Higher Risk for Colorectal Cancer

The recommendations for people at average risk do not apply to people who have a personal or family history that elevates their risk for colorectal cancer (see chapter 2 for more information on risk factors). The American Cancer Society has special screening guidelines for people at higher risk (see Table 3.2 on page 52) and recommends earlier and more frequent surveillance for persons with any of the following:

- a personal history of adenomatous polyps
- a personal history of colorectal cancer
- a personal history of inflammatory bowel disease
- a family history of either colorectal cancer or colorectal adenomas
- a family history of (or genetic testing indicating the presence of) a hereditary syndrome such as familial adenomatous polyposis (FAP) or hereditary non-polyposis colorectal cancer (HNPCC), two syndromes described in chapter 2

Table 3.1 American Cancer Society Guidelines on Screening and Surveillance for the Early Detection of Colorectal Adenomas and Cancer—Average-Risk Women and Men Ages 50 and Older

These options are acceptable choices for colorectal cancer screening in average-risk adults. Since each of the following tests has inherent characteristics related to accuracy, prevention potential, costs, and risks, individuals should have an opportunity to make an informed decision when choosing a screening test.

Test	Interval (beginning at age 50)	Comment
Fecal Occult Blood Test (FOBT) & Flexible Sigmoidoscopy	FOBT annually and flexible sigmoidoscopy every 5 years	Flexible sigmoidoscopy together with FOBT is preferred compared with FOBT or flexible sigmoidoscopy alone. All positive tests should be followed up with colonoscopy.*
Flexible Sigmoidoscopy	Every 5 years	All positive tests should be followed up with colonoscopy.*
FOBT	Yearly	The recommended take-home multiple-sample method should be used. All positive tests should be followed up with colonoscopy.*
Colonoscopy	Every 10 years	Colonoscopy provides an opportunity to visualize, sample, and/or remove significant lesions.
Double-Contrast Barium Enema (DCBE)	Every 5 years	All positive tests should be followed up with colonoscopy

* If colonoscopy is unavailable, not feasible, or not desired by the patient, double-contrast barium enema alone or the combination of flexible sigmoidoscopy and double-contrast barium enema are acceptable alternatives.

Why Are These Tests So Important?

By now you should be aware that screening for colorectal cancer can help in two important ways: it can find polyps early, allowing the opportunity to remove them before they become cancerous, and it can find colorectal cancer at an earlier stage, when the disease is more easily treatable.

Too often, people don't get these important tests. Colorectal cancer can grow silently and become quite advanced before symptoms ever surface. By this time, the cancer may be difficult to treat and impossible to cure.

Table 3.2 American Cancer Society Guidelines on Screening and Surveillance for the Early Detection of Colorectal Adenomas and Cancer—Women and Men at Increased Risk or at High Risk

Risk Category	Age to Begin	Recommendation	Comments
INCREASED RISK			
People with a single, small (<1 cm) adenoma	3–6 years after the initial polypectomy	Colonoscopy*	If the exam is normal, the patient can thereafter be screened as per average risk guidelines.
People with a large (>1 cm) adenoma, multiple adenomas, or adenomas with high-grade dysplasia† or villous change.‡	Within 3 years after the initial polypectomy	Colonoscopy*	If normal, repeat examination in 3 years; if normal then, the patient can thereafter be screened as per average risk guidelines.
Personal history of curative-intent resection of colorectal cancer	Within 1 year after cancer resection	Colonoscopy*	If normal, repeat examination in 3 years; if normal then, repeat examination every 5 years.
Either colorectal cancer or adenomatous polyps, in any first-degree relative before age 60, or in two or more first-degree relatives at any age (if not a hereditary syndrome).	Age 40, or 10 years before the youngest case in the immediate family	Colonoscopy*	Every 5–10 years. Colorectal cancer in relatives more distant than first-degree does not increase risk substantially above the average risk group.
HIGH RISK			
Family history of familial adenomatous polyposis (FAP)	Puberty	Early surveillance with endoscopy, and counseling to consider genetic testing	If the genetic test is positive, colectomy is indicated. These patients are best referred to a center with experience in the management of FAP.
Family history of hereditary nonpolyposis colon cancer (HNPCC)	Age 21	Colonoscopy and counseling to consider genetic testing	If the genetic test is positive or if the patient has not had genetic testing, every 1–2 years until age 40, then annually. These patients are best referred to a center with experience in the management of HNPCC.
Inflammatory bowel disease (includes chronic ulcerative colitis and Crohn's disease)	Cancer risk begins to be significant 8 years after the onset of pancolitis,§ or 12–15 years after the onset of left-sided colitis	Colonoscopy with biopsies for dysplasia	Every 1–2 years. These patients are best referred to a center with experience in the surveillance and management of inflammatory bowel disease.

If colonoscopy is unavailable, not feasible, or not desired by the patient, double-contrast barium enema alone or the combination of flexible sigmoidoscopy and double-contrast barium enema are acceptable alternatives.
† Dysplasia: abnormal development or growth of cells and tissues; tissue changes that can lead to cancer.
‡ Villous change: change in the villi, the tiny fingerlike projections on the surface of the mucous membrane of the intestinal tract.
§ Pancolitis: inflammation of the entire colon as a result of inflammatory bowel disease.

Table 3.3 Basic Advantages and Limitations of Screening Tests*

Screening Test	Advantages	Limitations
Fecal Occult Blood Test (FOBT) † ‡	No direct risk to colon No bowel preparation Sampling done at home Low upfront costs Proven effective in clinical trials	Must be done annually May miss many polyps and some cancers May produce false-positive test results Some forms of FOBT have pre-test dietary restrictions Colonoscopy will be needed if abnormal
Flexible Sigmoidoscopy	Fairly quick and safe Can perform biopsies Does not require a specialist and can be performed by internists, physician assistants, nurse practitioners, and nurses Done every 5 years	An enema is required to clean out the lower colon Views only about one-third of the colon Detects only two-thirds of all polyps and cancers Very small risk of infection or perforation (bowel tear) May be uncomfortable Colonoscopy needed if polyps or cancer seen
Colonoscopy	Can usually view entire colon Can perform biopsies and remove polyps Can diagnose other diseases Done every 10 years	Requires full bowel preparation High upfront costs Requires sedation Small risk of bowel tear (perforation), bleeding, or infection Requires a chaperone to drive patient home after procedure Patient may miss a day of work
Barium Enema	Can usually view entire colon Relatively safe No sedation needed Done every 5 years	May miss many small polyps and some cancers Requires full bowel preparation May be uncomfortable May produce false-positive test results Cannot remove polyps during testing Colonoscopy needed if abnormal

* For a more technical discussion of the advantages and limitations of colorectal screening tests, please visit the web sites of the U.S. Preventive Services Task Force (http://www.ahcpr.gov/clinic/3rduspstf/colorectal/colotab1.htm) and the National Colorectal Cancer Roundtable (www.nccrt.org).
† In-office FOBT at time of digital rectal exam is not an adequate substitute for the recommended 3-card take-home test.
‡ Immunochemical Fecal Occult Blood Testing is a new alternative to traditional FOBT. It employs a complex reaction using antibodies to detect hemoglobin and is less likely than traditional tests to yield false-positive results. In addition, it does not require dietary restrictions.

Which Test Is Best?

Doctors don't have any evidence to suggest that any of the recommended screening methods is the "best test" to screen for colorectal cancer. *The only unacceptable option is not to screen for colorectal cancer at all.* The best test is the one that's right for you—the one that fits your risk profile, your personal preferences, your current medical conditions, and the resources available to you for follow up and testing.

> "*Early detection saved my life.*"
>
> —JOHN

Talk to your doctor about your screening options. Together, you can discuss the benefits as well as the potential risks of each screening method, their advantages and disadvantages, and how often testing should take place. Table 3.3 on page 53 can help you in your decision making.

CHAPTER FOUR

INITIAL EVALUATION

Alan G. Thorson, MD

What brings people to the doctor for an initial evaluation for colorectal cancer? Some people may experience symptoms that might indicate colorectal cancer. These symptoms could include blood in the stool or a change in bowel habits. Other people might not have any symptoms, but they may have received suspicious results from a routine screening test, such as a yearly fecal occult blood test (FOBT). A few might come to the doctor because a close family member had colorectal cancer, and they are worried about their own risk.

If there is any reason to suspect that you might have colorectal cancer, your doctor will take a complete medical history and perform a physical exam. This will help him or her learn more about your past health record (any previous diagnosis of cancer, for example), your family health history, your current lifestyle (including such things as whether you smoke, drink alcohol to excess, or eat heathfully and exercise regularly—factors that can affect your risk), and any symptoms you're currently experiencing. In addition, your doctor will order some tests to find out if there is evidence of cancer and if so, if it's in an early or advanced stage.

If you have already had a screening test that diagnosed colorectal cancer (a flexible sigmoidoscopy or colonoscopy, for example), your doctor will still take your medical history and record related information that may help treat your disease.

Your doctor will also do a physical exam and will probably order additional diagnostic tests to determine the extent and seriousness of the cancer using a system of stages and grades (see chapter 5).

In the first scenario, the doctor makes a diagnosis, and in the second scenario, the doctor evaluates a diagnosis that has already been made. Although the process may happen in a different order, the steps of this "work-up" are very much the same.

What Is a Medical History?

When your doctor "takes a history," he or she will ask you careful questions about symptoms that could be caused by colorectal cancer: abdominal pain, any recent change in your bowel habits, a feeling that you need to have a bowel movement that is not relieved by doing so, rectal bleeding, weakness or fatigue, loss of appetite, or weight loss. (We'll talk more about symptoms of colorectal cancer later in this chapter). Of course, many other medical conditions and situations can cause one or more of these symptoms. The initial evaluation is a way to determine the cause(s) of any symptoms you experience, so that colorectal cancer can be ruled out or the appropriate tests can be done and proper treatment can be chosen if a diagnosis of colorectal cancer is made.

Personal Health History and Current Health Status

If the doctor you are seeing is not familiar with your personal health history, you should discuss past major illnesses, including past history of colorectal polyps, colorectal cancer, or other cancers that might be related.

Your doctor will also ask you about your lifestyle to find out if your daily habits put you at added risk for developing the disease. (See chapter 2 for more information on risk factors). You should also discuss your current health status, including whether you are experiencing any of the symptoms mentioned in the following sections that might be associated with colorectal cancer.

Symptoms You May Be Experiencing

Symptoms associated with colorectal cancer are generally not very specific. This means that these symptoms may be due to colorectal cancer or to a variety of other causes.

Symptoms of colorectal cancer include abdominal pain and bloating, change in bowel habit, continuous feeling that you need to have a bowel movement, rectal bleeding, anemia, weakness, fatigue, loss of appetite, and weight loss. More often than not, these symptoms will be caused by something other than colorectal cancer— stomach ulcers, gallstones, hemorrhoids, or even an adverse reaction to something you ate, for example. However, because of the dangers of colorectal cancer, people with these symptoms should immediately discuss them with a doctor.

No Symptoms

You may or may not experience colorectal cancer symptoms before a diagnosis. In fact, many people with early stage colorectal cancer will not experience any symptoms at all before it is diagnosed, particularly if they learned they had colorectal cancer through a screening program (see chapter 3). Remember, screening refers to testing done on people who have no symptoms. This is why screening for colorectal cancer is so important. Screening is your best bet to diagnose a colorectal cancer early, when it is most likely to be curable.

Symptoms of colorectal cancer become more apparent as the disease gets more serious. This means that the more symptoms a person has, the more likely it is that their cancer will already be somewhat advanced. By the time someone with colorectal cancer experiences symptoms, the disease may be harder to treat or cure.

> *"Previous to the initial diagnosis I had not had any symptoms of anything unusual: no blood in the stool or any kind of bleeding or anything that would indicate I had colorectal cancer. I was totally asymptomatic."*
> —JOHN

Abdominal Pain

Abdominal pain has many causes. It can be the result of bloating, overactivity of the bowel (which can cause cramps), or irritation of the lining of the abdomen. Bloating and cramping can occur when a cancer in the bowel has grown large enough to cause a blockage or obstruction of the bowel. The lining of the abdomen can become irritated by infection, from a cancer that has perforated (produced a hole in) the bowel, or from a tumor growing through the wall of the bowel into the lining of the abdomen or other abdominal organs. Sometimes abdominal pain can result from bleeding into a large tumor; this can cause the cancer to swell rapidly and put pressure on surrounding organs or tissues. Cancers on the left side of the colon are more likely to result in abdominal pain.

Many other illnesses can cause such abdominal pain, including appendicitis, diverticulitis, irritable bowel syndrome, other benign and cancerous tumors, and conditions such as ovarian cysts, ovarian cancer, kidney stones, peptic ulcer disease, stomach cancer, liver cancer, gallstones or gall bladder cancer, and pancreatic cancer.

Change in Bowel Habit

Some people with colorectal cancer may experience changes in their bowel habits. This could be someone with regular bowel habits who suddenly becomes constipated or someone with a history of constipation who develops loose stool or diarrhea. Changes in bowel habit are more likely to be noted with rectal or left-sided colon cancer than with right-sided colon cancer. This is particularly true for constipation. Cancers on the left side of the colon and in the rectum more commonly grow in a way that causes narrowing of the colon and rectum. In addition, the stool in the left colon is more solid than in the right colon, where stool is usually quite liquid. Therefore, the left colon is more likely to produce symptoms associated with obstruction, such as bloating and cramping. Left-sided colon cancer is more likely than right-sided colon cancer to cause a change in bowel habits as well.

> *"I had mild abdominal pain, irregular bowel movements, and I knew something wasn't quite right. So I decided to see my doctor."*
> —EDDIE

Cancers that are associated with certain types of polyps may lead to diarrhea. Villous polyps (see chapter 1) sometimes secrete or ooze large amounts of mucus that can lead to diarrhea. Cancers in the right colon sometimes become very bulky and cause a partial blockage that will hold back liquid stool and cause cramping and bloating. Eventually the blockage may build up enough pressure to bypass the cancer with an "explosion" of stool. This sudden passage of stool beyond the tumor may result in diarrhea with relief from the cramping and bloating.

A Feeling You Need to Have a Bowel Movement That Is Not Relieved by Doing So

Rectal cancer can cause symptoms unique to its location. A cancer in the rectum may produce a sensation of fullness or pressure. This sensation may feel just like stool in the rectum. It may make you feel like you need to have a bowel movement even after you have just had one. Occasionally, a cancer of the rectum will grow to fill most of the rectal space so there is little room left for stool. If this happens, when stool does enter the rectum, there may be a feeling like you have to go to the bathroom "right now" and are unable to hold back the stool. This is called urgency. This is a feeling like you are about to have diarrhea all of the time. The sensation may not go away.

Sometimes a rectal cancer will grow through the wall of the rectum and enter the sphincter muscle and muscle of the rectal wall. This can result in spasm or cramping of the muscle, a condition called tenesmus. This is like having a "charley horse" of the rectum.

Rectal Bleeding

Bleeding is probably one of the most recognized signs of colorectal cancer and the one that causes the most fear. Although most rectal bleeding is caused by reasons other than cancer, any bleeding should be evaluated by a doctor as soon as possible to be sure there is no serious problem. Common causes of rectal bleeding other than cancer include hemorrhoids, anal fissures, colitis, and diverticulosis.

Visible rectal bleeding occurs more often with rectal and left-sided colon cancer. Bleeding from right-sided colon cancer is more often occult (invisible or hidden) because small amounts of blood from a right-sided cancer get mixed with the stool while being passed through the rest of the colon. Blood loss from cancer on the left side of the colon and the rectum has less chance to become mixed completely with the stool before being eliminated. As a result, it may be visible in a bowel movement.

Anemia, Weakness, and Fatigue

Anemia is a lower-than-normal number of red blood cells in the blood. A low red blood cell count means less oxygen is carried to the body's cells, which can make a person feel tired or weak.

When someone is diagnosed as anemic, finding out the type of anemia is important. If a low red blood cell count is associated with low levels of iron, an evaluation of the large intestine may be recommended to rule out a colorectal cancer. Although there are many causes of anemia, loss of blood from a tumor in the colon or rectum is a serious one.

Anemia occurs more frequently with cancer in the right colon. This is because right-sided colon cancers more frequently result in hidden or occult bleeding. Therefore, cancer of the right colon may bleed unnoticed for a long time, causing anemia. Because cancers of the left colon and rectum more frequently result in the passage of visible blood, they are more often detected before enough bleeding has occurred to cause anemia.

Anorexia and Weight Loss

Anorexia is a loss of appetite or poor appetite. It often results in weight loss. This symptom is most often seen with more advanced colorectal cancers.

The reason for the loss of appetite may be that the cancer is affecting the ability of food to move through the intestines (partial blockage). However, it is more common not to be able to explain the loss of appetite. Sometimes, as cancers become more advanced, a person's appetite just seems to disappear. Although the way in which advanced cancer causes anorexia is not yet completely understood, researchers have found a numbers of substances released by cancer cells that suppress the appetite.

Because cancers of the right colon tend to have fewer visible symptoms (less visible bleeding, less frequent changes in bowel habit, and fewer symptoms of blockage, as discussed above), they are more often discovered when they are advanced cancers. Therefore, weight loss and anorexia are more often seen with colon cancer on the right side of the body than with left-sided colon and rectal cancers.

Family Health History

An important next step is for your doctor to find out more about your family history. Because a small number of colorectal cancers may be hereditary—familial adenomatous polyposis (FAP) and hereditary nonpolyposis colorectal cancer (HNPCC) are two examples—it is important for your doctor to be aware of your family's health history. As the number of family members with colorectal cancer increase, your risk also increases (see Figure 4.1).

Table 4.1 Differences in Symptoms of Cancer in the Right and Left Colon	
Symptoms of Right-Sided Colon Cancer Typically diagnosed at a *more* advanced stage because of *less noticeable* symptoms	**Symptoms of Left-Sided Colon Cancer** Typically diagnosed at a *less* advanced stage because of *more noticeable* symptoms
• Pain less common or less intense	• Pain
• Anorexia/weight loss	• Anorexia/weight loss less common
• Occult (hidden) bleeding	• Rectal bleeding, bleeding tends to be more visible
• Anemia	• Anemia less common
• Obstructive symptoms less common	• Obstructive symptoms and signs
• Change in bowel habit less common	• Change in bowel habit

Note: Colorectal cancer may not cause any symptoms until the cancer is advanced. Lack of symptoms does not mean that no cancer is present.

Figure 4.1 A Person's Lifetime Risk* of Colorectal Cancer Based on Family History

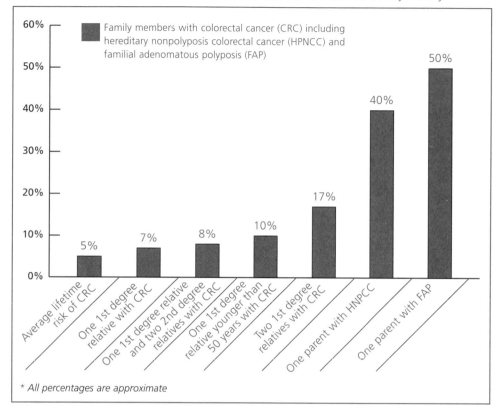

As you now know, your family history is a very important detail. You should do all you can to find out what types of cancers have occurred in your family, especially in first-degree relatives. First-degree relatives are your parents, siblings, and children. Second-degree relatives are grandparents and aunts and uncles. A history of colorectal cancer is most important to know about in terms of your own risk of colorectal cancer, but don't overlook cancers of the stomach, uterus, ovaries, kidneys, ureters, brain, and small bowel—these other cancers are also associated with some forms of hereditary colorectal cancer. If there is a history of *any* cancer in any of these relatives, your doctor may ask you for more detailed information about your grandparents, aunts, uncles, and cousins.

The age of family members who had cancer is very important too. You should tell your doctor of the ages of diagnosis of any family members with cancer and, if they are no longer living, at what ages they died.

Gathering this information about your family tree is important for *your* health, but it can also help ensure the continued good health of the ones you love. If your doctor tells you that your colorectal cancer may have a genetic or inherited component, you should talk candidly with your family members about their increased risk for the disease, and encourage them to follow the American Cancer Society guidelines for colorectal cancer screening for persons at high risk (reprinted in Table 3.2 on page 52).

Physical Examination

Your doctor will perform a simple physical exam in his or her office to add to the information gathered from your personal and family medical history.

The doctor will perform a digital rectal exam (DRE) to help determine if you have rectal cancer. When there is a cancer in the lower rectum just inside the anal opening, it is important for the doctor to examine the groin area for any evidence of enlarged lymph nodes, the small bean-shaped organs that make and store infection-fighting white blood cells. (Enlarged lymph nodes may suggest advanced cancer, although infection can also cause lymph nodes to enlarge.) Cancers higher up in the colon cannot be detected by a DRE.

The doctor will also feel your abdomen for masses, growths, or enlarged organs. (As colorectal cancer becomes more advanced, it may be possible to feel it as a mass in the lower abdomen. Enlargement of the liver, located in the right upper abdomen, is a possible sign of cancer that has metastasized, or spread.)

Your doctor will also do a general survey of the rest of your body. This assessment of your general health will help your doctor predict how well you will be able to tolerate potential treatments.

Diagnostic Tests

If the physical examination, your personal medical history, and/or your medical family history suggest to your doctor that colon or rectal cancer might be present, he or she may order a series of tests. The first test ordered is usually a colonoscopy, which can help evaluate the colon and rectum to see if there really is a cancer. If a growth is found during the colonoscopy, a biopsy can be taken at that time to confirm a diagnosis. Once a diagnosis of colon or rectal cancer is made, additional testing may be done. The tests your doctor orders will depend upon the location of the cancer and other factors that your doctor may consider. These tests are briefly described in the next section of this chapter.

Figure 4.2 Biopsy Showing Adenocarcinoma of the Colon

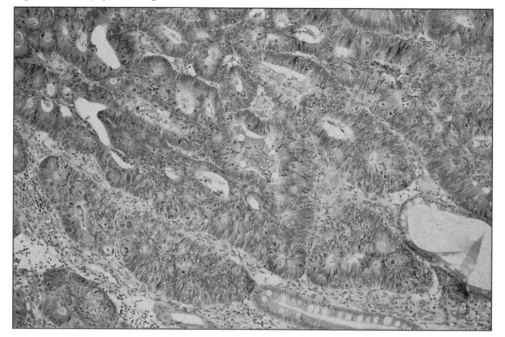

Source: Figure 5-12 from Willett CG. American Cancer Society Atlas of Clinical Oncology Cancer of the Lower Gastrointestinal Tract. *Hamilton, Ontario, Canada: BC Decker; 2001:61.*

Colonoscopy

A colonoscopy allows your doctor to look directly at the lining of the colon. Recall from chapter 3 that colonoscopy is a technique for looking at the colon or large bowel through a colonoscope, a lighted, flexible tube with a video camera at the end. This visual examination of the entire colon allows for a thorough inspection as well as tissue sampling, if necessary.

Biopsy of Lesion

One of the advantages of using colonoscopy for the examination at this time is the ability to biopsy any suspicious areas as soon as they are seen. A biopsy is the surgical removal of a small piece of tissue, which is then examined under a microscope to see if cancer cells are present (see Figure 4.2). Biopsies are performed using long instruments passed through the colonoscope.

Blood Tests

Certain blood tests, like a complete blood count (CBC), are sometimes used in the evaluation of colon and rectal cancer. In addition, other blood tests that look at how well your kidneys and liver are functioning are often used if you are receiving chemotherapy, because chemotherapy can sometimes affect kidney and liver function. In addition, large rectal tumors can block the ureters (the tubes that run between the kidneys and the bladder), which can interfere with kidney function.

Complete Blood Count

Some people with colorectal cancer may have anemia (see page 59). A CBC can help determine if this is the case. It can also help determine whether anemia is due to blood loss (which might indicate colorectal cancer) or to some other cause, such as leukemia or another chronic disease.

Imaging Tests

These tests are used to make images or pictures of the cancer and look for evidence of spread of the tumor. A number of different types of imaging tests are used in the evaluation of colorectal cancer. These include chest X-rays, ultrasound, computed tomography (CT), magnetic resonance imaging (MRI), positron emission tomography (PET), and angiography.

Chest X-Ray

X-rays use very short wavelengths of high-energy electromagnetic radiation to provide images of the body. X-rays are very common; almost everyone has had X-rays of their teeth in a dentist's office or has been given an X-ray to examine a broken bone in a hospital emergency room.

Chest X-rays are used to evaluate the lungs for possible metastases (spread) of colorectal cancer. If you have a chest X-ray that shows a spot suspicious for cancer, your doctor may order a CT scan of the chest to get more detail about it. If the spot can be seen on CT scan, it may need to be biopsied with a CT-guided needle.

Ultrasound

Ultrasound uses sound waves rather than X-rays to create images of the body. Many people are familiar with ultrasound from pregnancy or an evaluation of

Tumor Markers: CEA

Tumor markers are proteins or other substances that can signify the presence of cancer somewhere in the body. Carcinoembryonic antigen (CEA) is a tumor marker for colorectal cancer, especially advanced colorectal cancer. CEA can be detected with blood tests, but *these tests are not used to make a diagnosis of colorectal cancer* because CEA level is not elevated in all people with colorectal cancer. Several conditions other than colorectal cancer can raise the CEA level, which increases the likelihood of a false positive.

If this protein is elevated at the time of diagnosis, these blood tests can be used to follow the progress of therapy for colorectal cancer.

They can also be used to detect a recurrence of a colorectal cancer. They are most effective for this if they were elevated at the time of diagnosis and returned to normal after treatment. Then, if the level goes up again, doctors must consider a possible recurrence of the cancer. (See chapter 18 for a complete discussion of recurrence.)

the gallbladder. Ultrasound does not expose a person to radiation. In the case of colorectal cancer, ultrasound is used primarily in two situations: endorectal and intraoperative ultrasound.

Endorectal Ultrasound

Endorectal ultrasound (also known as transrectal ultrasound or TRUS) is used to evaluate how much a rectal cancer has grown into the wall of the rectum. It also evaluates lymph nodes in the rectal region. This information helps to determine the type of treatment that will be used to treat a rectal cancer.

Intraoperative Ultrasound

Intraoperative ultrasound is done with a special probe designed for use during an operation. Intraoperative ultrasound is most frequently used to evaluate the liver for evidence of metastases (cancer spread). Using an ultrasound probe directly on the surface of the liver during an operation is more accurate than using an ultrasound on the skin of the abdomen.

Intraoperative ultrasound can help to identify possible liver metastases that might be able to be removed during the operation. It can also identify metastases that might need to be treated with chemotherapy after an operation.

Computed Tomography

Computed tomography (CT, also called a "CAT scan") is a computerized X-ray procedure that produces cross-sectional images of the body layer by layer. This special radiology procedure takes X-ray pictures through a specific region of the body, which a computer then reconstructs to produce two- and three-dimensional images of your organs that are photographed for your doctor to study.

If you are told you have colon or rectal cancer, your doctor may order a CT scan of the abdomen and/or chest. Before the CT scan, you may be asked to drink "contrast" fluid or have "contrast" administered as an enema to help to identify your intestines on the X-ray picture. You may also have a needle inserted into a vein so that contrast material can be injected to help your doctor see your blood vessels.

The CT scan itself is not painful, although some people find the short tunnel or "doughnut" that the X-ray is done in to be uncomfortable, especially if they are claustrophobic. During the examination, you may hear whirring and clicking as the table you lie on moves through the "doughnut" and the X-ray tube spins around inside of the machine as it takes pictures from all sides of you. The examination may take from 5 to 30 minutes depending on how much of your body needs to be examined.

Not all people who have colorectal cancer need to have a CT scan. However, if you have rectal cancer, a CT scan may help determine if there is evidence of spread of the tumor to the lungs or the liver before starting radiation therapy.

Some medical centers are using special CT imaging to evaluate rectal cancers for the same information currently obtained by endorectal ultrasound. CT scans are also helpful in looking for a recurrence if you have a history of colorectal cancer and/or an increased level of CEA (see page 97).

Spiral CT

Spiral CT is done using a new generation of CT scanners designed to obtain a large volume of data by continuous scanning through a specific body area. The data are then stored in computer memory for later manipulation and interpretation so that specific areas of the body can be carefully analyzed without having to call someone back for more testing. Spiral CT means less examination time, less radiation exposure, faster test results, and less need for breath-holding. The evolving techniques of spiral or helical CT scanning have led to newer techniques such as CT colonography/virtual colonoscopy (see chapter 3).

CT-Guided Needle Biopsy

If you have an abnormal CT scan because of possible tumor spread, your doctor may order a CT-guided needle biopsy of the abnormality to determine if it is cancer. A CT-guided biopsy is a much less invasive way to get information about an abnormal X-ray than having an operation. It involves using a CT scan to re-identify the area in question. A small amount of local anesthetic is then used to numb the skin over the site, and a small needle is inserted. The CT scan is used to be sure the needle is placed in the spot that the doctor wants to examine more thoroughly. During CT-guided needle biopsy, a small amount of tissue can be brought out through the needle and sent to the laboratory to be analyzed under a microscope. This type of biopsy can be done for abnormal areas in the liver, the lungs, and sites in the abdomen and pelvis that can be viewed with the CT scan.

Magnetic Resonance Imaging

Magnetic resonance imaging (MRI) is a special type of imaging that does not use X-rays. Instead, by using a combination of radio waves and a strong magnet, differences in the atoms of various tissues can be identified and recorded. This information can then be made into pictures of the body.

Advantages of using MRI include the degree of detail that can be obtained in specific tissues and the fact that there is no radiation exposure. Some disadvantages are that you need to remain very still because motion can distort images, that MRI examinations generally take longer than CT scans, that the magnetic field prevents people with pacemakers from being scanned, and that metal objects must not be brought into the area of the scanner. The magnet in the machine can erase credit cards and other cards with a magnetic strip. There is a higher risk of claustrophobia than with CT scans, although newer generation "open" scanners greatly decrease this concern.

If you have colon or rectal cancer, MRI scans are sometimes used to examine tissues that are difficult to evaluate with CT scans. MRI is a particularly good technique to look at the brain and spine. Some centers are now using MRI to obtain information about rectal cancers similar to that provided by endorectal ultrasound.

Positron Emission Tomography

A positron emission tomography (PET) scan uses an entirely different method of imaging to evaluate a cancer. Generally, cancerous tissue has a higher metabolic rate than normal tissue. That is, cancer cells use more energy than normal cells. A PET scan takes advantage of this fact by using radioactive sugar injected into a vein. Because cancer cells use more energy than normal cells, they absorb more sugar. A special scanner can measure this increased absorption.

PET scans are generally used in combination with CT scans to better interpret abnormal findings, especially in people who may have had surgery for colorectal cancer (such as a resection of the colon, see chapter 10) in the past. Since a CT scan can only show shadows, it may be difficult to tell whether abnormal tissue on a CT scan is cancer or just scar tissue from a previous operation or cancer treatment.

If a PET scan shows that an abnormal area on a CT scan has higher-than-normal metabolic activity, it greatly increases the chance that the area is a cancer. PET scans can also help to find a cancer that has not been visible on other types of scanning, such as CT or MRI.

Angiography

Angiography is the process of X-raying blood vessels. If you have a colorectal cancer with metastases to the liver, and parts of the liver need to be removed (or resected), you may be given an angiogram. This test can help the doctor plan surgery on the liver so that as many healthy portions of the liver as possible can be saved and so that bleeding can be minimized. In many cancer centers, angiography is now being replaced by the newer generation CT and MRI scans.

If you have an angiography performed, an intravenous (IV) line will be inserted through your skin into a blood vessel. Depending upon what blood vessel your doctor wants to look at, you may have a longer catheter or tube passed into the blood vessel to near the point that needs to be studied. Contrast material is then injected into the blood vessel, and a rapid series of X-rays are taken. Pictures are then made of the images so that they can be reviewed and studied by your doctor.

Why Is All This Information Gathering Necessary?

During your initial evaluation for colorectal cancer, your doctor will gather a lot of information from you. He or she will record your personal and family health history to get a sense of the "big picture." Your doctor will also perform a short physical exam and will order a variety of diagnostic and imaging tests to learn more about your current condition.

All of this information plays a critical role in determining if you have colorectal cancer and, if you do, in helping to establish the extent and seriousness of your disease. The family medical history also provides clues about whether others you love may be at risk. The results of each of these tests supplies crucial information that will help you and your doctor work together to decide on the best course of treatment for your specific situation.

CHAPTER FIVE

DIAGNOSIS AND STAGING

David A. Rothenberger, MD
Robert P. Akbari MD
Rocco Ricciardi, MD

S ometimes an experienced doctor who performs colorectal cancer screening or diagnostic tests (see chapters 3 and 4) might be able to make a fairly confident diagnosis during an endoscopic examination based on the appearance of the tumor alone. At other times, the diagnosis of cancer is not as obvious and will be made based on additional test results, especially a biopsy of the abnormal area (see chapter 4). Sometimes, the diagnosis of colorectal cancer remains unknown until an operation is performed and the entire surgical specimen is studied.

Even when the diagnosis of cancer seems obvious, the doctor will almost always take a biopsy of the tumor. This allows a specially trained doctor called a pathologist to confirm the diagnosis and describe the cancer in greater detail to the rest of the health care team. This information about the nature of the cancer provided by the pathologist—how aggressive and widespread the cancer is, for example—is useful for determining which treatments may be most effective against the cancer.

The Role of the Pathologist

A pathologist is a doctor whose area of expertise is the study of diseases' effects on human tissues. Pathologists are experts in diagnosing cancer in tissue samples. They inspect the sample with the naked eye and then cut portions of it into very thin slices (sections) that are stained with special chemicals to help identify different structures and types of cells under the microscope.

The pathologist is an extremely important member of the health care team. The pathologist must carefully analyze tissue sample(s) to identify the presence of cancer cells, determine the type of cancer that is present, and evaluate the extent of cancer in the tissues. All of this information is reported to the doctors caring for the patient in the form of a pathology report, a document we'll talk more about later in this chapter (see page 82).

Initial Diagnosis

In the early phases of determining whether someone has cancer, the main task for the pathologist is to determine whether the tissue sample contains cancer. The thin slices of tissue are examined under the microscope to search for cancer cells. If cancer cells are present, the biopsy is considered malignant, and if no cancer cells are found, the biopsy is considered benign.

Of course, the pathologist can only interpret the findings of the tissue sample (biopsy) he or she is given. Therefore, if a biopsy is taken from an area just next to a cancer, the biopsy may show normal benign tissue. This does not mean that there is no cancer. Likewise, some tumors are made up of both benign and malignant tissue. A biopsy of a portion of the tumor may only include benign tissue even though malignant cells may be present only a fraction of an inch away.

"I had the colonoscopy, and when I was coming to, my doctor was standing next to the bed and he asked me if I was awake, and if I could hear him, and if I could understand what he was saying, and I said, 'Yes.' And he was holding a photo and he said, 'I'm sorry to tell you but we discovered you have a tumor on your colon. We took a biopsy, but I'm certain that it's colon cancer. You have to see a surgeon and you have to have surgery immediately.'"

—EDDIE

For these reasons, doctors often take multiple tissue samples so they can diagnose or rule out cancer with greater accuracy. If initial biopsies are benign but the doctor is highly suspicious that cancer is present because of the appearance or examination of the tissue, the doctor may insist on additional biopsies. Sometimes the entire abnormal growth is surgically removed so the pathologist can test it. This is called an excisional biopsy.

Tumor Type

The pathologist examines the specimen to determine the type of tumor. The vast majority of colorectal cancers are adenocarcinomas. Other types of malignancies such as carcinoid, lymphoma, squamous cell cancer, or melanoma can occur in the large intestine, but they are rare. (In this book, we focus on adenocarcinoma.)

Cancer cells can sometimes travel to other parts of the body, where they begin to grow and replace normal tissue. This process, called metastasis, occurs as the cancer cells get into the circulatory systems of the body. Because cancer can spread, the pathologist must also find the organ or tissue from which a cancer originally developed. For example, the pathologist may receive a biopsy of a suspicious growth in the liver of a patient who has a history of colorectal cancer. In this situation, the pathologist has to determine not only whether the biopsy is benign or malignant but also whether the cancer started in the colon and spread (metastasized) to the liver or if it is a "primary" liver cancer, meaning that the abnormal cells originated in the liver. (When cells from a cancer such as colorectal cancer spread to another organ, such as the liver, the cancer is still called colorectal cancer, not liver cancer.)

This distinction is important because it helps a doctor and patient to choose the best treatment. Sometimes, it is easy to tell the tissue of origin of the cancer biopsy; at other times, the pathologist has to do additional tests on the tissue to ensure the correct diagnosis. Some of these tests are called special stains because they use chemicals that "stain" or change the color of certain types of cells.

Stage and Grade of Cancer

In addition to making an initial diagnosis and determining the type of cancer, another important task for the pathologist is to provide grading and pathologic staging information to the doctor. The grading and staging systems are a kind of medical shorthand that tell health care professionals more about the nature of the cancer in simple terms. These numeric codes and systems also help doctors compare the results of treatment for similar forms of cancer.

Doctors use information about the cancer's characteristics to help determine the most appropriate treatment options, create a treatment plan, and predict a patient's prognosis. Since staging and grading information is so important, we'll return to these two topics later in this chapter to provide additional explanation (see page 75).

Permanent Section and Frozen Section Analysis

The pathologist also analyzes the slides of biopsied tissue, called sections. The process of creating a permanent section—the slides most medical centers rely on for a definitive diagnosis of cancer—typically takes one to three days. If there is an urgent need for pathology assessment, a frozen section can be done in a matter of minutes. However, a frozen section does not display the tissues as clearly as a permanent section, so the analysis may be less accurate.

The purpose of a frozen section analysis is to help the surgeon make an immediate decision about the extent of the operation before the procedure is completed. The term frozen section comes from the fact that the pathologist freezes the tissue sample and then makes thin slices from the frozen block of tissue for immediate study under the microscope to look for cancer. No special staining or other techniques are used to assess the sample, so the whole process takes only five to 15 minutes. The surgeon uses the information from a frozen section analysis to make an immediate decision about what should be done. If the pathologist finds cancer in the frozen section analysis, the surgeon may have to change the planned operation.

Most centers confirm the diagnosis made by the frozen section with a subsequent permanent section analysis.

Confirming Adequacy of Resection Margins

When surgically removing part of a diseased organ, the surgeon will remove some cancer-free tissue around the cancer to increase the chances of getting all the cancer cells out. This cancer-free tissue is called a margin.

During the surgical process of resection (see chapter 10), the surgeon may ask the pathologist to perform an immediate examination of the surgical specimen to confirm the adequacy of the resection margins (the amount of normal tissue that surrounds the cancer). As the size of the margin goes up, the likelihood of the cancer recurring in that location goes down. However, if the doctor takes too much tissue out, then the patient is at increased risk for complications after surgery.

The usual operations for colon cancer remove as much as a foot of normal-appearing colon tissue on either side of the cancer. Because there is still plenty of colon tissue remaining, this usually does not cause any problems for the patient. It is uncommon, therefore, for surgeons to request frozen sections to check the margins of a colon cancer. On the other hand, in removing rectal cancers, surgeons try to avoid damage to the muscles that control bowel movements. They need to be very precise about how much rectal tissue to remove, so frozen sections of margins are used more often.

Follow-Up Biopsies

After treatment of a colorectal cancer, there is a risk that the cancer could return (see chapter 18 for more information on recurrence). When cancer does recur, it can come back at the site of the original tumor or in other locations, like the liver or lungs. If a tumor recurrence is suspected, additional tests will be done, and a biopsy of the suspicious area is usually obtained. The pathologist then determines whether the biopsy contains tissue that has the same features as the original cancer.

Grading: How Aggressive Is the Cancer?

Grade (also called histologic grade; histology is the study of microscopic structures of tissue) is helpful in predicting the aggressiveness of the cancer. The grade is based on how the cancer cells appear under the microscope. More specifically, the grade describes how closely the tumor being examined resembles normal noncancerous tissue. In cancers that appear very similar to normal tissue, the pathologist can clearly see different cells grouped together; these are called well-differentiated cells and are classified as grade 1. The higher the grade of cancer, the less normal or more poorly differentiated the cells look.

A high grade means the cancer is more dangerous—that is, it is likely to grow fast and spread. For example, grade 1 (well-differentiated) cancers are the least aggressive, while grade 3 or 4 (poorly differentiated or undifferentiated) cancers are the most aggressive.

A simpler 2-tiered system of histology grading is becoming popular, with the phrase "low grade cancer" being used to describe grade 1 or 2 cancers, while "high grade cancer" is the term applied to cancers previously labeled grades 3 or 4.

The pathologist may use other terms to describe the histology of an aggressive adenocarcinoma. Talk to your doctor about the significance of these specific descriptions of your cancer.

Staging: How Widespread Is the Cancer?

Cancer staging is a process that doctors use to determine how widespread a cancer may be. In the case of colorectal cancer, they want to know if the cancer is contained to a small area, if it has grown locally and involved the lymph nodes, or if it has spread (metastasized) to distant sites in the body.

Clinical Staging

As part of your initial evaluation and diagnosis, and before your treatment begins, your doctor will combine the information gathered from your examination, special imaging studies, the biopsy of your cancer, and other tests to establish a clinical stage. A clinical stage is established before a major surgery. If you have surgery for colorectal cancer, the doctors will use the tissue they remove during the operation to establish a pathologic stage (see next section).

Clinical staging of rectal cancer differs from staging of colon cancer. If you have rectal cancer, your doctor will order special tests (such as an ultrasound or MRI) to determine how deeply the cancer has penetrated into the wall of the rectum and whether the cancer has spread to nearby lymph nodes. This information is used to select the best treatment for your particular stage of rectal cancer. If you have colon cancer, clinical staging is less involved. However, for both colon and rectal cancer, your doctor will order tests to determine whether the cancer may have spread to other sites in your body.

Why is clinical staging so important? Because the clinical stage is one of the key factors that your doctor uses to make a recommendation for a specific treatment plan. In addition, the clinical stage is the basis for a realistic discussion of the prognosis or likely outcome after your treatment (see chapter 6).

Pathologic Staging

After surgery for colorectal cancer, the pathologist examines all tissues that were removed by the surgeon to determine the pathologic stage. Sometimes the pre-treatment clinical stage is different from the final pathologic stage.

Your doctor will talk to you about both the clinical and pathologic stage of your disease. If the final pathologic stage is different from the pretreatment clinical stage, it may be necessary to adjust your treatment plan. You should feel free to discuss any changes with your doctor.

Staging Systems

A staging system is a standardized classification scheme that describes the extent of a cancer. As noted earlier, staging systems use codes to allow doctors to quickly and accurately describe a particular cancer using a universal language that all specialists can understand. Staging systems also help doctors compare the results of treatment of similar forms of cancer.

Over the years, a number of staging systems have been used to classify colorectal cancers. All systems describe the extent of colorectal cancer in terms of penetration

Table 5.1 Comparison of Colorectal Cancer Staging Systems

TNM	TNM Stage	Dukes	Astler-Coller
Tis	0	—	—
T1-2, N0, M0	I	A	A, B1
T3-4, N0, M0	II	B	B2, B3
T(any), N(1 or 2), M0	III	C	C1, C2, C3
T(any), N(any), M1	IV	—	D

Source: Table A1.3, Comparison of Dukes and TNM Stages, from Levin B. Colorectal Cancer: A Thorough and Compassionate Resource for Patients and Their Families. *Atlanta, GA: American Cancer Society; 1999:226.*

into the wall of the large intestine, spread to nearby lymph nodes, and spread to distant parts of the body.

The Dukes staging system, devised in the 1930s, uses the letters A, B, and C to describe the stage of the cancer. It was the most widely used classification until recently. As our knowledge of colorectal cancer increased, several modifications of the Dukes system were recommended. The most popular of these was the Astler-Coller staging system, which uses letters A through D as a code for the extent of the cancer.

In 1987, the American Joint Committee on Cancer (AJCC) developed a new classification for colorectal cancer, the TNM system. The TNM staging system is more precise than the other systems and is consistent with the way many other types of cancers are staged, making it easier for health care professionals to remember and use. As a result, it has become the most frequently used system for staging colorectal cancer in the United States and much of the rest of the world. It was recently modified to allow for an even more accurate picture of the extent of colorectal cancer. (See page 79 for a detailed explanation of the AJCC/TNM staging system.)

If your cancer stage is reported using the Dukes or Astler-Coller system, Table 5.1 will allow you to find the matching AJCC/TNM stage.

Growth and Spread of Colorectal Cancer

To understand the staging systems more completely, it is useful to review the way colorectal cancer grows and spreads. Cancers of the colon and rectum usually begin as nonmalignant tumors called polyps that grow from the inner lining

Figure 5.1 Layers of the Colon Wall

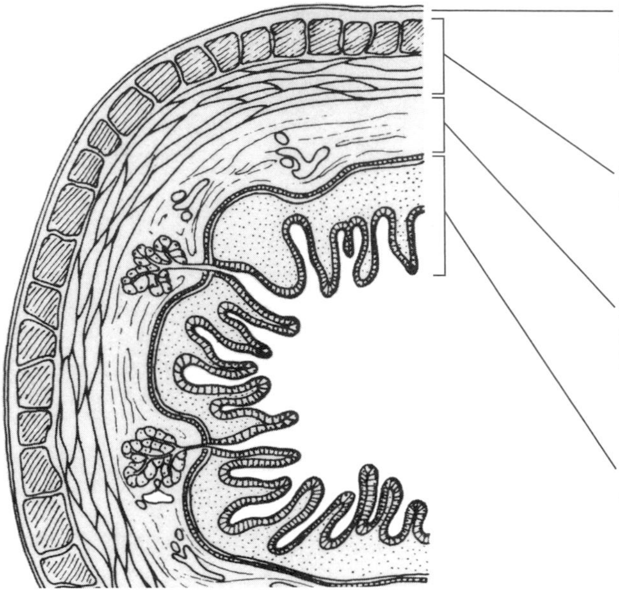

SEROSA
(outer covering of the
intestine, includes subserosa)

MUSCULARIS PROPRIA
(muscle layer)

SUBMUCOSA
(connective tissue containing
lymph and blood vessels)

MUCOSA
(includes muscularis mucosa,
lamina propria, and epithelium)

Source: Adapted from image courtesy of the National Cancer Institute.

(mucosa) of the intestine (see Figure 5.1). Over a period of many years, some of these benign polyps may undergo changes that ultimately lead to cancer. These changes involve a series of DNA mutations that cause the cells of the tumor to grow abnormally. At first, the growing mass of now malignant cells is contained entirely within an otherwise benign polyp. Later, these cells can spread through the benign tissue of the polyp and into the adjacent colorectal tissue. As the cancer grows slowly in three dimensions, it extends lengthwise along the inner lining of the intestine, radially around the circumference of the bowel (intestinal) wall, and deeply into and through the bowel wall. If the tumor penetrates the muscularis mucosa, which is a thin layer of muscle just next to the inner surface layer, it gains access to lymph channels and blood vessels in the submucosa of the intestine. The tumor can shed cancer cells into these channels and vessels, and the cancer cells can then flow through the lymph and blood systems to spread to other sites in the body. This process is called metastasis. A cancer that is confined to the muscle layer of the mucosa (muscularis mucosa) is never considered life-threatening (as long as it is treated promptly, before it spreads further) because it cannot spread to other sites. In contrast, a tumor that invades through the muscularis mucosa is considered a malignant tumor or cancer because it can metastasize.

Table 5.2 TNM Classification of Colorectal Cancer	
Tx	No description of the tumor's extent is possible because of incomplete information.
T0	No evidence of a primary tumor.
Tis	The cancer is in the earliest stage. It has not grown beyond the mucosa (inner layer) of the colon or rectum. This stage is also known as carcinoma in situ or intramucosal carcinoma.
T1	The cancer has grown through the mucosa and extends into the submucosa.
T2	The cancer has grown through the mucosa and the submucosa and extends into the thick muscle layer.
T3	The cancer has grown through the mucosa, the submucosa, and completely through the thick muscle layer. It has spread to the subserosa but not to any nearby organs or tissues.
T4	The cancer has spread completely through the wall of the colon or rectum into nearby tissues or organs.
Nx	No description of lymph node involvement is possible because of incomplete information.
N0	No lymph node involvement.
N1	Cancer cells found in one to three regional lymph nodes.
N2	Cancer cells found in four or more regional lymph nodes.
Mx	No description of distant spread is possible because of incomplete information.
M0	No distant spread.
M1	Distant spread is present.

Source: Used with the permission of the American Joint Committee on Cancer (AJCC), Chicago, Illinois. The original source for material is the AJCC Cancer Staging Manual, Sixth Edition (2002) published by Springer-Verlag, New York, www.springeronline.com.

TNM Staging System

In the TNM system, three elements are coded. T stands for the extent of the primary (main) colorectal tumor, N for the extent of lymph node involvement, and M for distant metastasis (spread) to other organs or tissues. Each of these letters is followed by a number that provides more details about that element; the higher the number, the more serious the state of each element in the system (see Table 5.2).

Although it is an important factor in staging other cancers, the size of the colorectal tumor does not affect its stage. Instead, the TNM system describes how deeply the cancer has penetrated the bowel lining and if the cancer has spread locally or to distant body parts.

T Stage

The T stage is the code used to describe the extent of tumor spread through the layers that form the wall of the large intestine. The T stage is extremely important because it correlates closely with the likelihood of spread to lymph nodes, distant spread to other sites, and patient survival. The higher the T stage, the worse the patient's prognosis.

N Stage

The N stage is the code used to signify spread of the colorectal cancer to the lymph nodes near the primary tumor. These lymph nodes are located near the major blood vessels that keep the large intestine alive. They are present in all people but do not normally contain cancer cells.

As a tumor penetrates the intestinal wall, cancer cells are shed into the lymph channels and then funneled into the nearby lymph nodes, where they grow. Depending on location, biopsies may be done to confirm the presence of cancer in lymph nodes. If cancer is found in the lymph nodes, this can affect the treatment plan.

Unfortunately, imaging technology is still not able to identify cancer in lymph nodes with total accuracy, so pretreatment clinical staging of the N status (the measure of the spread of colorectal cancer to the lymph nodes near the primary tumor) is often inaccurate. The final N stage is determined by the pathologist who identifies lymph nodes in the tissues removed by the surgeon and examines them under the microscope for the presence of cancer cells.

The pathologist should record the number of lymph nodes that are sampled from a specimen, since the accuracy of staging correlates with the number of nodes examined. Generally, seven to fourteen lymph nodes should be examined to confidently assess the N stage. N status is reported as N1 if one to three nodes are involved with cancer and N2 if four or more nodes are involved by cancer. N2 cancers have a worse prognosis than N1 cancers.

N stage does not include spread of cancer to the nodes around the liver, lungs, or other distant sites. Such distant spread is considered a metastasis and included in the M stage.

M Stage

The M stage is the code used to describe the spread of the colorectal cancer to other body organs or other distant sites. The liver and lungs are the most common sites of metastases from the colon and rectum. If distant metastases are present, the chances of long-term survival are lower than if no metastases are found.

Table 5.3 Stage Groupings

Stage	T	N	M	Explanation
0	Tis	0	0	Carcinoma in situ: cancer in its earliest stages that has not progressed beyond the inner surface of the colon
I	1 or 2	0	0	Cancer has grown into the wall of the colon, but it has not spread outside of the colon wall.
IIA	3	0	0	Cancer has grown through the wall of the colon but it has not spread in the lymph nodes or to distant sites.
IIB	4	0	0	Cancer has spread through the wall of the colon into nearby tissues but it has not spread in the lymph nodes or to distant sites.
IIIA	1 or 2	1	0	The primary cancer is confined to the bowel wall but it has spread to 1 to 3 regional lymph nodes. There is no distant spread.
IIIB	3 or 4	1	0	The primary cancer has spread through the bowel wall and may have spread into nearby tissues; 1 to 3 regional lymph nodes are involved but there is no distant spread.
IIIC	Any	2	0	The cancer has metastasized to 4 or more regional lymph nodes but there is no distant spread.
IV	Any	Any	1	Cancer has spread to other parts of the body (usually to the liver or lungs and rarely to bone, peritoneum, brain, adrenal glands, or kidney).

Source: Adapted from Levin B. Colorectal Cancer: A Thorough and Compassionate Resource for Patients and Their Families. Atlanta, GA: American Cancer Society; 1999:225; American Cancer Society and National Comprehensive Cancer Network, Colon and Rectal Cancer: Treatment Guidelines for Patients, version IV/February 2005, Atlanta, GA: American Cancer Society; 2005; and Greene FL. AJCC Cancer Staging Manual. 6th ed. New York: Springer-Verlag; 2002. Used with the permission of the American Joint Committee on Cancer (AJCC), Chicago, Illinois. The original source for material is the AJCC Cancer Staging Manual, Sixth Edition (2002) published by Springer-Verlag, New York, www.springeronline.com.

Overall Stage

After each element has been described, the TNM elements are combined to determine the overall stage of the cancer (see Table 5.3). The overall stage is described using roman numerals from 0 (in which the cancer is confined to the outermost portion of the colon wall) to stage IV (in which the cancer has spread to other areas of the body such as the liver and lungs). Letters A to C after the roman numerals provide additional information about the nature of the cancer spread.

This system of overall staging is being used more and more to select a specific treatment plan (also known as a protocol).

Molecular Profiling

The concept of molecular profiling of cancers is relatively new and is based on our current understanding of the genetic and cellular changes involved in the development, progression, and spread of cancer. We know that although colorectal cancers may look the same to the naked eye and may be almost identical microscopically, they differ at a molecular level. Each cancer is truly unique, just as each human has a unique fingerprint.

Despite doctors' best efforts, current staging systems are not able to predict outcomes with total reliability. They are a doctor's best guess about what will probably happen based on the information your doctor has at the time. But a small percentage of people with stage I disease will develop recurrence and even die of their cancer, while a small percentage of people with stage IV disease will beat the odds and survive over the long term. The reason for this difference in outcome from the expected prognosis is thought to reside in the "molecular fingerprinting" of the cancer.

In the future, molecular profiling may be able to help doctors more reliably predict a patient's outcome and possibly assist in treatment decisions.

The Pathology Report

The pathologist is responsible for clearly communicating the results of his or her analysis of all tissue samples to the doctors who are directly caring for the patient. These results are recorded in a document called a pathology report, which becomes a permanent part of the patient's medical record.

A pathology report includes the findings from the gross (visual) examination and the microscopic examination of frozen and/or permanent sections. The type of information included in the final pathology report depends on the situation. If the report is based on a small biopsy, the report will be quite limited; in contrast, if the report is based on analysis of an entire surgical specimen removed at the time of major surgery, more detailed information will be provided. This detailed information might include the length of bowel that was removed, the size of the cancer, how close the cancer is to the surgical margins, and how many lymph nodes are contained within the specimen.

In addition to information needed to properly identify the patient (such as name, date of birth, and social security or health record number), the pathology report may include the following information:

- *Specimen type.* Usually the pathology report includes the type of procedure performed to obtain the specimen and the tissue from which it was obtained. It should describe the size and visible (gross) characteristics of the submitted specimen.
- *Tumor site.* The location of the tumor (in the rectum or another section of the large intestine) should be stated.
- *Tumor size.* The size of the cancer is measured in three dimensions. This measurement is usually expressed in centimeters (1 inch = 2.54 centimeters).
- *Histology type and grade.* Recall that pathologists use a grading system (1–4 or low grade/high grade) to communicate how aggressive the cancer is based on how the cells appear under a microscope. The report will also include a type, which reflects whether the cancer is a typical adenocarcinoma or has certain distinctive features that indicate a special subtype (such as mucinous, medullary, signet ring, small cell, or undifferentiated carcinoma).
- *Tumor stage as described by the TNM system.* Recall that doctors use the TNM (tumor, nodes, metastasis) system developed by the American Joint Committee on Cancer (AJCC) to describe how widespread the cancer is. The TNM system tells whether the cancer is contained to the tumor, has grown locally into lymph nodes, or has spread (metastasized) to distant sites in the body.
- *Tumor margins.* When a surgeon attempts to remove cancer tissue from the colorectum, he or she also removes some normal tissue that surrounds the cancerous growths. This cuff of normal tissue is called the margin. If the surgeon has removed all known cancer and the gross and microscopic examinations show no cancer, the operation is considered "curative" and labeled an R0 resection. If the gross margins are free (no areas of cancer are seen at the margin with the naked eye) but the microscopic margins are positive (small deposits of cancer cells can be found under a microscope), the resection is labeled R1. If the gross margins are involved with cancer or gross disease remains after an incomplete resection, the resection is labeled R2. The risk of cancer recurrence is higher and the prognosis is worse for R2 resections compared with R1 resections.

(continued on page 86)

Figure 5.2 Sample Pathology Report

CASE: U12-12345 MR#: 123-34-6789
Patient Name: Smith, John
Collected: 1/1/01   Received: 1/1/01   Reported: 1/4/01
Ordering Physician: Mary Jones, MD

Specimen(s):
A: Right colectomy
B: Terminal ileum

Final Diagnosis:
A: Right colectomy:
  -Adenocarcinoma, moderately differentiated (low grade)
  -Tumor size: 6 × 5 × 3.1cm
  -Stage: T3N1Mx (stage III)
  -Bowel wall invasion: present
      a. Extent into serosa
  -Mucosal resection margins: clear
      a. Nearest distance to closest mucosal margin: 5.5cm
      b. Radial soft tissue margin: clear
  -Angiolymphatic invasion: present, extramural
  -Perineural invasion: absent
  -Invasion of adjacent structure: absent
  -Lymph nodes: Number of nodes: 15; Number of positive nodes: 2
  -Appendix with no evidence of malignancy
B: Terminal ileum:
  -No pathologic diagnosis

Gross:
Specimens received with patient's name and medical record number.
Specimen A is designated "right colectomy" and consists of a segment of colon and cecum
    measuring 19cm in length and 6.1cm in diameter with attached mesentery, measuring 9 cm in
    width and 1.3 cm in thickness.
Specimen B is designated "terminal ileum" and consists of a segment of small bowel measuring
    5cm in length and 3.1cm in diameter with attached mesentery, measuring 3cm in width and
    1.1cm in thickness.

Summary of Sections:

-A-1, cecal margin	-A-14, lymph node	-A-20, lymph node
-A-2, distal colon margin	-A-15, lymph node	-A-21, lymph node
-A-3-10, tumor	-A-16, lymph node	-A-22, lymph node
-A-11, appendix	-A-17, lymph node	-B-1, distal margin
-A-12, ileocecal valve	-A-18, lymph node	-B-2, proximal margin
-A-13, random colon	-A-19, lymph node	-B-3, random ileum

Signed out by:
Frank Glass, MD

Comments:

Patient, specimen, and physician information.

Essential information that ensures the proper recording of your pathology. It includes your pathology number, the type of tissue that was removed, when it was received, and when the report was finalized.

Final Diagnosis.

This includes the "bottom line" diagnosis. It includes the type, grade, and size of the cancer as well as the final stage of the tumor. The report includes particulars such as how much normal tissue was found between the tumor and the cut end of the bowel, the number of lymph nodes, and prognostic indicators such as lymphatic and neural invasion.

Gross.

This portion of the document tells you what the tumor looks like without the aid of a microscope. It is broken down by each type of tissue removed.

Summary of Sections.

This section describes the actual slides taken of the tumor. It is an itemized account of every slide made with the removed tissues.

Signed out by.

This is the name of the pathologist who analyzed your specimen.

Questions to Ask Your Doctor About Your Pathology Report

- What type of colorectal cancer did you find?
- What is the grade of my cancer?
- Were the margins of the resection adequate? If not, what is the recommended next step?
- What is the stage of my cancer?
- Was there any involvement in the lymphatic or blood vessels? How many lymph nodes did the pathologist find for analysis?
- Was there any sign of spread of the cancer to other tissues or organs? If so, do I need other treatment than what we initially planned?
- Can you recommend someone who can offer a second opinion?
- Are there any other tests I should consider having?
- Does my type and stage of cancer typically require additional treatments?
- What follow up do I need if I do not need further treatment right now?

- *Spread via the blood vessels or lymphatic system.* Cancer can spread to other areas by way of the lymphatic system (the tissues and organs that produce and store cells that fight infection as well as the channels that carry lymphatic fluid) or the blood vessels (arteries, veins, and capillaries). Cancer that has spread to the lymph system is defined as lymphatic invasion and coded with an L. If cancer cannot be seen with the naked eye but is detected in the blood vessels using a microscope, it is labeled V1; if cancer is visible to the naked eye, it is labeled V2. Cancers coded L, V1, and V2 are associated with a worse prognosis.

Getting a Second Pathologist's Opinion

Pathology reports of colorectal cancer generally provide an objective assessment. However, there are subjective elements involved in interpreting the specimen. Pathologists have different levels of experience, interest, and expertise. For this reason, pathologists often seek the opinions of their own colleagues if there is an unusual feature such as margin clearance that is not clear.

Second opinions are especially important if a different interpretation by a second pathologist would change the treatment decisions you might make.

When you seek out a second opinion, do not have the second doctor re-interpret the existing pathology report. Request that your permanent section slides or pathology "blocks" (small pieces of tissue that have been preserved within small rectangular blocks of wax) be sent to the second doctor, so he or she can perform his or her own independent assessment of the situation and provide an unbiased second opinion.

CHAPTER SIX

UNDERSTANDING YOUR PROGNOSIS

Edward W. Greeno, MD

Prognosis is a prediction of your outcome, or how well you will do with your cancer. Prognosis is usually expressed in terms of how long you are likely to survive. As painful as it can sometimes be to hear, this knowledge is crucial to your understanding of your disease. How much you need to know will depend on your personal circumstances and how you can cope with the information.

Knowing your prognosis helps you make plans for the future. You can also make better treatment decisions if you know how your prognosis changes with various therapy options. Don't be afraid to talk with your doctor about this, and in particular make sure he or she understands how much you want to know. Always ask more questions if you don't understand the answers you are getting.

Prognosis

As you talk about your prognosis, understanding the different elements of this prediction about your future health status will help make the picture clearer to you. Your prognosis can be expressed as the probability of being cured or as the probability of surviving a certain length of time. Which of these categories is most relevant to you will depend on your particular situation.

Your Prognosis Is Only a Prediction

Your prognosis is just a prediction, not a guarantee. Occasionally, even the person with the worst prognosis sometimes does quite well. The numbers we talk about apply quite accurately to groups of people, but your outcome will be unique.

> *"The latest oncologist came in and reviewed my situation and said, 'As far as I can tell, you've defied all the odds, normally speaking, with the way you look and where you're at. You shouldn't even be here.' And so I said, 'Well, I'll just keep defying all the odds, as long as I possibly can.'"*
>
> —CARL

If you are in a group with a 60 percent cure rate, you won't be 60 percent cured. For you, the answer will be 0 percent or 100 percent, but that answer can only be obtained by the test of time. For this group of people, however, we can use scientific data to estimate that 60 of 100 people in this group will be cured, and 40 won't. Likewise, if you are in a group with an expected survival of two years, it is highly unlikely that you will survive exactly two years to the day. That is just a likely estimate based on the scientific data collected about people with health profiles similar to your own. For you, the time of survival will be either more or less than two years. Again, only time will tell.

Your Prognosis Can Change

Another factor to keep in mind about your prognosis is that it can change with the passage of time and the occurrence of various events. Surgical procedures may reveal that the extent of your tumor is more or less than expected. An excellent response to chemotherapy may shift you into a group with a better prognosis.

Even the simple passage of time changes your prognosis. We know that for people with advanced disease, the longer a person survives, the better the prognosis gets. A person with advanced disease whose initial expected survival was 18 months and has now survived for those 18 months has an expected survival of another two years. If that person survives another two years, the expected survival after that would be another five years.

The passage of time plays another role in improving prognosis because of the development of new therapies. New surgical techniques may allow effective local control of previously untreatable types of colorectal cancer. New nonsurgical therapies may lead to better control of colorectal cancer that is considered inoperable, increasing potential survival time.

Doctors' understanding of survival times is based on the outcomes of people diagnosed in the past, and those survival times do not reflect the benefits of recent therapeutic advances. In the past 30 years, the five-year survival rate of all people with colorectal cancer has increased from 50 percent to about 64 percent overall, and the survival of the average person diagnosed today can be expected to be even better than that.

Understanding Five-Year Survival Rates

One of the most commonly used statistics for understanding outcomes is the five-year survival rate. Doctors use this statistic to help provide the simplest picture of what you may expect. This statistical measure also gives health care professionals and researchers an easy way to compare the prognoses among different groups or over the course of a specific period.

The five-year survival rate refers to the percentage of people diagnosed with colorectal cancer who live at least 5 years after the cancer is diagnosed. The five-year *relative* survival rate also refers to the percentage of people diagnosed with colorectal cancer who live at least five years after cancer is diagnosed, but it excludes from the calculation anyone who has died of causes unrelated to colorectal cancer. Because they look specifically at colorectal cancer and exclude other causes, the five-year relative survival rates are considered to be a more accurate way than standard five-year survival rates to describe the prognosis for people with colorectal cancer. For people diagnosed with colorectal cancer between 1995 and 2001, the overall relative five-year survival rate has been 64.1 percent. That means that after five years, about 64 people of every 100 diagnosed with colorectal cancer will still be alive.

> *"I told my doctor, 'I won't talk about survival rates or statistics because I'm a person, not a number.'"*
> —EDDIE

Patients can find information that is slightly more relevant to their particular circumstance if they examine the corresponding five-year relative survival rate by the stage of their cancer at the time of diagnosis. See Figure 6.1 on page 92 and Table 6.1 on page 93 for two estimates of five-year relative survival based on stage at diagnosis. The earlier your cancer is diagnosed, the better your odds of survival. Figure 6.1 uses the terms local, regional, and distant to describe how widespread the cancer is. Table 6.1 uses the AJCC staging system.

Other Measures of Survival

You may read or hear other measures of survival that can provide answers to somewhat different questions. The five-year survival rate is close to the cure rate, but the two are not exactly the same, because some people who are five-year survivors

Figure 6.1 Five-year Relative Survival Rates for Colorectal Cancer by Stage at Diagnosis, 1995-2000

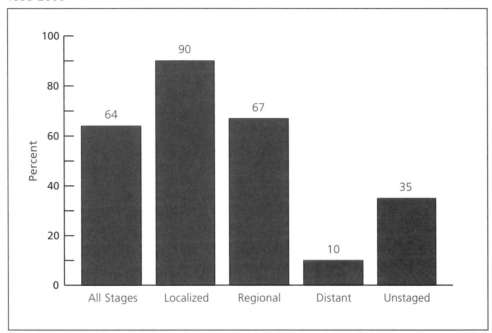

Data from: Surveillance, Epidemiology and End Results (SEER) program (www.seer.gov) SEER Stat Database: Incidence—SEER 9 Registries (1973–2001), SEER 11 Registries plus Alaska Public-Use, Nov 2003 Sub for Expanded Races (1992–2001), National Cancer Institute, DCCPS, Surveillance Research Program, Cancer Statistics Branch, Released April 2004, based on the November 2003 submission.

Source: American Cancer Society, Colorectal Cancer Facts and Figures, *Special Ed., 2005. Atlanta, GA: American Cancer Society; 2005:5.*

may still eventually die of colorectal cancer, so the relative survival will drop a few percentage points after the first five years.

As a result, 10-year survival rates are sometimes used to more accurately approximate cure rates. To get the most rapid estimate of prognosis rates from research studies, the three-year disease-free survival rate is sometimes used. This number reflects the percentage of people who are still alive and don't have any evidence of cancer three years after initial diagnosis.

As an example, in a study of chemotherapy after surgery for people with stage II and III colorectal cancer, the measures of survival could be expressed in any of the following ways:

- three-year disease-free survival was 65 percent
- five-year cancer-specific survival was 64 percent

Table 6.1 Five-Year Relative Survival Rates by AJCC Stage at Diagnosis

These numbers reflect the percentage of people who are alive five years or more after being diagnosed with colon cancer, depending on what stage they were in when they were diagnosed. The survival for rectal cancer, stage for stage, is about the same.*

Stage	Survival Rate
I	93%
IIA	85%
IIB	72%
IIIA	83%
IIIB	64%
IIIC	44%
IV	8%

* NCDB Commission on Cancer

Data from: O'Connell JB, Maggard MA, Ko CY. Colon cancer survival rates with the new American Joint Committee on Cancer sixth edition staging. J Natl Cancer Inst. 2004;96:1420-1425.

- five-year overall survival was 64 percent
- ten-year cancer-specific survival was 59 percent
- overall survival was 46 percent

The answers we get from these different measures generally fall within a few percentage points of the five-year survival rates. However, in the future, as we get better at treating advanced disease, it is likely that more people who aren't cured of their disease will live well beyond the five-year mark.

For people with advanced disease that is unlikely to be cured, the use of median survival statistics may be more relevant. The median survival is the length of time that half the patients in a group will live. This is the statistic most commonly meant when you hear someone has an expected survival expressed in terms of a number of months. Because half the people will survive less than this time and half will live longer, the predicted number of months is rarely correct for any individual patient. The median survival of advanced colorectal cancer has been improving rapidly in recent years because of many treatment advances. A decade ago, the median survival of colorectal cancer that could not be surgically removed was about eight to 12 months. In 2004, the median survival rate approached two years and is expected to improve further.

What Combination of Factors Predict Outcome?

All of the numbers and percentages we have talked about so far represent an average of all patients, each of whom has a very different prognosis. So how do you use this information to get information tailored to you? You can gather additional information about your particular cancer and your personal health profile to help give you a more precise prediction. We'll look at the factors that may influence your personal colorectal cancer outcome in the next few sections.

Stage

The single most important prognostic factor is the stage of your colorectal cancer at diagnosis.

Patients with localized disease that has not yet grown through the bowel wall (stage I disease) have a better than 90 percent chance of surviving five years if they receive appropriate therapy.

For regional disease in which the cancer has spread through the bowel wall or to local lymph nodes (stage II disease), the chances of survival go down to 67 percent. Within this group, the prognosis can be further refined. For those with minimal invasion through the bowel and no lymph node involvement (stage IIA disease), five-year survival is 85 percent, whereas for those with involvement of more than three lymph nodes (stage IIIC disease), survival is 44 percent.

The worst outcome occurs if the cancer has spread to distant sites, such as the liver or lungs (stage IV disease), when the chance of surviving five years is less than 10 percent. However, even within this advanced stage, we can identify some patients with much better prognoses. Those with only a few sites of distant spread that can be completely removed surgically still have a 25 to 30 percent chance of surviving five years.

Age and Life Expectancy

Many expect the very elderly and the very young to do poorly with cancer. In fact, outcomes directly related to colorectal cancer are only indirectly affected by age.

For people younger than 40 years old, colorectal cancer is often diagnosed at a more advanced stage because the diagnosis is not suspected for a long time in such a young person. When outcomes are corrected for the stage at diagnosis, the seemingly worse outcomes are much less apparent.

For the very elderly, the belief that they may not tolerate therapy can lead to less treatment and thus worse outcomes. In fact, the effectiveness of therapy for colorectal cancer can be just as good in the healthy elderly as any other group.

Ethnicity and Outcomes

Outcomes in colorectal cancer vary significantly based on ethnicity. Since racial designations are largely determined by social rather than biological factors, the differences in outcomes are likely to be a function of socioeconomic rather than biological differences between groups.

As noted earlier, the death rates for colorectal cancer are highest for African Americans at 29 per 100,000 persons per year, compared with 21 for white Americans and 15 for Hispanic and other American minority groups. These differences in death rates in part reflect differences in the rate of developing colorectal cancer. African Americans have the highest incidence of colorectal cancer of the above groups, probably because of differences in diet, exercise, and other risk factors for colorectal cancer, as well as access to appropriate medical services (see chapter 2).

However, even after controlling for the rate of colorectal cancer development, there are still differences in outcomes. For African Americans diagnosed with colorectal cancer, five-year survival rates are approximately 57 percent, whereas white people have a higher survival rate of about 64 percent. For other ethnic groups, colorectal cancer survival is also worse compared with whites, though only by about 1 to 2 percent.

This disparity appears in part because of differences in when the cancer is diagnosed. The difference in stage at diagnosis is due in part to lower rates of screening in minority groups. There may also be delays in seeking evaluation of symptoms in minority groups on the part of both patients themselves and their doctors.

Even after a cancer is detected and adjustments for stage are made, the differences persist to a degree. Some studies suggest that minority patients are less likely to receive aggressive care for their cancer. The reasons for these disparities are complex and not fully understood, reflecting a mixture of factors. These factors include problems with access to care because of insurance, education, and social issues (such as access to treatment facilities). Other medical problems that people may have can also influence their ability or willingness to go forward with treatment. In addition, the beliefs of patients and doctors about health care and acceptance of cancer therapies may affect decision making.

Although some elderly people have a number of serious health problems and are quite frail, many others are in excellent health and quite able to tolerate the usual treatment for colorectal cancer. For this reason, treatment decisions should be based on a person's overall health status rather than his or her age. Since colorectal cancer delivers most of its impact on survival in the first five years after diagnosis, and all but the extremely aged can be expected to survive more than five years (aside from the colorectal cancer), the outcomes of therapy should be the same as in younger people.

Pathology of the Tumor

The appearance of your tumor under the microscope can provide a little more information about how your cancer might be expected to behave. Tumors that are better differentiated (they look more like normal cells) tend to behave less aggressively than those that are poorly differentiated. Tumors that can be seen invading blood or lymph vessels are more likely to have spread to distant areas of the body via blood or lymph. The presence of such features can refine the prognosis to a small degree but usually don't make enough difference to affect treatment decisions.

Tumor Volume

Unlike most other cancers, the size of the primary tumor has very little impact on outcomes in colorectal cancer.

Surgical Margins

The surgical margin is the distance between the edge of the tumor and the point where the surgeon cut. Usually the surgeon will try to cut at least 1 cm (about a half-inch) away from all edges of the tumor. The chances of a local recurrence of the tumor increase markedly if the margins are very small, and especially if the margin is positive—meaning tumor cells are present right up to the edge of the specimen. Usually margins are much more than one centimeter because the surgeon removes adjacent lymph glands.

General Health

Your general health can have an important impact on your prognosis. If you have serious heart or lung disease, performing needed surgeries might be much riskier. Other health problems with specific organs such as the liver or kidney may interfere with the administration of chemotherapy. In general, if your health is so poor that you must spend most of your time in bed, the risks of treatments will outweigh the benefits.

Serum CEA Level

Carcinoembryonic antigen (CEA) is a substance that can be measured in your bloodstream. We all have some CEA in our blood, but people with colorectal cancer will often have higher levels. If the CEA level is increased before surgery, and particularly if it does not return to normal after surgery, the risk of recurrence is much greater.

CHAPTER SEVEN

COPING WITH YOUR DIAGNOSIS

Simon Kung, MD
Pamela J. Netzel, MD
Teresa A. Rummans, MD

What were the first emotions you felt when your doctor said, "You have colorectal cancer"? People experience a wide range of feelings upon receiving the diagnosis of cancer. Oftentimes, these feelings are so strong that hearing the rest of what the doctor had to say during that visit is difficult. As the news sinks in, managing these emotions may feel like riding a roller coaster.

> *"There are plenty of people like me who are proof you can get through this."*
> —BECKY

In this chapter, we'll talk about some things you can do to regain your sense of control and maintain your sense of well being as you weigh your options and begin your cancer treatment.

Consider Your Whole Self

Receiving a diagnosis of cancer can make you feel as though the affected body part is the most important piece of who you are right now. Because of your diagnosis, your health care team will be paying close attention to your colon and rectum, asking you many questions, and performing a variety of tests to find out more about your colorectal health and habits.

But your health isn't just about a single body part. It's about you—the total package.

Recognize that cancer affects your whole self. The diagnosis of colorectal cancer will probably affect all areas of your life somehow: not only your physical health, but your social life, spiritual existence, mental state, and emotional well being too. Paying attention to all of these areas can help you to better cope with your cancer and maintain your quality of life throughout treatment.

There are an increasing number of options for medical treatment of colorectal cancer (see chapters 9–14), but other factors can also improve your feeling of well being and physical functioning. These factors include getting regular exercise, eating a balanced diet, and avoiding alcohol and nicotine. Consider walking, riding your bike, or any other activity that you can do comfortably. (Discuss any new exercise plan with your doctor.)

It is easy to feel isolated when you receive a diagnosis like cancer, so try to remain socially connected to family, friends, and others whose company you enjoy. Support groups with others who can relate to your feelings can also be helpful. If you feel limited in your ability to visit with others, consider other ways of maintaining communication such as the telephone or by writing letters or e-mails. The American Cancer Society Cancer Survivors Network is one such source of support for people with cancer and their families and friends. To participate, visit http://www.acscsn.org.

It is also important to take care of yourself emotionally. Doing so will help you to better deal with the challenges of having cancer. Learn to pamper yourself. Think about things that you enjoy and find a way to make them part of your daily life. Maybe it's watching a movie, preparing a meal, listening to music, drawing, or reading. Discovering new hobbies and interests can also help your self-esteem. Don't beat yourself up; cancer is hard enough to face without any added stressors. Be good to yourself.

When new or upsetting emotions like anger or depression crop up, don't bury them or pretend they don't exist. Acknowledging your feelings is the first step in coming to terms with them. We'll talk more about coping with specific emotions such as anger and depression in the next part of the chapter.

> *"I think men in our society are supposed to be strong and stoic and not show emotions. When you have cancer, it's a time to just let it all out. There were certainly times when I was just a basket case, especially the first few weeks. I think the danger is if we don't let out our emotion, it's only going to get bottled up and that can only make our health worse. I think it's so important just to let out the emotion, either with a family member or with a therapist or support group. Don't hold all that emotion in, because it only makes things worse."*
>
> —EDDIE

The most important thing to remember is that each person will have unique concerns and responses to cancer. These feelings will probably change over time. There is no one right way of coping, so experiment to find what works best for you, your personality, and your unique situation.

Coping With Emotions

It is important to know that your first emotions upon receiving the diagnosis of cancer—unpleasant, unfamiliar, and/or distressing as they may seem—are totally normal. Dealing with these emotional effects of cancer is as important to your well being as managing the physical effects of the disease.

As you adjust to the diagnosis of cancer, you will develop different emotions along the way. You may even find, as many people with cancer do, that your diagnosis eventually leads you to new insights and a different perspective on life.

But first, how can you cope with these initial emotions? Everyone has a different coping style, but in general, identifying and talking about these feelings is a good first step.

> *"Everyone has a different reaction to being given a diagnosis of cancer. In Sheryl's case, my partner, here's a woman who's very capable, was extremely successful at two careers so far in life, and one of her reactions to being handed the diagnosis was denial. She knew that she had a very serious life-threatening illness, but for whatever reason, she was paralyzed."*
> —SUSAN

Disbelief and Denial

Disbelief and shock are common first reactions when receiving the diagnosis of cancer. Some people might think, "Maybe there was a mix-up with the test results, and it's someone else who really has the diagnosis." Usually the results are correct, and additional testing will provide confirmation. You might even seek a second opinion, only to hear the same diagnosis. The disbelief and denial will wear off as you uncover more information about your situation.

Anger

After the disbelief and shock of having cancer wears off, feelings of anger might arise. You might ask, "Why me?" Many factors contribute to the development of colorectal cancer, including age, genetic predisposition, and other medical conditions (see chapter 2 on risk factors). It is difficult to identify one factor that is solely responsible. However, you should not feel that you have cancer because you have been a bad person or have done something wrong.

Anger itself is not a bad thing; how you handle it is the key. Anger can be a productive emotion. Try redirecting your anger into constructive action, such as making positive changes in aspects of your life and cancer care that you can control.

Persistent and unresolved anger will distract you from your number one goal: treatment and recovery. If your anger is directed at certain people and you find yourself lashing out, try talking to these persons. Seeking the help of a counselor/therapist is also a wise move when you feel like anger or other emotions are out of control.

If your anger results in a spiritual crisis, talk to your religious leader.

Grief

Don't be surprised if you experience feelings of grief after receiving your diagnosis. It is not uncommon for people with cancer to mourn the loss of their former, healthier selves, and to grieve over lost opportunities or "what might have been."

> "We went and saw my daughter's pre-K graduation, and I looked at her and was just in tears, thinking, 'Will I be here for her high school graduation?' Now that's not a daily thing, but that's something that can creep into my thoughts."
>
> —COLLEEN

Allow yourself time to adjust. Perceiving yourself in a new context—accepting your diagnosis and taking steps to make the best of your new situation—is the next stage and an essential part of coping with your disease.

Fear

Cancer is a frightening diagnosis because of the uncertainty that lies ahead. "What will happen to me? What will happen to my family?"

Years ago, people thought of cancer as a death sentence. However, with advances in diagnosis and treatment, there are now almost 10 million cancer survivors in the United States. The overall five-year survival rate for colorectal cancer is approximately 64 percent and is as high as 90 percent when colorectal cancer is diagnosed at an early, localized stage.

Part of fear is the unknown, and as you learn more about your own situation, the fear will lessen. For example, you may be concerned about what chemotherapy will be like, but after receiving your first chemotherapy, you will know what to expect for future chemotherapies. The more you learn, the more you will feel a sense of control, and that will decrease your worry.

Stress and Anxiety

Stress and anxiety are related to fear in many ways. For example, fear of what chemotherapy might be like could lead to stress and anxiety. Other causes of stress and anxiety might pertain to practical matters, such as financial questions. (Financial issues are discussed in chapter 17.)

If not addressed, stress, and anxiety can lead to disabling problems such as panic attacks or constant anxiety that can prevent you from leading your daily life. These problems may appear in the form of physical symptoms, such as fast heartbeat or muscle tension. In these situations, mental health professionals such as psychiatrists and psychologists can help with combinations of medications and/or counseling. In addition, behavioral techniques such as relaxation therapy can also decrease stress and anxiety.

> *"It's a roller coaster ride. Some days are good, some are not so good."*
> —PETE

Remember that whatever your concern, you are not alone. There will always be someone or some organization that can provide assistance. Don't be afraid to ask for help.

Depression

Depression may occur by itself or in conjunction with anxiety. Doctors estimate that 25 percent of people with cancer will experience depression during the diagnosis and treatment of cancer.

Sadness is a normal and common reaction to a diagnosis of cancer, and part of that is grieving for the loss of your previously healthier self. However, prolonged sadness might lead to a clinical depression. If you find yourself feeling sad and depressed for more than two weeks, with changes in your sleep patterns or appetite, decreased energy or concentration, decreased interest in activities you used to enjoy, ruminating guilt about past or present events, agitation or moping, or thoughts of not wanting to be alive, seek help from a mental health professional. Also, tell your primary care doctor or oncologist.

As with anxiety problems, mental health professionals can use a combination of medications and/or counseling to relieve problems with depression. These interventions are usually very effective. See chapter 15 on coping with symptoms and side effects for specific strategies for dealing with depression.

Isolation and Withdrawal

When you receive your diagnosis, you might feel totally alone. However, if you look around, you are not alone. You have family and friends who will continue to support you, and you now have a community of fellow patients and survivors of colorectal cancer.

Beware of isolating yourself, withdrawing from life, and avoiding the activities that usually bring you pleasure, because that might lead to depression or other problems. Respect cancer for what it is, and take the appropriate time off during the diagnosis and treatment. However, try to lead the life you would like to lead. If you enjoy working, try to continue to work; that will help maintain your self-esteem. If you enjoy going to the movie theater or having poker night with your pals, try keeping up those activities as well—rent movies instead of going out and have your friends come over to your house for games. Life doesn't come to a halt with the diagnosis of cancer.

Taking Action

Sometimes, there's no better way to cope with a problem than to do something about it. You may not be able to make your cancer disappear, but there are many things you can do to take control of your situation and cope with your disease.

Educate Yourself

Oftentimes, we are scared of what we don't understand. Learning as much as you can about colorectal cancer may help you and your family deal with your fears.

Don't hesitate to ask your doctors, nurses, and other health care providers if there is something you want to know. Don't be embarrassed to ask the doctor to repeat or explain something or spell unfamiliar words. Don't worry that your doctor will be upset if you question his or her treatment recommendations. Most health care professionals know that coping with treatment is easier when people with cancer understand what is happening and why.

There are many sources from which you can gather information to complement the information you receive from your healthcare providers. The American Cancer Society (800-ACS-2345/800-227-2345 and http://www.cancer.org) and the National Cancer Institute (800-4-CANCER/800-422-6237 and http://www.cancer.gov) can provide educational materials and resources regarding support services.

You may also find it helpful to talk with other people who have cancer about their perspective. If you have concerns about specific aspects of the treatment, search out information about it. For example, if you are curious about the appearance or the care of a colostomy, it may be helpful for you to talk with a nurse or doctor about it, or perhaps others who have a colostomy would be willing to share their experiences with you.

Educating yourself about your cancer can help you to regain a sense of control and may help you to feel less overwhelmed. Keep in mind that different people need different amounts of information to feel comfortable. Some people prefer to know as much as possible about the details of their care, and others find that it only increases their stress. Likewise, some people prefer to manage decisions on their own with their doctors, and others find it reassuring to have a family member or friend as the facilitator of communication regarding medical decisions. It is important for you to communicate your wishes to your health care team so they can better understand the approach that is most helpful for you.

Take an Active Role in Your Treatment and Care

Taking an active part in your care can help you regain a sense of control. There are many ways to get involved. For example, do what you can to keep your doctor informed. Make notes about your symptoms and report how you feel. If problems arise, describe them as specifically as possible. Ask your health care team to share all options with you, even complementary methods or the possibility of participating in research studies and clinical trials (see chapters 14 and 13, respectively). Tell your health care team that you want be involved in making decisions. This will help give you a sense of autonomy.

Maintain Your Physical Health

Despite your recently diagnosed colorectal cancer, you can still make a conscious effort to live healthfully.

Eat a variety of healthy foods, stay active, and get an adequate amount of rest. Continuing to make the effort to live healthfully can help you combat the stress of your illness and can help boost your spirits and heighten your energy level. Challenge yourself to carry on these good habits after treatment to improve your quality of life after cancer.

> *"You have to really participate in your own illness. You have to ask questions. You have to be active. You have to go on the Internet and find out what are all the newest medicines? What are the clinical trials? What kind of chemotherapy? What blends of chemotherapy are better? You have to be an advocate in your own illness, and not just be told what to do. And once you're sick, you have to fight to get well, and not be passive about it."*
> —BARBARA

Plan Ahead

Planning ahead can reduce uncertainty and can help redirect negative emotions like anger and fear toward productive ends. It can also play an important role in maintaining a positive, hopeful outlook.

For example, use this time to plan your treatment schedule. Your health care team can help you plan your treatments around your routine (administering chemotherapy on a Friday so you can use the weekend to recover if being back at work on Monday is a priority for you) or around important events (a family reunion or special anniversary, for example). You or a loved one may also want to coordinate the efforts of people who have volunteered to pitch in during your illness.

This is a good time to think about other aspects of your life that could benefit from some forethought and planning. For example, you may want or need to revisit your financial situation and ensure your insurance and financial resources are in place before beginning treatment (see chapter 17 for more information on money matters).

If your treatment involves surgery or a hospital stay, you will probably be asked about your advance directives (sometimes called a living will), a document that specifies your preferences about how you would like to be cared for if you become unable to speak for yourself (see chapter 17).

Cancer may also encourage you to reflect on your family, your life achievements, and the assets you have gathered during your life journey. At this point, you may want to consider drawing up a will to ensure your loved ones are looked after in the event that you can no longer do so. Don't consider these types of plans morbid—think of them as activities that reaffirm to those around you how much you care about their continued well being.

Talking About Your Cancer

Talking about your cancer can be difficult. Talk about your cancer only when you are ready, and keep it at your own pace and based on the information that you know to be true. Try to find a good listener among your family and friends with whom you can communicate openly.

Decide Whom to Tell

You may not want to tell the whole world that you have cancer, so it's time to think about whom you want to tell. Usually you will want to share the diagnosis with your family and friends, as they will be an important source of support in the upcoming weeks and months. If you have family members with whom you are at odds, this might be an opportunity to re-establish a relationship with them.

If you work, whether to tell your employer is up to you. You will need to take time away from work for your treatment and recovery, and your employer and coworkers might be an important source of support. At some point, there may be side effects of treatment that will make it difficult to hide the fact that you have a serious medical condition.

As a person with cancer, you have specific rights under the Americans with Disabilities Act (ADA), so if you feel you are being treated unfairly at work because of your illness, call the Equal Employment Opportunity Commission (EEOC) at 800-514-0301.

Family and Loved Ones

Your family will probably be the first people you tell about your cancer. Many people don't understand cancer and may be afraid of your illness or worried that they will say something that will upset you. Reassure them that you want to speak openly and honestly about your cancer, and set a good example by being open with your loved ones about your own feeling and fears. Then ask what feelings and fears they have. Keeping the lines of communication open will help reduce later misunderstandings and friction.

Don't hesitate to ask your nurse, social worker, counselor, or religious leader to help bring family members together to talk.

TALKING TO CHILDREN

When talking with children and adolescents about cancer, be truthful and keep it simple. Provide as much information as is appropriate given their age and level of maturity. Children and adolescents can recognize when they are being told something that doesn't seem right. As with other family members, they will have their own feelings and fears about cancer. Try to spend extra time with them to let them know that although you are ill, your relationship with them will still be basically the same. The American Cancer Society has information on talking with children about cancer that can be accessed on the web site (http://www.cancer.org) or by calling 800-ACS-2345/800-227-2345.

> *"We thought it was particularly important to talk to my daughter about the fact that there are a lot of kinds of cancer, that not everyone who has cancer dies. That many, many people have cancer and survive and are very healthy and have long active lives.... We would try to answer [her questions] to the best of our ability. We wanted to give her factual information that would reassure her, not alarm her, but also not gloss things over."*
>
> —SUSAN

Friends

Our lives consist of family and friends, so you'll probably share your cancer diagnosis with friends as well. Remember that different people will have different reactions when hearing about someone with cancer. Most people are encouraging and supportive, but there might be some who mean well but say the wrong things or are uncomfortable and don't know what to say. They may have their own fears and issues with cancer that come out in the wrong ways. For example, someone might say to you, "Oh, your cancer can be easily treated," with the intention of cheering you up about your prognosis. However, to you, it might seem that they are viewing your cancer lightly, and your cancer, as you know, is a serious subject.

> *"Be willing to admit you need help... this has been a hard thing for me. Let people help you. It helps them when they can help you. It makes them feel that they have an active part in helping you get well."*
> —JACY

Good friends want to feel helpful to us, so if it does make your treatment and recovery easier, take them up on their offers of help. Delegate specific tasks to those who offer to help, like asking them to prepare a meal for your family for next Tuesday, or picking up the children/grandchildren from school the day of your next treatment.

Cancer's Effects on the Family

Cancer has a profound effect on the family and is one of the most stressful events a family can experience. It forces the family to face mortality and results in a re-examination of life and life goals. There may be many ups and downs during the cancer journey, and different family members may have different limits on how many ups and downs each can withstand. Some family members may be unrealistically optimistic or pessimistic, leading to misgivings or misunderstandings.

Family counseling is often available to help families weather the cancer experience and to improve family relations whatever the outcome.

Building Your Support Network

Coping with a diagnosis of colorectal cancer requires a good support network. Some people turn to family members or a few close friends, while others prefer to seek support that is more widespread. You support network does not need to be extensive; it just needs to be the right size for you.

Whom Can You Turn to for Support?

Who should be on your support team? Your health care providers, consisting of your doctors and nurses and other medical personnel, are there to explain your cancer and treatment. Don't feel shy about asking them questions; that's their job. They should also be the ones you call when you have questions about medications, side effects, or other symptoms.

For emotional and practical support throughout your treatments, look toward your family and friends. For example, have someone accompany you to your appointments; you'll have the advantage of two sets of ears listening to the health care providers giving you instructions, your companion will feel helpful, and you won't feel alone. If you are having difficulty coping or handling your emotions, a psychiatrist, psychologist, or licensed counselor can help.

If you have a faith community, it can be another source of support for you. Spirituality can bring meaning and purpose to your life and provide strength during times of crisis, illness, and suffering. Spirituality has a wide range of meanings to different people and can be expressed in a variety of ways. For many, it comes from religious experiences, but it can also be discovered through a connection with nature or other higher power. Meditation, prayer, and relaxation techniques can nurture your sense of spiritual well being and help you to better cope.

For other practical matters such as finances or drawing up legal documents, ask your health care team to involve a social worker in your care. He or she can help directly or provide referrals to someone who can.

Support Services and Groups

There are many support services and groups available to persons with cancer. A partial list is shown at the end of this book in the Resources section. Further resources can be found through the American Cancer Society (800-ACS-2345/800-227-2345 and http://www.cancer.org). Government health organizations, such as the National Cancer Institute (800-4-CANCER/800-422-6237 and http://www.cancer.gov), can also be of use. There are other online cancer web sites, but be aware that the quality and type of information can vary. Some web sites might include postings from people about their own experiences or their own investigations into complementary or alternative treatments. If you have any questions about the reliability of cancer information you find online, ask your health care team.

> *"I went to a men's support group here locally and that support group really helped tremendously. I was able to meet others that were in similar situations, and that really kind of pulled me through some very difficult mental and emotional times."*
> —CARL

Large hospitals and medical centers will also have materials and resources (including web sites) that can provide support and help you cope. Your health care team can refer you to local resources as well.

"I think you have to look at cancer as something that happened to you, and you go on from there. I'm fortunate enough that it isn't the end of my life, you know. I'm two years out and I feel fine and I'm working full time and doing the things I want to do, and I think you just have to realize that you need to go on with your life. You can't let the cancer diagnosis stop you. You can't just crawl into a hole and give up and say, 'I've been diagnosed with cancer, therefore I can't do anything.' You just have to look forward and build that future that you anticipate will be there."

—PATTI

Looking Ahead

Immediately after your diagnosis, all of your attention may be focused on dealing with and treating cancer while the other parts of your life are excluded. You may wonder if your life will ever feel normal again. Although your life has changed and there will continue to be difficult times, most people find they are able to return to many of their usual activities. The good news is that these days, most people diagnosed with colorectal cancer—especially those whose cancer is caught early—can look forward to a healthy future.

In addition, many people with cancer or other serious illnesses find that their experience eventually causes them to develop a new perspective of life and what is important to them. Your colorectal cancer experience may inspire you to re-evaluate your priorities and discover a renewed appreciation of the things you may have taken for granted before your diagnosis. Having cancer may encourage you to positively re-evaluate your relationships, your spiritual faith, your work, and many other aspects of your life.

CHAPTER EIGHT

MAKING THE MEDICAL SYSTEM WORK FOR YOU

Catherine Tomeo Ryan, MPH

Being diagnosed with colorectal cancer can be an overwhelming experience, and dealing with the medical system is no small part of that. It's easy to feel like you've been put in a strange place where you don't know the people, the language, or what's expected of you. To help you navigate this unfamiliar terrain, this chapter will familiarize you with your health care team and what they do, and will offer suggestions to help you get the best care possible.

Building Your Health Care Team

Building a qualified and supportive health care team can increase your chances of having a positive experience with colorectal cancer treatment and recovery. Although you might sometimes feel overwhelmed by the number of health care professionals you meet after your diagnosis, you can also be reassured by the sheer number of people who are available to help you, including doctors, nurses, social workers, and counselors. Some of these people will focus on treating your cancer medically, while others will put more emphasis on meeting your emotional needs and ensuring your quality of life.

Knowing the role of each person can help you feel more comfortable asking questions and getting the information you need. Below is an alphabetical list of the health care professionals that you might encounter during your colorectal cancer treatment. You may see some of these people daily, while others may be seen infrequently or not at all.

Dietitian

A dietitian is specially trained to help you make diet choices before, during, and after cancer treatment. A registered dietitian (RD) has at least a bachelor's degree and has passed a national competency exam.

Gastroenterologist

Gastroenterologists are doctors who specialize in diseases of the digestive tract (also called the gastrointestinal tract). Most people with colorectal cancer receive their diagnosis from a gastroenterologist based on the results of their colonoscopy. After a diagnosis, the gastroenterologist will usually talk with your primary care physician to identify a surgeon and/or oncologist for you. He or she may arrange for tests to determine how far the cancer has spread and may also help you manage any changes in your bowel habits.

The gastroenterologist's main role in your care, though, is to give you regular check-ups after you finish your treatments. These check-ups will include routine colonoscopies to make sure that your colon and rectum remain cancer-free.

Genetic Counselor

A genetic counselor is a health professional trained to help people through the process of genetic testing. If you or a family member is considering genetic testing, your genetic counselor can explain the available tests to you, discuss the pros and cons, and address any concerns you might have. If you decide to have a genetic test, your counselor will arrange for it and then help you interpret the results. (See page 21 for more information on genetic testing.)

Radiologist

Radiologists are doctors who use imaging techniques (such as X-rays) to see inside the body. Sometimes procedures are performed using imaging techniques. The images help guide the doctors as they pass very small tubes or instruments through the body to diagnose or treat disease.

Figure 8.1 The Members of Your Health Care Team

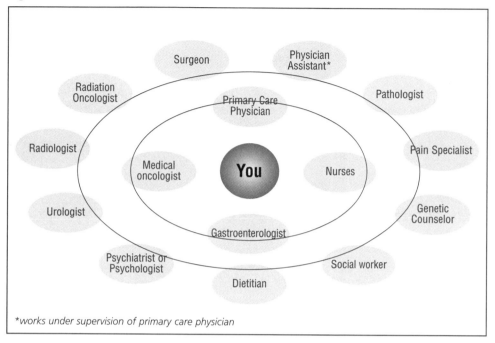

*works under supervision of primary care physician

Some radiologists, called interventional radiologists, perform procedures that would otherwise require invasive surgery. For example, with a CT-guided needle biopsy, a CT scan is used to direct the placement of the needle for a biopsy.

Medical Oncologist

Oncology is the field of medicine concerned with the diagnosis, treatment, and study of cancer. A medical oncologist is a doctor who is specially trained to diagnose and treat cancer with chemotherapy and other medicines. Your medical oncologist will probably be your main doctor during cancer treatment and will coordinate the care you receive from other doctors. He or she will have complete knowledge of your clinical information and will keep in contact with the rest of your health care team to ensure that you are receiving the best treatment possible. Most medical oncologists work closely with registered nurses, clinical nurse specialists, nurse practitioners, and physician assistants.

Nurses

Nurses are health professionals who can monitor your condition, administer treatment, provide information, and help you adjust physically and emotionally to your cancer diagnosis. You will probably receive care from many different types of nurses.

A registered nurse (RN) has an associate's or bachelor's degree in nursing or a diploma from a hospital-based program. He or she has also passed a state licensing exam. A nurse practitioner (NP) is a registered nurse who also has a master's or doctoral degree. Nurse practitioners are licensed to diagnose conditions, prescribe medications, and order diagnostic tests. Clinical nurse specialists (CNS) have a master's degree in nursing and specialize in such areas as oncology, psychiatry, and critical care nursing.

Oncology-certified nurses (OCN) are registered nurses who have demonstrated an in-depth knowledge of cancer care. They have passed a certification exam and can be found in all areas of oncology (cancer) practice. AOCNs, AOCNSs, and AOCNPs have achieved advanced-level oncology certification.

Some people with colorectal cancer also receive care from an ostomy nurse (also called a wound, ostomy, and continence nurse (WOCN) or an enterostomal therapist (ET) nurse). These nurses are specially trained to teach people how to care for an ostomy, which is a temporary or permanent opening that is sometimes created in the abdomen during colorectal cancer surgery (see chapter 16). If you have an ostomy, an ostomy nurse will help you take care of it while you're in the hospital and teach you how to care for it at home. He or she will also help you choose and order ostomy supplies, such as pouches and skin care products.

Pain Specialist

Pain specialists are doctors, nurses, and pharmacists who are experts in managing pain. They can help you find pain control methods that are effective and allow you to maintain your quality of life. Since only some doctors and nurses are trained in pain care, you may have to request a pain specialist if your pain relief needs are not being met. (See chapter 15 on managing your symptoms and side effects.)

Pathologist

As discussed in chapter 5, a pathologist is a medical doctor specially trained in diagnosing disease based on the examination of microscopic tissue and fluid samples. He or she will determine the classification (cell type) of your cancer, help determine the stage (extent) and grade (estimate of aggressiveness) of your cancer, and issue a pathology report so that you and your doctor can decide on treatment options.

Physician Assistant

Physician assistants (PAs) are health care professionals licensed to practice medicine with physician supervision. Physician assistants practice in the areas of primary care medicine (family medicine, internal medicine, pediatrics, and obstetrics and gynecology) as well as in surgery and the surgical subspecialties. Under the supervision of a doctor, they can diagnose and treat medical problems and in most states can also prescribe medications.

Primary Care Physician

Your primary care physician is the doctor who takes care of your general health needs. He or she may be a family doctor, internist, general practitioner, or gynecologist.

Even though you will see many specialists during your cancer care, your primary care doctor will continue to be an important and active member of your health care team. He or she will discuss your diagnosis with you, be involved in your care, and refer you to specialists. He or she may also communicate regularly with your specialists, providing them with details about your medical history and getting routine updates from them.

Psychiatrist or Psychologist

Many people with cancer have a psychiatrist on their health care team to help them deal with any depression or anxiety they are experiencing. Psychiatrists are medical doctors who specialize in mental health and behavioral disorders. They can counsel you during your cancer care and prescribe medication if necessary. Psychologists have doctoral degrees in mental health and behavior disorders.

Radiation Oncologist

Radiation oncologists are medical doctors who specialize in treating cancer with radiation (see chapter 11). They can help you make decisions about radiation therapy and, if necessary, determine the type and amount of radiation you should receive. Radiation oncologists are usually assisted by radiation therapists. They also work with radiation physicists, who are trained to ensure that you receive the right dose of radiation treatment. Radiation physicists are assisted by dosimetrists, who help plan and calculate the dosage, number, and length of your radiation treatments.

Social Worker

A social worker is a trained specialist in the social, emotional, and financial needs of individuals and families. Medical social workers are health specialists with master's degrees in social work and, in most cases, are licensed or certified by the state in which they work.

They can help you deal with a range of practical issues, such as finances, child care, transportation, and problems with the health care system. If your social worker is trained to work with cancer patients, he or she can also counsel you about your fears and concerns, answer questions about your diagnosis and treatment, and lead cancer support groups.

Surgeon

Several different types of surgeons provide treatment for colorectal cancer. A general surgeon is trained to operate on all parts of the body, including the digestive tract. A surgical oncologist is a surgeon who has had advanced training in the surgical treatment of people with cancer. A colorectal surgeon is trained in general surgery but also has advanced training in the treatment of colon and rectal problems including colorectal cancers. Cancer centers usually have one or more such individuals on their staff.

Although each type of surgeon has a different area of expertise, each plays the same role in treating people with colorectal cancer. If you require surgery as part of your treatment (see chapter 10), the surgeon will perform the operation and then manage any side effects you might have. He or she will also issue a report to your other doctors to help determine the rest of your treatment plan.

Urologist

A urologist is a doctor that specializes in treating problems of the urinary tract in men and women and of the genital area in men.

Colorectal cancer treatments occasionally cause side effects that require the expertise of a urologist. For example, radiation therapy can cause the bladder to become irritated, and some types of colorectal surgery can affect sexual function. If you experience these types of side effects, your doctors will probably consult with a urologist to address these conditions.

Choosing a Doctor

Soon after your cancer is diagnosed, you'll need to choose a surgeon and/or oncologist. This is a very important decision because doctors vary not only in their bedside manner but also in their level of expertise and the quality of care they provide. You'll want to choose a doctor who is an expert in treating colorectal cancer, is easy for you to talk to, and is someone you can trust.

(Sometimes, because of your financial or health insurance situation or your geographic location, you may not be able to choose your doctor or treatment facility. If that is the case, jump ahead to the section later in this chapter on working with your health care team and ensuring good communication (pages 123–127). These strategies can help you make the best of your situation even if your choices are limited.)

Going through this process can take several weeks, and many people are tempted to rush through it to start their treatment sooner. Keep in mind, though, that most people with cancer can afford to take some extra time to ensure that they get the best care possible. *Ask the doctor who diagnosed your cancer whether your situation requires immediate action or if you can take a short but reasonable amount of time to investigate your options.*

Choosing a good surgeon and/or oncologist now will benefit you for years to come, since your relationship will extend past treatment into long-term follow-up care. The Agency for Healthcare Research and Quality has outlined the following steps for finding a good doctor.

Step 1: Decide What You Want and Need in a Doctor

Before you start searching for a surgeon or oncologist, think about the qualities that you want your doctor to have. A few ideas are listed below, but you may want to add others.

> *"A lot was happening and I was involved and not involved. I was given a surgeon and… they scheduled me for surgery. And there was very little choice, it seemed, at the time, and everything was just sort of happening around me rather than happening as part of me. … I didn't have a choice in the surgeon and I think I was pretty lucky in the surgeon who was chosen for me, but I decided that since I was going to be working so closely with an oncologist I really wanted to like that person. I feel that's really important to have a good relationship with your oncologist, because if you want to take an active role like I did, you need to have somebody that you can talk to. So I interviewed a couple of different ones and I chose a doctor I really liked and I felt like I could talk to."*
>
> —ADELE

- You need a doctor who has experience with colorectal cancer. Studies show that doctors have better success treating a condition if they have a lot of experience with it.
- You need a doctor who is part of your health plan and/or accepts your health insurance. Otherwise, you need to be prepared to pay for your health care yourself.
- You want a doctor who has privileges (is permitted to practice) at a hospital that you find acceptable. Doctors can only treat patients in facilities where they have admitting privileges.
- You want a doctor that you feel comfortable with. Although some people prefer their doctors to have a business-like manner, many people with long-term illness value a physician who can attend to both their emotional health and medical needs.

Step 2: Make a List of Doctors Who Might Be a Good Fit

One of the best ways to identify a surgeon and/or oncologist is to get referrals from people you trust, like your primary care doctor. You might also try to get recommendations from other people in your community who have been treated for colorectal cancer. Check with your hospital, local American Cancer Society, or United Ostomy Association chapter to see if they can help you get in touch with these people.

The following organizations (contact information is listed in the Resources section at the end of this book) may also provide helpful information about a doctor's credentials: the American Board of Medical Specialties, the American Medical Association, the American Society of Clinical Oncologists, the American College of Surgeons, and the American Society of Therapeutic Radiology and Oncology. If you're in a health plan, be sure to review their list of doctors too, which is usually available online or by calling the member services hotline. Advocacy organizations such as the Colon Cancer Alliance or Colon Cancer Coalition may also be helpful.

Step 3: Call the Doctors' Offices and Make Appointments

Once you've identified doctors that seem like a good fit for you, call their offices and find out whether they're covered by your health plan and are taking new patients. You may also want to find out which hospitals they're affiliated with, if that's important to you.

The next step is to schedule appointments with a few doctors. The most important question to ask them is whether they have experience treating your type of cancer. If you're meeting with surgeons, find out how often they perform the type of surgery you need, how many of these surgeries they've performed before, and what their success rate is.

Studies suggest that patients with colorectal cancer may do better after surgery if their surgeon specializes in colorectal cancer and/or does colorectal surgery on a regular basis. This may be particularly true for people with rectal cancer, because the surgery is more challenging and may carry a greater risk of permanent colostomy. Look for someone who has done more than a handful of your type of surgery in the past year, is board-certified in colorectal surgery by the American Board of Colon and Rectal Surgery, and is a member of the American Society of Colon and Rectal Surgeons.

In addition to finding out your doctor's medical qualifications, take note of how comfortable you are with him or her. One way to gauge this is to ask yourself the following questions after your appointment.

- Did the doctor give you a chance to ask questions?
- Did you feel like the doctor was listening to you?
- Did the doctor seem comfortable answering your questions?
- Did the doctor talk to you in a way that you could understand?
- Did you feel like the doctor respected you?
- Did the doctor ask your preferences about different kinds of treatments?
- Did you feel like the doctor spent enough time with you?

Trust yourself when deciding whether a doctor is right for you. Keep in mind, though, that relationships take time, and it might take more than one visit for you and your doctor to get to know each other.

Choosing a Treatment Facility

Choosing a high-quality treatment facility or hospital is another way to ensure that you get the best cancer care possible. Since good doctors are rarely affiliated with substandard hospitals, the easiest way to informally assess the quality of a hospital is to determine which well-respected doctors work there. After you've selected skilled doctors that you trust and respect, the choice of a hospital usually follows automatically.

If you do have a choice in your treatment facility, make sure that you choose one that is covered by your health plan and where your doctor has admitting privileges. Below are several other key questions suggested by the Agency for Healthcare Research and Quality.

Does the Facility Have Experience and Success in Treating Colorectal Cancer?

Studies suggest that people with colorectal cancer may fare better if they receive their surgical care at a hospital that routinely treats people with their condition. For example, they may be less likely to have a permanent ostomy or to have their cancer come back after treatment.

Does the Facility Actively Evaluate and Work to Improve Its Quality of Care?

A growing number of hospitals are trying to evaluate and improve their quality of care. For example, they may keep track of how successful they are with certain procedures or chart the rate of infections that occur in the hospital. Check with a hospital's quality improvement department to find out how exactly how they monitor their care. You can also ask to see any reports they have available, including patient satisfaction surveys.

Have State or Consumer Groups Rated the Facility Highly for Its Quality of Care?

Many states and consumer groups develop report cards to grade the quality of care being delivered by local hospitals. These tools have been shown to help consumers make informed decisions and encourage hospitals to improve their quality of care. Find out if these resources are available in your area by calling your state department of health or your state hospital association.

Has the Facility Been Approved by a Nationally Recognized Accrediting Body?

At the very least, your hospital should be accredited by the Joint Commission on Accreditation of Healthcare Organizations (JCAHO). Receiving this accreditation means that the hospital is providing at least a minimum standard of care in terms of quality and safety. To check a hospital's JCAHO accreditation status, visit http://www.qualitycheck.org or call 630-792-5800.

Although JCAHO accreditation is a good *general* measure of quality of care, it does not evaluate *cancer care* specifically. This is done by the Commission on Cancer of the American College of Surgeons. If a hospital has what the Commission calls an "Approved Cancer Program," you'll know that it meets stringent standards and offers total cancer care, including lifetime follow-up. You'll also know that your hospital's ability to deliver quality cancer care is under close scrutiny, whether it's

Understanding Your Rights as a Patient

According to the American Hospital Association's Patient Care Partnership, you have specific rights as a patient. These include the rights to:

- high-quality health care and a clean and safe environment
- be involved in your care, including receiving understandable information about diagnosis, treatment, and prognosis, and the opportunity to discuss and make decisions about these things
- know the identity of those involved in your care
- have your privacy protected
- have your goals and beliefs taken into account as much as possible
- consent or decline to participate in clinical studies
- know the immediate and long-term implications of treatment choices, including financial implications
- receive help with your bill and with filing claims
- receive information and resources to prepare you for care and coping after you leave the hospital

If you feel that these rights are not being met, bring it to the attention of your health care team.

---

a large well-known facility or a small community hospital. To find an Approved Cancer Program near you, visit the American Cancer Society Web site at http://www.cancer.org and search under Hospital Locator.

If your doctors expect your treatment plan to be complex, you should strongly consider a hospital that has been designated by the National Cancer Institute (NCI) as a "comprehensive cancer center" or "clinical cancer center." These hospitals have consistently demonstrated their expertise both in conducting rigorous research and providing high-quality care. To get a list of NCI-designated cancer centers, visit http://cis.nci.nih.gov/fact/1_2.htm or call 800-4-CANCER/800-422-6237.

Establishing Your Role on Your Health Care Team

Once you have built your health care team and chosen a treatment facility, think about your own role on the team. Each team member has a unique area of expertise, but it's important to remember that you also have a certain expertise. You are the only one who knows how your body truly feels and what is most important to you about your treatment and recovery.

Your health care team will rely on you to share your preferences with them and be an active partner in your care. At a minimum, this means going to scheduled appointments, taking your medications, and reporting any side effects. Beyond these responsibilities, you should feel free to choose how much or how little you want to be involved in your care. In making this choice, ask yourself two key questions: How much do I want to know about my diagnosis and treatment, and how involved do I want to be in making medical decisions?

How Much Do I Want to Know About My Diagnosis and Treatment?

As a patient with cancer, you can learn a lot about your diagnosis and treatment, but you don't have to. Some people like to know all the details of their medical care because it helps them feel in control of the situation. Others are overwhelmed or uncomfortable with the details and prefer to just get the basics. Let your health care team know your preferences, so that you can get the amount of information that is right for you.

How Involved Do I Want to Be in Making Decisions About My Care?

People with colorectal cancer often find that they have several decisions to make about their care. For example, they might need to decide whether to see a general surgeon or a surgeon who specializes in colorectal cancer. They might also need to make decisions about whether to have chemotherapy or radiation therapy, depending on how advanced their cancer is. How each person approaches these types of decisions is a matter of personal preference. What's important is that you be involved in making decisions to the extent that you want to be. Studies show that not being involved the way you want (whether too little or too much) can lead to less satisfaction with your care and more anxiety.

Many people with colorectal cancer—particularly men and older people—prefer to leave the medical decisions to their doctors. They usually feel that their health care team has more skill and knowledge to make these decisions than they do, or they may prefer to focus on their daily lives rather than their medical care.

Other people choose to make medical decisions themselves because they feel it gives them more control over what is happening to them. If you opt for this approach, make sure your decisions are well informed. Get all of the information you need from your health care team to make a sound decision (for example, the pros and cons of any treatment options you're considering), and evaluate the information carefully. You may also want to get second opinions about which treatment is best for you (see page 126).

Communicating With Your Health Care Team

Communicating with the members of your health care team is an essential part of receiving good care. They can answer your questions, provide support, refer you to community resources, and tell you where to look for information about your cancer treatment. Give yourself permission to take this information in at your own pace and to be as involved in your care as you want to be.

Remember that communication is a two-way street: just as you will be counting on your health care team to keep you informed, they will be relying on you to keep them up to date about your condition.

Giving Information

Talking honestly and openly with your doctors and nurses is one of the best ways to feel confident in your treatment. It will also help them provide you with the best care possible. Below are some key pieces of information to share with them.

- Throughout the treatment process (and afterward), make note of any changes you experience in your bodily functions, from sleep and bowel habits to headaches and nausea. (Keeping a diary can be a very helpful way to keep track of these changes; it's easy to forget details from one day to the next.) Report these to your health care team as accurately and thoroughly as you can, so that they can help you find relief.
- Be honest about your lifestyle habits (things like smoking, drinking alcohol, or using illicit drugs), even if you're not proud of them. Something you think is minor could affect your treatment, and something you think is serious might not.

- Bring your medications list with you to every doctor's appointment, and be prepared to say how often and how long you've been taking each medicine. If you're having any allergies or reactions to your medications, let your doctor know.
- Talk to your doctor if you're considering or already using any complementary therapies, such as dietary supplements, herbal extracts, massage therapy, or acupuncture. Although some of these therapies can be used safely to relieve symptoms and side effects, others are known to interfere with conventional cancer treatments. For this reason, you should keep your doctor informed about any therapies that you're using or considering using, even if your doctor doesn't ask you about them. Since complementary medicine is still an area that many doctors are unfamiliar with, approach this issue in a non-confrontational manner. If you're considering a complementary therapy, let your doctor know that you want to make sure it will not interfere with the treatment he or she has prescribed. If you're taking dietary supplements, give your doctor a complete list of the doses you're taking, and be sure to report any side effects you're experiencing. (See chapter 14 for more information.)

> "I think you need somebody else in the room with you and you need to be taking notes, and don't let a doctor, he or she, put a hand on the doorknob to leave until you're through. You're the customer, and you ask all the questions and make sure you get them answered in a layperson's language so you can comprehend what they're saying."
>
> —KEITH

Getting Information

During meetings with your health care team, a large amount of detailed information will probably be exchanged. Processing and documenting all of this information can be challenging if you feel anxious or are unfamiliar with the terms beings used. Below are several ways to help ensure that you understand and accurately remember what your health care team tells you.

- If you don't understand something, ask to have it repeated or rephrased. You might say, "I'm having trouble grasping what you just said. Would you mind telling me again, or could you put it another way?" Another tactic is to repeat what was said and ask for confirmation: "Let me see if I have this right. You're saying that…" You might also ask your doctor or nurse to draw pictures to help you understand certain concepts.
- Write down information as you get it. When you can, get information in writing rather than verbally so that you can refer to it later. Many hospitals prepare handouts to help people understand common treatments or perform at-home care.

- Don't be afraid to ask questions. It shows that you're eager to learn and take an active role in your care. Write down your questions ahead of time, and ask the most important ones first. If your doctor or nurse doesn't have time to answer all of your questions during your appointment, ask when a good time would be to finish your conversation or if other resources are available.
- Bring a family member or friend to your doctor's appointments. Having another person there can help you communicate better and relieve a great deal of your stress. Choose someone you trust who listens well and will be available when you need them.
- Tape-record your doctor's appointments and phone conversations if your doctor allows it. This will help you remember the details of the discussions and allow you to share them with your loved ones.

Taking Enough Time

In an ideal world, health care providers would have more than enough time to answer your questions and explain things perfectly. In reality, though, patients often feel that their doctors are rushed. If you feel this way, talk to your doctor or nurse about it, and find creative ways to get the information you need. Below are some suggestions.

- Ask your doctor or nurse when the best time is to call with questions. Every practice has its own way of handling phone calls, and it's helpful to know this up front. For example, some doctors have a special time to return calls; others prefer to return their calls throughout the workday. You should expect your doctor to call you back, but remember that a quick response isn't always possible.

> *"You need to have a physician or nurse, whoever you're working with, who is looking out for your best interest and your total interests. If it's somebody that you're not comfortable talking with, then you need to go find somebody that you are comfortable talking with. You really do have to manage your own medical care. You can't just turn it over to some physician and say, 'Here, take care of me.' Talk about how you're feeling. Talk about what you're scared of, talk about what you want your future to be. You've got to communicate with people."*
>
> —GLENDA

- Find out which situations warrant an immediate call to your doctor or nurse. Some side effects and symptoms need to be reported right away, while others can wait until your next appointment—or at least until regular business hours.
- Ask your doctor if he or she responds to e-mail. A small but growing number of doctors use e-mail to communicate with patients, and it can be a convenient way to get your questions answered in writing.

Keeping Your Family Informed

If you would like your doctors and nurses to keep certain family members and friends informed about your illness and treatment, make sure to let them know.

Health care providers are bound by law to keep patients' health information confidential, and so they cannot share your information unless you permit them to. Let your health care team know exactly who may be contacting them and with whom they can share your information.

Keep in mind that while most health care providers are happy to talk to your family if you permit them to, it helps if you designate a family spokesperson.

- Ask your doctor or nurse to recommend brochures, videotapes, and web sites that can provide you with sound information. Many hospitals have resource areas to assist you.

Resolving Communication Problems With Your Doctor

If you have a problem talking with your doctor, there are often ways to improve the situation. First, state your concern as honestly and openly as possible. Here are some opening statements to consider:

- "I'm concerned that we aren't communicating well, and here's why..."
- "I need to be able to talk with you about _____, and I feel like I can't. Can we discuss this?"
- "I realize that you're very busy, but I very much need to discuss _____ at more length. Can we schedule a time to do that?"
- "I'm having trouble understanding _____. Can you help me?"

Even if you feel frustrated or angry, try to avoid being hostile or accusatory toward your doctor. People usually become defensive or withdraw if they feel attacked, and this type of response will not help you in the long run. Try to state your concerns as clearly and honestly as you can without making any accusations.

If you feel you've done your part but the situation hasn't improved, consider talking to a third party about the problem. For example, some hospitals have patient advocates or social workers on staff to help with these kinds of issues, or your primary care provider may be willing to intervene. Sometimes this is less stressful than facing your doctor directly and can help improve the situation. If not, it might be time to find a new doctor.

Getting a Second Opinion

Once you've chosen a doctor, you shouldn't feel that he or she has to be the sole source of your cancer care. Throughout your diagnosis and treatment, there may be critical points when you want to see other doctors for second opinions. By all means, do so. Colorectal cancer is a serious condition, and you should feel confident that you're getting the best care possible. Although some people with colorectal cancer need to begin their treatment without delay, most can take a few weeks to meet with other doctors and consider all of their options before moving forward.

> *"Obtain as MANY opinions as possible, with various experts in different treatment modalities, at the time of initial diagnosis, before a definitive treatment plan is decided upon. Because of varying experience and expertise, an expert in one type of treatment (such as surgical oncology) is not necessarily the most qualified to make a decision about the necessity for additional or other types of treatments."*
> —GARY

Some people hesitate to get second opinions because they worry about offending their doctors. This is an understandable concern, but rest assured that second opinions are well accepted within the medical community. Your doctor will understand that you need confirmation about your treatment plan and may be willing to arrange an appointment for you with another doctor. Consider seeing the person that your doctor recommends, but you may also want to see another doctor, just to ensure that you get an independent second opinion.

In terms of health insurance, second opinions are often covered—and even required. Before you seek a second opinion, though, contact your insurance company to find out exactly what your policy covers. They may require that your second opinion come from a doctor who is associated with your health plan.

When you make an appointment for a second opinion, ask what information the doctor needs and how quickly he or she needs it. Most doctors will want to review your medical information before your appointment, so that they can be fully prepared to discuss it with you. They typically want to see your medical records, pathology slides, medication list, and the results of any tests or diagnostic studies you've had (such as X-rays, CT scans, PET scans, bone scans, or MRIs).

Maintaining Your Medical Information

Maintaining a comprehensive record of your medical information can help ensure that the people involved in your treatment—including yourself—are as informed as possible. A good way to organize this information is to get a three-ring binder or accordion file and divide it into the following categories.

Ongoing Treatment Log

Maintain a detailed diary of events and information related to your cancer care. For each doctor's visit, list the following:
* the name of the doctor and facility you visited
* the names of those in the office with whom you had contact

Figure 8.2 Sample Treatment Log

Your Name: Martha Hill Bartels
Your Date of Birth: 02/09/40
Diagnosis Date: 07/21/01
Diagnosis: Adenocarcinoma of the Colon, Stage IIIA
Surgeon(s), Surgery(ies), Date(s): AP Resection, 8/12/01
Chemotherapy Treatments, Dates: 5-FU and leucovorin × 6 cycles (10/1/01 – 11/21/01)
Radiation Treatments, Dates: no radiation therapy
Other Related Procedures, Dates: follow-up CEA every 6 months; yearly colonoscopy; last colonoscopy on 8/15/03 was normal; last CEA on 2/15/04 was normal
Medications, Dosages, and Instructions: on no medications

Primary Care Physician, Nurse, Physician's Assistant, or Office Manager: Dr. Stephanie Rowlands/Suzanne or Thomas
Phone 404-555-1234
Fax 404-555-1235

Surgeon, Nurse or Office Manager: Dr. Robert Gonzalez/Deanna
Phone 404-555-1236
Fax 404-555-1237

Oncologist, Nurse or Office Manager: Dr. Clifford Sprenger/Lakeesha
Phone 404-555-1238
Fax 404-555-1239

- the date of the visit
- any information you received about your cancer or your care

For all biopsies, procedures, and treatments, note the dates and specific details, such as:
- the name and dose of any medication, including chemotherapy, you receive
- the total amount of any radiation you receive
- the exact location of the radiation treatment field
- the dates when treatments began and ended

You can also record your symptoms here and make notes about problems or side effects you experience.

Health Care Team Directory

Collect information from your health care team, making sure you know the names, office addresses, phone numbers, and fax numbers of all of your doctors, present and past. You might use a plastic business-card holder to organize this information. As you meet new members of your health care team, ask them for their information and organize it in your file. Copy this section of your binder and give it to the various members of your health care team so that they can easily reach one another. You may also want to share this information with the family members and friends involved in your care.

Personal Information Directory

Compile a list of all of your personal information such as:
- your date of birth and social security number
- your contact information (including home, work, and cell numbers)
- the contact information of any family or friends involved in your care
- the names and phone numbers of people to call in an emergency
- the contact information for anyone you might need to reach in a pinch
- a brief summary of your medical history

Insurance Information

File the following insurance information so that it will be handy when you need it:
- your insurance policy number
- the address and phone number of your insurance company
- the names of the people you've had contact with at the insurance company
- a copy of your health insurance policy or certificate

Figure 8.3 Sample Personal Information Directory

Personal Information
Your Name: Martha Hill Bartels
Social Security Number: 000-000-0000
Health Record or Insurance ID Number: SPN89577
Allergies: Penicillin

Brief Medical History:
- appendix removed 2/75
- history of high blood pressure
- mother had uterine cancer
- AP resection of colon for colon cancer 8/12/01; treated with adjuvant therapy of 5-FU/leucovorin × 6 cycles

Personal Contact Information
Home Address: 1217 Shady Oak Lane, Atlanta, GA 30329
Home Phone: 770-555-0123
Employer: Shady Oak Elementary School
Work Phone: 917-555-0123
Cell Phone: 404-555-0123

Spouse's Information
Spouse's Name: Bill Bartels
Bill's Work Phone: 917-555-3210
Bill's Cell Phone: 404-555-3210

Martha's Health Care Team
Dr. Stephanie Rowlands, primary care physician: 404-555-1234
Dr. Robert Gonzalez, surgeon: 404-555-1236
Dr. Clifford Sprenger, oncologist: 404-555-1238

Call in an Emergency:
Jenny and Russell Jeffries (daughter and son-in-law): 404-555-3211
Caroline Robinson (sister): 404-555-3212

Miscellaneous:
Alice and Daniel Schultz (neighbors): 404-555-3213
Shady Oak Kennels (boarding for pets): 404-555-3214
Shady Oak Neighborhood Pharmacy: 404-555-3215

- your benefits booklet and explanation of benefits
- copies of materials you received when you enrolled in the plan and updates you've received since then
- copies of any correspondence you've had with your insurance company
- bills, payment records, and statements

Reports

Keep your test results and procedure reports in this section, including:
- the name of the exact kind of cancer you have
- the date you were first diagnosed
- dated reports of blood work
- dated reports from all surgeries and procedures
- dated pathology reports

Medicines

Maintain a complete and up-to-date list of the medications you're taking, including prescribed medications and any vitamins, herbs, or over-the-counter medicines. Include the following details:
- the names of your medicines
- the dates they were prescribed (or that you started taking them)
- notes about when you're supposed to take them
- doses
- notes about what each medication is meant to do
- the side effects that should be monitored
- the problems that you should report immediately, and to whom

Calendar

A one-year calendar on a single page allows you to see at a glance the overall progress of your treatment. It shows you the larger picture—for example, when your surgery, radiation, and/or chemotherapy treatments are—and helps you to schedule vacations, business trips, and other obligations between treatments.

Potential Problems

Ask members of your health care team about short- and long-term risks or problems that may result from your cancer or treatment. Take notes about what you can do to prevent or be alert about these potential problems and record them in this section of your binder.

Community Resources

File the addresses, phone numbers, and web sites of organizations that could be helpful to you in your cancer care. Include news, advice, and tips you've received from these organizations and pages you've printed out from the Internet. The American Cancer Society can provide you with information, support, and contacts in your local community; call 800-ACS-2345/800-227-2345 or visit http://www.cancer.org. The Resources section of this book is another good place to start.

Questions

Keep a record of the questions you have about your care and the answers you receive. Date each entry for future reference.

Maintaining Your Health

This is the place for information or hints about staying well or caring for yourself before, during, and after treatments. For example, you might want to include information on preventing the nausea that often results from chemotherapy, or you could include tips for caring for an ostomy after surgery.

In addition, file general wellness plans and any suggestions from your health care team about diet and exercise.

Follow Up

After your treatment, you will continue to see your doctors regularly for follow-up care (see chapter 18). In this section, record any recommendations from your health care team about your follow-up schedule, including which procedures you need to have and when.

Getting the Best Care Possible

Dealing with cancer is never a pleasant experience, but every person with colorectal cancer deserves to receive the best care possible. Navigating the medical system successfully and understanding your choices not only helps ensure excellent care but can save you time and trouble, give you peace of mind, and allow you to focus your energies on your recovery.

CHAPTER NINE

MAKING INFORMED DECISIONS ABOUT TREATMENT OPTIONS

Marilyn Mulay, RN, MS, OCN

A diagnosis of colorectal cancer immediately plunges you into an unfamiliar world of medical specialists and confusing language. You are asked to make decisions based on new and sometimes confusing information, and those decisions may have life-altering consequences.

As we discussed in chapter 7, the emotional impact of learning that you have cancer or that your cancer has returned or has grown is complex. Your mind may be in a whirl about what your future holds. You may feel anxious and vulnerable. You may feel angry or sad. You may even feel paralyzed by the news and unable to cope.

Amidst all of these emotions and new experiences, what can you do to become a knowledgeable healthcare consumer? What can you do to make the important decisions you're facing with confidence? This chapter is designed to help you organize your thoughts and enable you to make well-informed decisions. It will also provide you with some general information about the standard of care for treating both colon and rectal cancers.

Treating Your Colorectal Cancer: You Have Choices

Making decisions in cancer treatment is not a one-time experience. Instead, people with cancer travel along a decision-making continuum throughout the course of their illness. At every decision-making point, a person with cancer must make one of three choices.

One option is to do nothing at all. With some cancers that progress very slowly, such as prostate cancer, this is a more common option, especially for older men. In other cases, such as when cancer is advanced, people with metastatic disease may choose to spend their remaining time focusing on quality of life rather than receiving aggressive cancer treatment that may have unpleasant side effects. In most cases, though, it is in your best interest to treat your cancer.

Once you decide to have treatment, the next choice is to select conventional therapy. Conventional treatments have been tested through clinical studies and subjected to peer review to determine the validity and reliability of the information. Drugs and methods used in conventional therapy have been tested and deemed safe and effective by the US Food and Drug Administration (FDA). Information about how the treatments work, the response rates, and side effects is readily available.

As part of this decision, you will need to select from among your treatment options. Depending on your situation, your doctor may recommend multimodal treatment, a combination of different therapies, each having a specific purpose in the treatment of your cancer, such as radiation to shrink the tumor followed by surgery to remove it. You can also add complementary therapy (supportive treatments such as acupuncture, massage, and yoga that do not cure cancer but may help control symptoms and improve well being) to your treatment. Always ask your doctor before undertaking any complementary therapy. See chapter 14 for more information.

The third choice is experimental therapy. Experimental therapies show promise but have not yet been approved by the FDA for routine use. Drugs and interventions are tested in several phases of clinical trials, with each answering questions about the new treatment or combination of treatments. How much is known about experimental drugs and interventions depends on what phase of testing the drug is in. Clinical trials will be discussed in more detail in chapter 13.

Another avenue you may be curious about—*one we do not recommend under any circumstances*—is to pursue alternative therapies. Alternative therapy is unconventional treatment used *instead of* conventional medicine. Because alternative therapies have not been tested in clinical trials, oncologists cannot verify their worth. These therapies are often peddled on the Internet and may promise "miracle cures." Be wary of spectacular claims because these treatments can be expensive and may be harmful despite their favorable claims. In addition to this danger, people who choose alternative treatments lose the proven benefits of conventional anticancer therapies. See chapter 14 for more information on alternative medicine.

The Standard of Care

The standard of care is a term health care professionals use to describe the recommended treatment for a certain health condition that is generally recognized by the profession as the best practice or the treatment most likely to ensure the most positive outcome. These recommendations are based on evidence gathered from research and clinical trials.

The standards of care for both colon and rectal cancer are outlined by stage in the following sections and include brief mentions of surgery, radiation, chemotherapy, and other treatment options. Each of these treatment modalities is discussed in detail in its own chapter (see chapter 10 for information on surgery, chapter 11 for radiation therapy, chapter 12 for chemotherapy, chapter 13 for clinical trials and emerging therapies, and chapter 14 for complementary treatments).

Of course, it is critically important to realize that every person's body is different, and your situation or circumstances may dictate that your medical team depart from the standard of care in order to provide the best outcome for you. Therefore, the information that follows should only be used as a general reference.

If the treatment your doctor recommends is different from what is listed here, and you are concerned about this, talk to your doctor so that he or she can address your questions and explain why in your particular situation a different approach might be best.

Treatment by Stage of Colon Cancer

Recall from chapter 5 that cancer is classified by stage depending on how widespread it is. For all but stage IV colon cancer, surgery to remove the tumor is the primary or first treatment. Adjuvant therapy (additional treatments) may also be used.

- Stage 0: The cancer has not grown beyond the inner lining of the colon, so surgery to take out the cancer is all that is needed. This may be accomplished in many cases by polypectomy or local excision through the colonoscope. Surgical resection may be necessary if your tumor is too big to be removed by local excision.

- Stage I: The cancer has grown through several layers of the colon, but it has not spread outside the colon wall itself. Surgical resection to remove the cancer is the standard treatment. Additional therapy is not needed.
- Stage II: The cancer has grown through the wall of the colon and may extend into nearby tissue. It has not yet spread to the lymph nodes. Surgical resection is usually the only treatment needed. If the cancer is likely to come back because of its appearance under the microscope or because it was growing into other tissues, radiation therapy or chemotherapy may be recommended. Chemotherapy is not standard treatment for stage II colon cancer, but many doctors recommend it if the risk of recurrence seems high. Special tests are being developed to evaluate the risk of recurrence or spread.
- Stage III: The cancer has spread to nearby lymph nodes, but it has not yet spread to other parts of the body. Surgical resection is the first treatment. Chemotherapy is also given. Radiation therapy is added as well if the cancer was large enough to grow into adjacent tissues.
- Stage IV: The cancer has spread to distant organs and tissues. Surgery in stage IV is usually not done with the expectation of curing the colon cancer. The goal of surgery in this stage is usually to relieve blockage of the colon and to prevent other complications such as bleeding or perforation. If the cancer is small and the patient's health is poor, doctors may avoid surgery. Chemotherapy or radiation therapy (or both) may also be given to relieve, delay, or prevent symptoms. If only a few small metastases are present in the liver and can be completely removed along with the colon cancer, surgery can help the person live longer and might even cure the cancer. Chemotherapy might also be given after this surgery.
- Recurrent colon cancer: Recurrent cancer means that the cancer has returned after treatment. Surgery to remove local recurrences can sometimes help a patient live longer. As with stage IV colon cancer, surgery to remove metastases can also sometimes help and, along with chemotherapy, can still be curative. If the metastases can't be removed, chemotherapy is the main treatment. Doctors may also recommend clinical trials at this point.

Treatment by Stage of Rectal Cancer

Except for some patients with stage IV cancer, surgery to remove the rectal cancer is the first treatment. Adjuvant therapy (additional treatments) may also be used.
- Stage 0: The cancer has not grown beyond the inner lining of the rectum. Removing or destroying the cancer is all that is needed.

- Stage I: The cancer has grown through the first layer of the rectum into deeper layers but has not spread outside the rectal wall itself. Surgery is performed and no further treatment is needed. If a patient is too sick or elderly to withstand surgery, he or she may be treated only with radiation therapy; however, this has not been proven to be as effective as surgery.
- Stage II: The cancer has grown through the wall of the rectum into nearby tissue. It has not yet spread to the lymph nodes. Stage II rectal cancers are usually treated by surgical resection, along with both chemotherapy and radiation therapy. Radiation may be given either before or after the surgery. Most doctors now favor giving the radiation therapy along with chemotherapy before surgery. In addition, many doctors now favor giving chemotherapy after surgery.
- Stage III: The cancer has spread to nearby lymph nodes but not to other parts of the body. The rectal tumor is usually removed by surgical resection. Radiation therapy is given before or after surgery. As in stage II, many doctors now prefer to give radiation therapy along with chemotherapy before surgery. Chemotherapy will usually be given after surgery.
- Stage IV: The cancer has spread to distant organs and tissues such as the liver or lungs. The goal of surgery in this stage is to relieve or prevent blockage of the rectum by the cancer and to prevent local complications such as bleeding. The cancer usually cannot be cured by rectal surgery because it has spread. However, in some cases, it may be possible to use a combination of surgery, radiation, and/or chemotherapy to help a patient live longer, contain metastasis, and/or relieve some of the patient's symptoms.
- Recurrent rectal cancer: Recurrent cancer means that the cancer has returned after treatment. It may come back locally (near the area of the initial rectal tumor) or in distant organs. As with stage IV cancer, it may be possible to use a combination of surgery, radiation, and/or chemotherapy to help a patient live longer, contain metastasis, and/or relieve some of the patient's symptoms. Your doctor may also suggest appropriate clinical trials.

Your Role in Decision Making

Consider your role in the decision-making process. Will participating in decisions about your treatment and care help relieve your fear or worry, or will it add to your stress? You may be the type of person who wants to and needs to take an active role in decisions. On the other hand, you may want to be more passive, deferring the decisions to a doctor, family member, or trusted friend.

Table 9.1 What Is Your Preferred Role in Decision Making?

Model	What Role You Want	What You Might Say to the Doctor
Paternalistic	Doctor is primary decision maker	"I would like you to make a clear recommendation."
Informative / Consumer	Shared decision making between you and your doctor	"I would like you to tell me about the treatment options so I can think about the risks and benefits, and then I would like us to make a decision together."
Deliberate	You are the primary decision maker	"I would like to hear about the treatment options, so that I can make a decision about what would be best for me."

There are many models for making decisions (see Table 9.1). In the paternalistic model, the oncologist is the primary decision maker. This model assumes that the doctor knows best and will decide for the patient. Patients in this model are often passive during the decision-making process but later may feel that their value system was not considered.

In another model, sometimes called the informative or consumer model, the doctor presents the information and works together with the patient to make the decision. Although the patient can assert his or her values, he or she often does not want the sole responsibility of making the decision—particularly if there is a chance of an unfavorable outcome.

> "The atmosphere in which medicine occurs now is different than it was 20 years ago, in that doctors are very accustomed to patients asking questions and wanting to be more involved in the process of their health care."
>
> —ERNESTINE

In the deliberate model, the doctor and patient review the patient's values and discuss how these values will affect treatment choices. The patient makes the final choice of treatment.

Clearly, not every doctor/patient exchange fits neatly into one of these models but will fall somewhere in between. All of the models require that the patient understands and is able to express his or her values. There is no best approach—only the one that makes you the most comfortable.

Styles of doctor communication also vary. Some doctors give very detailed medical information and ask closed-ended questions that require the patient to answer only with a yes or no. In a more consumerist style, the patient asks questions and the doctor provides information. The most effective communication between doctor and patient seems to be when the doctor is allowed to present his or her findings and recommendations and the patient then asks questions. Over time, a patient forms a relationship with his or her doctor. The doctor understands the patient's values, making open exchanges of information and collaborative decision making easier.

Other Factors Affecting Decision Making

Your decisions will probably be driven by your individual value system. For example, your religion may dictate a specific stance on certain types of medical intervention. Because each person's value system is unique, you should make your values known and feel comfortable that your doctor will respect and honor their decisions. You are the expert about you and what you value.

Time is another factor that may limit your choices or affect your decision. How quickly do you need to make a decision? You should take time to become familiar with your options. Share the information you have collected with those whose opinion you trust—perhaps a spouse, a sibling, a friend, or your primary care doctor. Although you should not make snap decisions, you should move forward as soon as you can. If you are delaying making a decision, ask yourself if you need more information or if you simply do not want to face the decision.

> *"I immediately did as much research as I could about colon cancer. Especially hereditary colon cancer, since that's what I had. I did a lot of research and a lot of reading. I talked to associates, and doctors, and other cancer survivors to get their experiences. So, I learned. I feel that knowledge is power. The more you know, the better you are able to be your own advocate."*
>
> —LOU

Gathering Additional Information

Gathering and understanding information can be a daunting task. Your individual learning style dictates the best way for you to get information. Do you retain more information if you read it or see it in a chart or graph? If so, you are a visual learner and will get more from printed material. Do you prefer to hear things explained to you? If so, you are an auditory learner.

Many patients ask the help of a family member or friend who can research printed material or attend consultations. Sharing the process may make information gathering easier for you.

Your Health Care Team

The health care team is the best source of information. It is important that you are comfortable with your doctors and their staff members and feel that you can communicate well when questions or problems arise.

As we noted in the previous chapter, you will probably have many medical professionals involved in your care. The doctors may include a gastroenterologist, a surgeon, a medical oncologist, a radiation oncologist, and a pathologist. In addition, nurses, social workers, and other health care professionals may also be involved in your care. Each part of the health care team is a valuable source of information for you and your family.

Nonprofit Organizations

The American Cancer Society is the nation's largest nonprofit organization dedicated to eliminating cancer as a major health problem by preventing cancer, saving lives, and diminishing suffering from cancer through research, education, advocacy, and service. The Society provides information, services, and support to anyone facing cancer, including family members and caregivers. Call 800-ACS-2345/800-227-2345 any time of day, any day of the week, or visit the web site at http://www.cancer.org. You can also use these information channels to find your local American Cancer Society unit.

Other organizations that are good resources for patients with colorectal cancer are the Colon Cancer Alliance, Colorectal Cancer Coalition, and Colorectal Cancer Network. The Resources section of this book has information on how to contact these and other reliable organizations. Some of these organizations provide a service that allows you to speak with another colorectal cancer patient about doctors, drugs, side effects, and other issues that may be of concern.

Printed Materials

Books and pamphlets can also be a valuable source of information and are available through a variety of sources.

This book is one example of the many types of printed material available from the American Cancer Society. The American Cancer Society has a comprehensive collection of free information on all aspects of cancer, including clinical trials, that can be customized to your information needs and delivered to your mailbox or viewed online. Call 800-ACS-2345/800-227-2345 or visit the American Cancer Society web site at http://www.cancer.org.

Don't overlook your local public library. Libraries are good sources of free information and are staffed by librarians who are trained in locating helpful resources.

Because of the delay in getting current information published, books may not contain the latest information about treatment options. Although every effort is made to provide literature in a timely manner, it still takes some time to publish a book. The most up-to-date information about treatment options is published in medical journals, but these articles can be like reading a foreign language to a person who hasn't gone to medical school.

Significant studies are often reported in the popular press so you may find information in the newspaper or news magazines. However, journalists may exaggerate the importance of a particular finding or study result to make the piece seem more newsworthy, so if you encounter some information in the popular press that you think might affect your cancer treatment, be sure to discuss it with your healthcare team.

ACS/NCCN Colon and Rectal Cancer Treatment Guidelines for Patients

Together with the American Cancer Society, the National Comprehensive Cancer Network (NCCN) publishes a comprehensive booklet on colorectal cancer that contains useful information and treatment guidelines. Portions of these guidelines are referenced throughout this book and are generally considered the standard of care for persons facing colorectal cancer. These guidelines include valuable "decision trees" to help patients make informed decisions about treatment based on cancer grade, stage, and specific situation. To receive a copy of this booklet, contact the American Cancer Society (800-ACS-2345/800-227-2345 or http://www.cancer.org) or the NCCN (888-909-NCCN/888-909-6226 or http://www.nccn.org) and ask for the *Colon and Rectal Cancer Treatment Guidelines for Patients*.

The Internet

The Internet can be a terrific source of high-quality, free cancer information to those who know where to look. In addition to the American Cancer Society web site (http://www.cancer.org), the federal government's National Cancer Institute (http://www.cancer.gov) is a reliable source for information online; their PDQ information summaries designed specifically for patients are especially helpful. Medline, a service of the US National Library of Medicine for medical professionals, has now established a service for consumers called Medline Plus. It is not specific to cancer, but has good cancer information and can be found at http://www.medlineplus.com.

Information about treatments, the risks and benefits, side effects, and outcomes are often published online by pharmaceutical companies and academic medical centers. The Internet also can be used to access information on doctors, cancer centers, and hospitals. Current clinical trials can be accessed there as well.

A wide variety of excellent web sites are listed in the Resources section at the end of this book.

Dangers of the Internet

The Internet can be an excellent source of information and an effective way for patients to access free health information and online support. However, it can also be a source of rumors, misinformation, and half-truths. Do not take everything you read there as the absolute truth. Anyone can post a claim without having to substantiate it, because publication of information on the Internet is not subject to peer review or regulation.

> "When doing online research, we have to make sure that we are reading legitimate research because unfortunately in the cancer care field, there are people who make wild claims about eating certain things or doing a certain procedure. So we have to make sure we're getting legitimate information from sources like the National Cancer Institute and the American Cancer Society."
>
> —EDDIE

Several organizations have web sites with chat rooms or message boards where patients can share information or concerns. Remember that each patient is an individual and not everyone will have the same response to treatment or experience the same side effects. A patient with an atypical reaction to a drug or who is angry about something may post a statement in a chat room that conveys an erroneous message. On the other hand, these forums can be valuable place to share concerns with others in similar situations.

Look at the source of the information to assure that the information can be trusted. If in doubt, ask your healthcare team. See Figure 9.1 for tips on finding quality information on the Internet.

Drug Information

The American Cancer Society has a cancer drug database that can be accessed on the Internet at http://www.cancer.org. (Type the generic or trade name of the drug in the search box or go directly to http://www.cancer.org/docroot/CDG/cdg_0.asp for the entire online cancer drug guide.) Another comprehensive web site called Cancer Tools is offered at http://www.fda.gov/cder/cancer. The following web sites also provide reliable information about cancer drugs:

Finding Quality Information on the Internet

- Choose a web site from an organization that you trust (a national nonprofit organization, a government agency, or a large university or hospital)
- Use several different web sites to compare information
- Check to see that authors' credentials as well as affiliations and financial interest are clearly stated
- Look for sources—are they clearly referenced and acknowledged?
- Make sure that the information has been recently updated
- Be wary of any doctor or institution who proposes to diagnose or treat you without examination and consultation
- Be wary of any web site that sells products to treat your cancer
- Read the web site's privacy statement to assure that any information you supply will be kept confidential.
- Use your common sense!

- US Food and Drug Administration home page at http://www.fda.gov
- FDA Cancer Liaison Program home page at http://www.fda.gov/oashi/cancer/cancer.html
- US Food and Drug Administration Center for Drug Evaluation and Research at http://www.fda.gov/cder/cancer/index.htm
- Physician's Data Query of the National Cancer Institute at http://www.nci.nih.gov/cancerinfo

For FDA-approved drugs, you can usually find package inserts for the particular drug on the Internet by typing http://www.[drugname].com.

Be particularly careful about information about drugs you find on the Internet. Many testimonials for "miracle cures" or alternative cancer therapies are posted on the Internet. Most of these are schemes that will take your money and may even do you harm.

Advice From Family and Friends

Well-meaning family and friends will often share stories about other patients "just like you" who have the "same" diagnosis. It can alarm you or make you second-guess your decisions when you learn that another patient with colorectal cancer is receiving something different than has been recommended for you.

It is important to realize that there is no other patient "just like you." Not everyone with colorectal cancer will receive the same treatment. A doctor's recommendations for treatment are based on a wide variety of factors including the site of the primary tumor, lymph node involvement, whether the cancer has spread to distant areas of the body, prior treatment history, prior medical history and, most importantly, you, the unique patient.

Each patient and his or her situation require and deserve consideration of the individual aspects of his or her cancer. Your doctor will make recommendations that fit your specific situation and health profile.

Getting the Most From Your Doctor's Appointments

Bringing someone along to doctor's appointments and medical consultations is always a good idea. Be prepared to take notes. Also, ask if audio-taping the consultation is allowed, because there will be a great deal of information given at that time, and it may be impossible to recall it all later. Your doctor may even have patient information sheets or brochures to share with you. You will probably repeat the details of the consultation multiple times to various family members and friends, and it is important to have the correct information.

When seeing the doctor for the primary consultation, you should bring along all available information about your diagnosis and treatment to date. It is useful to begin a notebook to keep all of the important documents over the course of your treatment (see chapter 8). That way, you will have all pertinent information handy if you need to see a new doctor.

Sometimes, the doctor may want to see your pathology slides or actual CT films, so ask if you need to bring those things before the visit. By bringing the information at the time of the visit, the physician will have all necessary data to make informed recommendations and time will not be wasted waiting to gather reports from various sources.

Questions to Ask About Your Treatment Options

- What are my treatment options?
- What are the advantages and disadvantages of each treatment option?
- What treatment plan do you recommend and why?
- Is the goal of this treatment plan to cure the cancer or control my symptoms?
- Will this treatment extend my life? How will it improve the quality of my life?
- How successful is this treatment for the type and stage of cancer I have?
- How will you evaluate how well this treatment is working?
- What options will be available to me if this treatment does not work?
- What are the possible immediate, short-term, and long-term side effects of the treatment? Can anything be done to prevent or lessen these side effects?
- If we decide on a multimodal approach, will the first treatment have side effects that may affect the second treatment? For example, if I get radiation first, will I have to delay surgery? For how long? How will it affect my recovery?
- What is the timetable for treatments? If I receive a combination of treatments, how long will I wait between treatments? How long will the whole plan take?
- Will I have to be hospitalized? Can any of the treatments be done on an outpatient basis?
- What will my energy level be like?
- How will this treatment affect my life? What changes should I expect to make in my work, family life, and leisure time?
- How much will my treatment cost? Is my treatment plan covered by my insurance?

Be sure to tell your doctor about all of your medications, including over-the-counter drugs. Some of these compounds are not as harmless as they may seem and could interfere with your treatment or even be harmful to you.

Be prepared with a list of questions. Many of them may be answered by the time the doctor finishes the consultation, but if you have a list, nothing will be forgotten.

Comparing Your Options

The worksheet in Figure 9.1 on page 147 may help to organize the information and assist in making informed decisions.

Your treatment plan may be multimodal, which means it will include a combination of therapies. (For example, many patients have surgery followed by chemotherapy with a combination of drugs.) For combination therapies, you may need one sheet for each method of treatment. For chemotherapy treatments involving several medications, you may need one sheet for each drug in the treatment regimen. Write down all of the issues that you can think of about the treatment: what are the pros and cons, the risks and the benefits, how long will it take, what are the side effects, and anything else that comes to mind.

> *"The bottom line for me was I wanted to treat my cancer aggressively. I'm a young man. I thought I had a lot of life left, so I wanted to treat my cancer with everything that I possibly could, regardless of how sick I got or how bad it was."*
>
> —KEN

All treatments have potential side effects. No one can predict if you will experience a certain side effect. Some patients have a mild response to one drug and a strong response to another. Some patients recover more quickly from surgery than others. Some patients experience none of the side effects of cancer treatment and others experience all of them. Most patients are somewhere in the middle. Drug or radiation doses can be modified (lowered) if you have a severe reaction; in an extreme case, the treatment can be stopped. Knowing the potential side effects of a treatment may help to decide on the right option for you.

Understand Your Options

Understanding exactly what the doctor is saying can be difficult if he or she uses technical terms. When discussing various treatment options, terms like response rate, time to progression, and time to survival help to define the options. If at any time your doctor uses terms that you do not understand, stop and ask for an explanation. Hearing the information and understanding it can be two different things. Remember, the only dumb questions are the ones that are not asked.

Getting a Second Opinion

As was mentioned in the chapter on diagnosis, patients may want to consider getting another opinion to gain confidence that the recommended treatment is

Figure 9.1 Treatment Worksheet

Treatment Worksheet

Method of Treatment:

Names of Drugs Used:

Frequency of Treatment:

Route of Treatment (IV or oral):

Preparations Needed Before Treatment:

Arrangements Needed During Treatment:

Duration of Treatment:

How Will We Know If the Treatment Is Working?:

How Well Has the Treatment Worked for Other Cancer Patients with Diagnoses Similar to My Own?:

How Long Will the Cancer-Fighting Effects of This Treatment Last?:

Short-Term Side Effects:

Long-Term Side Effects:

Benefits:

Cost of the Treatment:

My Questions:

---

appropriate or to help in making a treatment choice. Patients should not feel that the doctor would resent it if they sought another opinion and therefore be afraid to pursue one. A second opinion is a very good idea when treating a serious problem like colorectal cancer, especially if you need to choose among several options.

Your Personal Treatment Plan

One of the most serious concerns of cancer patients is that they will lose control over their lives. The diagnosis and treatment of your cancer will undoubtedly change your life forever. However, participating in the development of your personal treatment plan—to the extent that you feel comfortable—can help restore your sense of control.

Studies have shown that patients who participate in making decisions about their treatments are more compliant with their care. They also have better outcomes.

The next few chapters will describe the primary approaches doctors use to treat colorectal cancer, including surgery (with special attention to colostomies), radiation therapy, chemotherapy, emerging therapies, clinical trials, and complementary and alternative therapies. These chapters will familiarize you with each procedure and will introduce the potential benefits and disadvantages of each option. Your health care team can supplement the information with information that is specific to your individual situation.

Once you've weighed all the options, commit to a personal treatment plan and be sure that the members of your health care team and your support network are all on board. Ask any questions you have before your therapy begins.

Making the Best Decision...for You

Today, there are many approaches to treating colorectal cancer. Information gives people with cancer a certain degree of power over their situations and helps them to maintain their autonomy. A knowledgeable patient can make well-informed decisions and is more likely to feel confident and optimistic when treatment begins.

Questions to Ask Your Medical Team About Your Personal Treatment Plan

HOW DO I PREPARE FOR THIS TREATMENT?

- How long will this treatment last? How is treatment given?
- Will I be hospitalized during this treatment? If so, for how long? What is the average recovery time for people receiving this treatment?
- Should I follow a special diet before, during, or after treatment?
- What medicines or vitamins should I avoid during treatment?
- How will my treatment be evaluated?
- How will you know that my treatment is working?
- What are the chances that my cancer may recur after the treatment programs we have discussed?
- What will my checkup schedule be after treatment?
- What tests will I undergo at my checkups?

HOW DO I PAY FOR THIS TREATMENT?

- Is this treatment covered by most insurance or health care plans? Is it covered by my plan? How will I be billed? For example, will I receive separate bills from the hospital, surgeon, anesthesiologist, pathologist, and radiologist?
- How much does this treatment cost?

WHO IS ON MY TREATMENT TEAM?

- Do the members of my treatment team agree on the details of the proposed plan?
- Who will coordinate and monitor my treatment? What other specialists will take part in my care? Will they all be involved throughout my treatment?
- Whom should I call with questions? When is the best time to call? Will this person communicate with the rest of my treatment team?
- Who will be in charge of monitoring my health after I've finished treatment?
- Can I speak to someone who has undergone this treatment under your care?

149

CHAPTER TEN

SURGERY

David A. Rothenberger, MD

Surgery is the primary form of treatment for colon and rectal cancer. The surgery needed by a person with colorectal cancer may vary from a minor outpatient procedure to a complex operation performed by a team of surgeons. Often, surgery is combined with other treatments such as radiation and chemotherapy. (This is called multimodal treatment.) Sometimes colon or rectal surgery is combined with other types of surgery if the cancer has spread to other organs such as the liver.

Your treatment plan will be based on the clinical stage of your cancer (see chapter 5), your current overall health status, your health care team's recommendations, and your own personal preferences and unique situation.

Most often, the goal of surgery is to cure the cancer. There are times when cure is not possible, but doctors recommend an operation to relieve current symptoms or prevent major problems from developing in the near future (see the statement about palliative treatment at the bottom of page 182). Your surgeon will discuss the options with you and make a recommendation for treatment.

It is important that you are comfortable with your treatment plan and with your surgeon. Usually you can take your time to think about your choices and make an informed decision. (Your health care team will let you know if your situation requires immediate action.) You may want to ask for a second opinion to provide more information and to help you feel more confident about the treatment you choose.

Sometimes, even with the best planning, unexpected events may require a change in the treatment plan; for example, more extensive cancer may be discovered or problems such as major bleeding are encountered during surgery. It is important that you choose a surgeon you trust to make decisions on your behalf in case such situations unexpectedly arise.

In this chapter, we'll talk about the different procedures used for colorectal cancer surgery. Although we usually discuss colon and rectal cancer together in this book, because the surgical techniques and treatment for the colon and rectal cancer are different in very important ways, in this chapter, we'll discuss the two separately. First, we'll look at the process of colon cancer surgery and the techniques surgeons use, and then we'll look at rectal cancer surgery.

The Process of Elective Radical Colon Surgery

You may be wondering what surgery on your colon will involve. In the next few sections, we'll talk about what you can expect when you choose to undergo surgery to treat colon cancer. Next, we'll discuss specific procedures surgeons use to treat colon cancer.

Later in this chapter, we'll discuss surgery for rectal cancer (see page 172).

Preparing for Surgery

You will need to prepare your bowels the day before your colon surgery. This involves following specific instructions your doctor will give you and may require eating a modified diet and taking laxatives or a liquid to cleanse the large intestine. This preparation is necessary to remove the contents of the colon and reduce the number of bacteria so infection is less likely to develop. You may also be instructed to take oral antibiotics to further reduce the risk of infection.

"I had surgery on August 26, 1999, and the doctors removed the right portion of my colon, which is known as the ascending colon. They also removed my appendix and part of my small intestine and they removed all the lymph nodes in the area."

—EDDIE

Most patients are admitted to the hospital on the day of surgery. It is important not to eat or drink anything for six to eight hours before the operation unless your doctor has specifically given you permission to do so. In the preoperative area, you will meet other members of the operating team including the anesthesiologist, a doctor with special training in safely providing you with anesthesia (medication that reduces feeling, such as pain) during the operation. The anesthesiologist and his assistants will talk with you about what to expect as you are taken into the operating room and will review all of your medications and any allergies that you may have. They will answer any questions you have about anesthesia.

An intravenous line (IV) is started to provide you with fluids and the medicines needed to assure a safe and painless operation, including the anesthetic and possibly an antibiotic. You may also be asked to wear special devices to decrease the risk of blood clots forming in your legs and pelvic veins.

Most often, the operation is done under a general anesthetic so you are unconscious and will be pain-free (general anesthesia produces an overall sleep-like state; regional anesthesia numbs a specific body part). When you are unconscious, the anesthesiologist must control your breathing; this is done by placing a tube through your mouth into your windpipe. Oxygen is given through the tube directly into your lungs. Your heart, lungs, and other vital functions will be monitored carefully during the operation.

During the Surgery

After anesthesia is given, you will be positioned on the operating table. Usually a member of your health care team will place a tube called a catheter into your bladder; this allows the team to monitor your urine output during the operation. The catheter may be left in place for a few days after the operation. After the skin of your abdomen is washed with a special antibacterial solution and other preparations are made, the surgeon begins the operation.

The operation is typically done through an open incision, but laparoscopic approaches (see page 154) are being used more and more often. Once the incision is made and the abdomen is opened up, the surgeon will assess the contents of the abdominal cavity to confirm the preoperative clinical staging (the stage assigned to the cancer before surgery; see chapter 5) and to exclude other unforeseen abnormalities or circumstances. If necessary, the health care team will modify the operative plan to fit any new findings.

The surgeon will remove the cancer itself, as well as a segment of normal large intestine on either side of the tumor, and the adjacent soft tissues (called the mesentery) that contain the blood vessels and lymph nodes from that segment of colon. This entire specimen is sent to the pathologist for further study and to assess the adequacy of the cancer-free margins. Next, the surgeon will connect the two ends of intestine left after the cancerous tissue is removed. The place where the two parts of the intestinal tract are joined is called the anastomosis. There are many ways to do an anastomosis, including hand-suturing and surgical stapling. Your surgeon will choose a technique that fits your situation and his or her preference.

ON THE HORIZON

Laparoscopic Surgery

Surgery on the colon or rectum to treat cancer traditionally involves a surgeon making a large cut (incision) through the skin and muscles of abdomen, which may be painful during recovery, may become infected, and may take a long time to heal. However, with a newer technique called laparoscopic surgery, it is sometimes possible to remove segments of diseased colon and nearby lymph nodes that are affected in a much less invasive way.

To perform laparoscopic surgery on the colon, the surgeon, instead of cutting an opening in the abdomen large enough to work in, makes a handful of small incisions (less than a half-inch) in the patient, through which a video camera and miniature versions of the usual surgical instruments are passed. The surgical team then performs the colectomy (removal of a portion of the

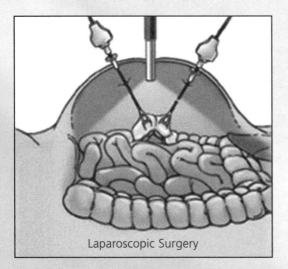

Laparoscopic Surgery

In laparoscopic colorectal surgery for cancer, the abdomen is filled with gas. Thin, specially designed instruments and a magnifying video camera are placed into the abdomen and used for dissection.

Source: Figure 1 from Weiser MR. Laparoscopic colorectal surgery for cancer: is it ready for prime time? Available at http://www.cancernews.com/articles/laparoscopiccancersurgery.htm. Accessed September 16, 2004. Copyright © 2002 Memorial Sloan-Kettering Cancer Center.

Regardless of the technique used, the surgeon must make sure that the blood supply to the ends of bowel used to connect the intestines is adequate and that there is no tension pulling on the anastomosis. Otherwise, it will not heal.

After the anastomosis, the patient's abdomen is washed with a sterile solution and the incision is closed with sutures (stitches), staples, or both.

colon) entirely inside the abdomen. The portion of bowel that needs to be removed is inserted into a special specimen bag and pulled through one of the incisions that has been enlarged just enough to pull the diseased tissue out. The colectomy is the same, but the patient is left with three to four small incisions and possibly one larger incision several inches long rather than one eight- to twelve-inch incision.

Applying this technique to colorectal cancer surgery is fairly new (less than 15 years old). The National Comprehensive Cancer Network (NCCN) guidelines have recently been updated to include laparoscopic colectomy as another option because clinical trials have shown that laparoscopic colectomy is as effective as traditional abdominal colectomy in treating colorectal cancer.

Surgeons who perform colorectal laparoscopy say patients typically experience less pain and return to normal intestinal and overall physical activity more quickly after this type of operation, but not all studies have shown this to be the case. Laparoscopy has its downsides, too: the limited area of vision means the surgeon might miss something, the procedure usually takes longer, and it may be more expensive. And we don't have much evidence about the success of using laparoscopy to remove lymph nodes—an important part of many colorectal surgeries.

If you are considering this procedure, gather as much information as you can about the pros and cons of laparoscopy for colorectal cancer and ensure that your surgeon is very experienced, because there is a significant "learning curve" for laparoscopic colectomy. Minimally invasive surgery for colorectal cancer is an evolving field. Be sure to discuss this option with your surgeon if you are interested in it, as research in this area is ongoing.

Postoperative Recovery

Once the surgery is completed, the anesthesiologist will stop the anesthetic and remove the tube from your windpipe so you can breathe on your own. You will be moved to a recovery room for close monitoring for one to three hours. When you are more alert, you will be moved to a nursing station in the hospital to continue your recovery.

Patients typically stay in the hospital from three to eight days while they regain their bowel function and strength. By the time of discharge, you will be eating regular food and will be up and about. You will be having bowel movements and you are likely to experience some cramping and variability in bowel function. Gradually, over a month or two, your bowel function will return to a normal pattern. Convalescence and recovery at home takes several more weeks and you should plan to combine mild exercise such as walking with periods of rest. Most surgeons instruct you not do strenuous activity or heavy lifting for about six weeks after the operation (doing so increases the risk of developing a hernia or rupture in the wound).

> "I was very sore and in pain after the surgery and was put on a morphine drip for two and a half days. I was in the hospital for a total of six days. When I got home, I followed my doctors' orders and I began to gain strength: and in time I began to feel like my usual self. Every day I did a little more with the encouragement of my family. It took me approximately three months to be myself again."
>
> —EILEEN

Before your discharge from the hospital, your surgeon will tell you whether there were any unusual findings or problems that developed at the time of surgery that made a change in operative plan necessary. Your surgeon can tell you whether spread to other organs such as the liver was found and whether the operation was considered curative or palliative. The surgeon often provides you with an informal assessment of margins of clearance of the tumor, but he or she may wait for the final pathology report.

The pathologist will assess all of the removed tissue to determine the pathologic stage of the cancer (see chapter 5). The final pathology report will explain whether the resection was complete or incomplete using the numbers 0 to 2. This information should be shared with you so you understand your current situation and prognosis.

- Cancer resections are labeled as R0 if a complete resection of the cancer was done and if all margins are clear and there is no known residual cancer.
- An R1 resection means the cancer removal was incomplete because microscopic tumor was found at the margins even though all visible tumor was removed.
- An R2 resection is incomplete because margins are involved or visible tumor remains despite the resection.

Postoperative Treatments

You and your surgeon will discuss your treatment plan in light of the pathology report. Sometimes no other treatments are needed and the surgeon will move directly to developing a plan for long-term follow up (see chapter 18). For an R1 resection, your surgeon may decide to perform additional surgery to remove residual cancer, but this is rare. If chemotherapy or other treatments are advised, you will be referred to a medical oncologist or other appropriate specialist. These additional treatments will begin after you have recovered from the operation.

Your surgeon will give you more specific instructions and realistic expectations for your recovery based on knowledge of your particular situation. You will need to attend follow-up appointments with the surgeon to be sure your recovery goes smoothly.

Overview of Colon Surgery

Depending on the type and seriousness of your colon cancer, your doctor will recommend one of several different surgical options.

It is possible to surgically remove some very early colon cancers or cancerous polyps using a procedure called a polypectomy. Local excision is a procedure that removes superficial cancers and a small amount of nearby tissue. Polypectomy and local excision can often be done using a colonoscope and are not considered major surgery because the surgeon does not have to cut into the abdomen. (See chapter 3 for more detailed information on colonoscopy and removal of suspicious growths during this procedure.)

For more advanced colon cancers, your surgeon may perform an operation called a segmental resection or partial colectomy. During this type of surgery—the most common treatment for colorectal cancer—a length of normal tissue on either side of the cancer as well as the nearby lymph nodes are removed (resected). Then the remaining sections of the colon are attached back together (anastomosed). There are many different types of colectomies that can be performed, depending on the location and extent of the cancer. Segmental resection or partial colectomy is considered a major surgery.

> *"Surgery does bring some downtime for recovery and I'll wear my belly scars for life. It goes without saying that this is a small price to pay to be cancer-free."*
> —DICK

Sometimes, the removal of portions of the colon or the presence of a tumor in the colon blocking the flow of feces may require re-routing of the colon. This procedure, in which an opening is created between

Terminology of Colorectal Cancer Surgery

A complete glossary of colorectal cancer terms is featured at the back of this book. Here are some key terms you may encounter in this chapter.

Anastomosis: the technique used to reconnect the ends of intestine after removal of a segment containing a cancer.

Colectomy: an operation to resect a portion of the colon (large intestine).

Colon: large intestine consisting of the ascending colon (right segment), transverse colon (middle section), the descending colon (left segment) and the sigmoid colon (S-shaped segment just above the rectum).

Colostomy: an operation that brings the large intestine through a hole in the abdominal muscles and sews an open end of the colon to the abdominal skin so the body's wastes (feces and gas) can be eliminated into a special pouch.

Ileostomy: an operation that brings the ileum (last part of the small intestine) through a hole in the abdominal muscles and sews an open end of the ileum to the abdominal skin so the body's wastes (feces and gas) can be eliminated into a special pouch.

Laparoscopic surgery: a minimally invasive surgical approach performed through multiple small incisions using specially-designed surgical instruments and viewed through a laparoscope, or surgical telescope.

Local excision: an operation that removes superficial cancers and a small amount of nearby tissue without making a major abdominal incision.

Mesentery: the soft tissues that surround the intestine that house blood vessels and lymph nodes.

Polypectomy: surgical removal of a polyp. May be a piece-meal polypectomy or a snare polypectomy, depending on whether the polyp is pedunculated or sessile.

Proctectomy: an operation to remove the rectum.

Radical resection: a resection operation that also includes removal of the adjacent mesentery.

Resection: an operation in which a length of normal tissue on either side of the cancer is removed and then the remaining sections of the colon are joined back together (anastomosed).

the colon and the outside of the abdomen to allow for the elimination of feces outside the body, is called a colostomy. An ileostomy is an opening in the abdominal wall to allow the ileum (the part of the small intestine above the colon) to empty directly outside of the body. Both colostomies and ileostomies require the person to wear a collection pouch to trap stool and gas (see chapter 16 for more information on ostomies). We'll examine the variety of surgical procedures for colon cancer in greater detail in the next few sections.

Polypectomy and Local Excision

Cancer of the colon usually develops from a benign (noncancerous) polyp. Colon polyps grow in two shapes. Some polyps grow on stems or stalks (called pedicles), causing them to look like mushrooms. These are called pedunculated polyps. When they grow directly onto the inner wall of the colon—like spilled paint—they are called sessile polyps (see Figure 10.1 on page 160).

During a colonoscopy, if a doctor finds a growth, he or she will assess its location, size, extent of attachment to the wall of the colon (sessile or pedunculated), and its chance of being malignant. If the growth looks cancerous, the doctor will collect tissue samples (biopsies) so the pathologist can confirm the diagnosis.

If the growth looks like a noncancerous polyp, it is removed by a process called snare polypectomy. In a polypectomy, the doctor passes a wire through a chamber in the colonoscope and loops or snares the polyp. The polyp is removed with electrocautery, a surgical technique that uses electrical current to cauterize (burn) the tissues while it cuts to seal the blood vessels cut by the wire (see Figure 10.2 on page 161). The polyp is then retrieved by the doctor and sent to the pathologist for analysis.

If the pathologist finds that the polyp contains a cancer, the next step is to figure out how widespread the cancer is. If the cancer is confined to the mucosa (that is, if it is in situ or noninvasive cancer, also called stage "Tis") or if it is an invasive stage T1 cancer confined to the head, neck, or stalk of a pedunculated polyp and the margins are free, snare polypectomy alone is adequate. If the tumor is more widespread—if the margins are not clean or if the cancer extends into the submucosa—your doctor will probably recommend additional treatment.

If the growth appears to be a superficial mucosal cancer (Tis), a benign tumor such as a villous adenoma, or if the person with colon cancer has other medical problems that make the risk of undergoing major colon surgery excessive, the doctor may decide to remove a moderate-sized, sessile colon growth by doing a local excision of the area using a technique called piece-meal polypectomy. This technique involves repeatedly using a snare to cut into and remove the inner lining of the colon containing the tumor. The tumor is removed in pieces that are later

Figure 10.1 Pedunculated and Sessile Polyps

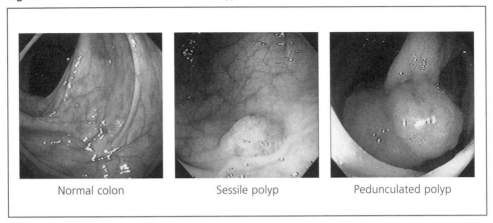

| Normal colon | Sessile polyp | Pedunculated polyp |

analyzed by the pathologist. This technique has some risks; it can cause bleeding or perforation, and it usually requires several follow-up colonoscopy sessions. It is not an ideal way to treat invasive cancers of the colon because only the lining of the colon is removed and no lymph nodes are sampled. But benign tumors and very early stage cancers can be cured by a local excision of the lining of the colon, and if the patient is medically fragile, the doctor may believe it would be less risky to remove the tumor in pieces than to subject the patient to an unnecessary major colon operation.

Major Surgery

Your doctor may determine that your cancer is too serious or widespread to treat with polypectomy or local excision. In this case, you will probably need to undergo major surgery. See page 162 for a list of questions to ask your doctor about surgery.

Colon cancer is almost always treated with major surgery and without any other preoperative treatment. (Other cancers, including rectal cancers, are sometimes treated with radiation or chemotherapy first, followed by surgery.) Colon cancer surgery is usually a scheduled, two- to four-hour elective procedure, although sometimes surgery is needed on an urgent or emergency basis (see page 169).

The standard elective operation performed for most colon cancers is a segmental resection or partial colectomy. This involves removal of a foot or more of the colon along with the adjacent mesentery (tissue that contains the blood vessels that nourish that segment of intestine as well as the lymph nodes that drain the area).

Figure 10.2 Snare Polypectomy of a Pedunculated Polyp

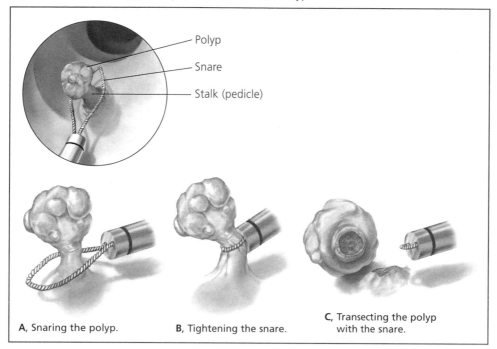

Polyp

Snare

Stalk (pedicle)

A, Snaring the polyp.   B, Tightening the snare.   C, Transecting the polyp with the snare.

The main view is of a polyp on the inner lining of the intestine, as seen through the colon. The polyp is about to be transected with a snare.

In special circumstances, the surgeon may do a more extensive colon removal, called subtotal or total colectomy.

In general, after any of the elective operations for colon cancer, the remaining ends of the intestine are connected by a process called an anastomosis (see Figure 10.3 on page 163). If an anastomosis is done, a permanent colostomy or ileostomy is unnecessary. However, on occasion, the surgeon will perform a temporary ileostomy upstream from the anastomosis to let it heal before allowing the colon to return to functioning normally.

Radical Resections

Recall that the colon is about six feet long and takes the general shape of an upside-down U. Each of the different parts of the colon has a specific name; these parts are labeled in Figure 10.4 on page 164.

You may wonder why surgeons remove so much tissue when the typical colon tumor is less than three to five inches in size. Surgeons do this to remove segments

Questions to Ask Your Medical Team About Surgery

- What did the biopsy show? Is that what you expected?
- What is the stage of my disease? Is there any spread to other sites? How confident are you that the stage is accurate?
- What is the name of the operation you are planning for me? Can you show me a drawing with the location of my cancer and indicate the part of the intestine you are planning to remove?
- After you remove the tumor, can the colon be reconnected or will a colostomy or ileostomy be necessary? If so, is it permanent or can it be reversed?
- Is the surgery likely to cure me of my cancer?
- Will surgery be combined with other treatments such as radiation or chemotherapy?
- Is there a reasonable alternative for me to consider? What about local treatments?
- What is my risk of dying or having major complications?
- Will the operation affect my bowel function? Urinary function? Sexual function?
- How many operations for this type of cancer have you performed? How many do you perform each year? Will you have assistance?
- Will you follow my condition after the surgery or does someone else do that?
- Should I get a second opinion?

of tissue where the tumor may have begun to spread microscopically in the lymphatic and blood vessels that run through the wall of the intestine and then into the nearby mesentery. To remove this potential spread, surgeons cut the tissues and divide the blood vessels some distance from the obvious cancer. The exact length of colon that is removed on either side of the cancer is determined primarily by the blood supply of the colon. When the main blood vessels feeding a segment of colon are divided near their origin, the blood supply to a whole length of colon

Figure 10.3 Colon Anastomosis

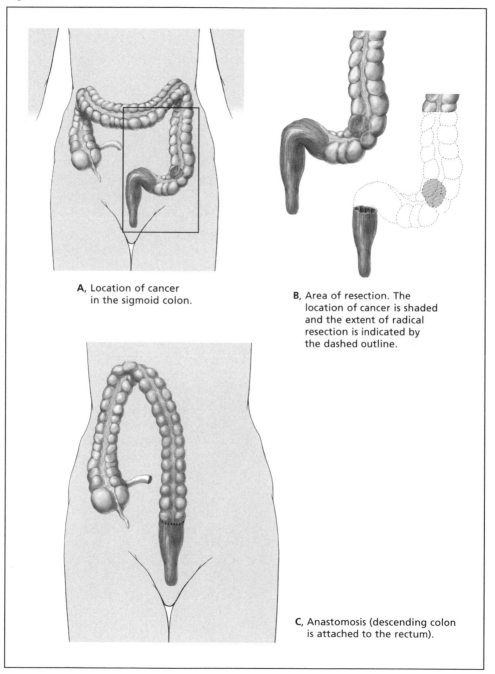

A, Location of cancer in the sigmoid colon.

B, Area of resection. The location of cancer is shaded and the extent of radical resection is indicated by the dashed outline.

C, Anastomosis (descending colon is attached to the rectum).

Figure 10.4 Parts of the Colon and Rectum

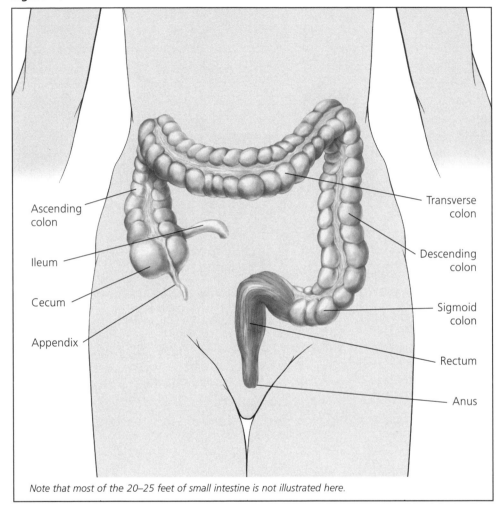

Ascending colon

Ileum

Cecum

Appendix

Transverse colon

Descending colon

Sigmoid colon

Rectum

Anus

Note that most of the 20–25 feet of small intestine is not illustrated here.

is interrupted and that segment will die. It must be resected (an operation in which a length of normal tissue on either side of the cancer is removed, and then the remaining sections of the colon are joined back together).

The practice of removing an appropriately long segment of the colon and the adjacent mesentery is called a "radical" resection and is the usual treatment for colorectal cancer. The term "radical" means that the surgeon removes not only the cancer but also a length of bowel above and below the tumor after dividing the feeding vessels near their origin from the aorta and the adjacent mesentery that contains those vessels and the draining lymph nodes.

Figure 10.5 Types of Colectomy

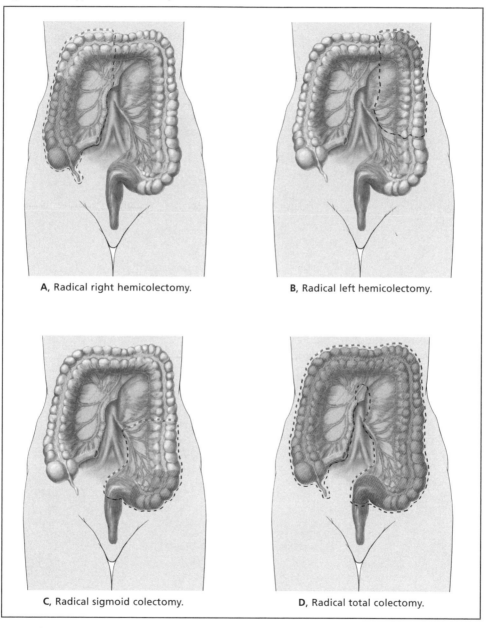

A, Radical right hemicolectomy.

B, Radical left hemicolectomy.

C, Radical sigmoid colectomy.

D, Radical total colectomy.

Types of colectomy are shown (area of the cancer is shaded; the extent of radical resection of the adjacent mesentery is indicated by the dashed line).

Table 10.1 Summary of Types of Colectomy

Procedure Name	Location(s) of Cancer the Procedure Is Used to Treat	Parts of the Colon Removed (associated mesentery also removed)	Name of the Anastomosis	Anastomosis Connects the Following Parts	Notes
Radical right hemicolectomy	Cecum or ascending colon	Right half of colon	Ileocolostomy or ileocolic anastomosis	Ileum to mid-transverse colon	*Shown in Figure 10.5A*
Extended radical right hemicolectomy	Hepatic flexure or right transverse colon	Right half of colon plus left side of transverse colon, including left branch of middle colic artery	Ileocolostomy or ileocolic anastomosis	Ileum to left transverse colon	Similar to radical right hemicolectomy
Transverse colectomy	Middle portion of the transverse colon	Middle portion of transverse colon	Colocolostomy or colocolic anastomosis	Hepatic flexure to splenic flexure	Extended right, extended left, or subtotal colectomy generally preferred over this procedure
Radical left colectomy	Splenic flexure and descending colon	Left half of transverse colon and descending colon	Colocolostomy or colocolic anastomosis	Middle portion of the transverse colon to sigmoid colon	*Shown in Figure 10.5B*
Extended radical left colectomy	Left transverse colon	Left half of colon plus right side of transverse colon, including right branch of middle colic artery	Colocolostomy or colocolic anastomosis	Right transverse colon to descending or sigmoid colon	Similar to radical left colectomy
Radical sigmoid colectomy	Sigmoid	Sigmoid colon	Colorectal anastomosis	Descending colon to upper rectum	*Shown in Figure 10.5C*
Radical subtotal colectomy	Multiple locations of cancer or polyps throughout colon	Right, transverse, descending plus or minus a portion of sigmoid colon	Ileosigmoidostomy or ileosigmoid anastomosis	Ileum to sigmoid	Similar to total colectomy
Radical total colectomy	Multiple locations of cancer, polyps throughout colon, or hereditary nonpolyposis colon cancer (HNPCC)	Entire colon: right, transverse, descending, and sigmoid colon	Ileorectal anastomosis	Ileum to rectum	*Shown in Figure 10.5D*; similar to subtotal colectomy

The term "segmental" or "partial" means that a portion or segment of the intestine is removed. This is in contrast to a "total" or "subtotal" colectomy, in which most or all of it is removed.

Several types of radical segmental colon resections are commonly performed (see Figure 10.5 A–D on page 165), and a summary of all of these colectomy procedures can be found in Table 10.1. Each procedure is described in detail in the sections that follow.

The location of your cancer in the colon determines the type that is appropriate for you. The extent of removed tissue (shown by the dotted lines in the drawings) may vary slightly depending on where your cancer is located and other factors.

Radical Right Hemicolectomy

Radical right hemicolectomy (see Figure 10.5A on page 165) is used for cancers in the cecum or ascending colon (parts of the colon in the right half of the abdomen) and removes the right half ("hemi" means half) of the colon. After the colectomy, the last part of the small intestine (ileum) and the mid-transverse colon are connected in an anastomosis procedure. This is sometimes called an ileocolostomy or ileocolic anastomosis.

Extended Radical Right Hemicolectomy

The extended radical right hemicolectomy operation is often used for cancers in the hepatic flexure or right transverse colon. It is similar to the radical right hemicolectomy but is considered "extended" because it extends across to the left side of the transverse colon by dividing the left branch of the middle colic artery and resecting the associated additional mesentery. The anastomosis connects the ileum and the left transverse colon.

Transverse Colectomy

A transverse colectomy is occasionally used to treat a cancer growing in the middle portion of the transverse colon. After removing the cancer and the adjacent mesentery, the surgeon must free up both the hepatic and splenic flexures (the two "corners" of the colon) to bring the two ends of the colon together for an anastomosis. Most surgeons prefer an extended right, an extended left, or a subtotal colectomy for a cancer in the middle transverse colon.

Radical Left Colectomy

Cancers of the splenic flexure and descending colon are often treated by removal of the left half of the transverse colon and the descending colon, which is called a radical left colectomy (see Figure 10.5B on page 165). In this case, the anastomosis is between the middle portion of the transverse colon and the sigmoid colon. This is called a colocolostomy or a colocolic anastomosis.

Extended Radical Left Colectomy

An extended radical left colectomy may be used for cancers in the left transverse colon. This procedure extends the left colectomy to the right side of the transverse colon by dividing the right branch of the middle colic artery. The anastomosis connects the right transverse colon with the descending or sigmoid colon.

Radical Sigmoid Colectomy

Cancers in the sigmoid may be treated by a segmental resection of the sigmoid colon, called a radical sigmoid colectomy (see Figure 10.5C on page 165). Depending on the location of the tumor, the resection may include a portion of the descending colon or a portion of the upper rectum. The anastomosis is between the descending colon and the rectum. This is called a colocolostomy or colorectal anastomosis.

Radical Subtotal Colectomy

The procedure known as a radical subtotal colectomy involves removal of the right, transverse, and descending colon segments with the adjacent mesentery. This may be done if more than one cancer is present in different parts of the colon or if there are multiple polyps in other parts of the colon in addition to the colon cancer. The anastomosis is between the ileum and the sigmoid colon, called an ileosigmoidostomy or ileosigmoid anastomosis.

Radical Total Colectomy

A radical total colectomy (see Figure 10.5D on page 165) may be chosen instead of a radical subtotal colectomy if the person with colon cancer has a family history of certain inherited colorectal cancer syndromes (see chapter 2). Because the risk of developing additional cancers in the remaining colon is very high with HNPCC, the surgeon will remove the entire colon rather than just resecting the segment containing the cancer. This procedure is similar to the subtotal colectomy but also removes the sigmoid and its mesentery. The anastomosis between the ileum and the rectum is called an ileorectal anastomosis.

When Emergency and Urgent Colon Cancer Surgery May Be Needed

Although the vast majority of colon cancer operations are elective, surgery is occasionally needed on an emergency basis because of: complete blockage of the colon from the cancer; major infection and peritonitis (inflammation of the lining of the abdomen) caused by leakage of feces from a perforation caused by the cancer; or life-threatening bleeding resulting from the cancer eroding into a blood vessel. In such cases, the patient is usually so ill that evaluation in an emergency room is necessary. After the patient is stabilized with intravenous fluids, antibiotics, and blood if needed, the doctor will make a prompt diagnosis and undertake emergency surgery.

Staging an Operation

Emergency operations are always more risky than elective operations because the patient has not had a full medical assessment, preoperative staging of the cancer is incomplete, the bowel is not fully cleansed, and the person undergoing treatment has had no time to consider options. Not surprisingly, the surgical options for emergency colon surgery are more limited than for elective surgery. In many cases, what would have been done in one elective operation can only be done in two or sometimes three operations undertaken because of an emergency. This series of multiple surgeries is called staging an operation.

Fortunately, emergency surgery for colon cancer is rarely necessary. It is often possible to convert what seems like an emergency situation to one in which an urgent or even semielective operation can be done. In this way, staged operations can often be avoided. The surgeon will try to do this whenever possible.

Emergency and Urgent Surgical Procedures

Colon cancer can cause obstruction of the intestine, but often it is only a partial blockage. If so, the person with cancer may be hospitalized and fed with intravenous fluids while the bowel is decompressed with a suction tube in the stomach to remove secretions. Enemas or gentle laxatives may be given to cleanse the colon and slowly relieve the obstruction. Otherwise, the surgeon or a radiologist may place a stent into the colon at the site of narrowing from the cancer. (A stent is a device implanted in a body part to support its structure and help keep it open.)

This may relieve the obstruction so a full bowel cleansing can be done and the patient can be fully prepared for an urgent operation a few days later. This is another way the surgeon can avoid a staged operation.

To relieve a complete obstruction requiring emergency surgery, the surgeon has several options. A radical resection of the cancer is performed to try to cure the cancer whenever it can be done safely. On the other hand, if the cancer is extensive and it appears that it cannot be safely removed with clear margins, the surgeon may decide to perform a palliative "bypass" around the cancer. In this circumstance, the intestine upstream from the area of blockage caused by the unresectable cancer is connected to the bowel downstream from the colon cancer. A third option is to do a temporary colostomy or ileostomy upstream from the cancer. This is done by bringing a cut end of the intestine through a hole made in the abdominal wall and sewing the edge of the cut intestine to the skin. The patient then wears a pouch over the intestinal opening to collect feces and gas (see chapter 16). The cancer is left undisturbed until it can be resected during a later elective operation. This option is especially useful if the patient is unstable or the surgeon is uncomfortable proceeding with a major colon cancer resection in an emergency situation.

To control bleeding or infection caused by a perforation from a cancer, the surgeon often has to resect the cancer. If the surgery was done in an emergency, there was probably no time to do a bowel cleansing, so the colon may be filled with feces and distended with air. In addition, there may be extensive peritonitis and the patient's condition may be too fragile to go ahead with additional procedures. In such circumstances, it is not safe to do an anastomosis. Instead, the surgeon will make a temporary colostomy or ileostomy. The anastomosis will be performed at an elective operation after the patient has fully recovered from the emergency surgery.

The Process of Elective Radical Proctectomy

In the next few sections, we'll talk about what to expect when you choose to undergo elective radical proctectomy and how surgery on the rectum differs from colon surgery. Then we'll discuss some specific types of surgical procedures used to treat rectal cancer.

Preparing for Surgery

Before deciding to go ahead with any surgical procedure, you should speak with your medical team about possible complications and side effects—for example, patients with rectal cancer should be aware that a temporary or permanent colostomy may be necessary, and that damage to the nerves during certain types of rectal surgery may result in erectile dysfunction (impotence).

If it is likely that you will need a permanent or temporary colostomy (formed between the skin of your abdomen and your large bowel) or ileostomy (formed between the skin and small intestine), you may meet with a wound, ostomy, and continent nurse (WOCN) or enterostomal therapy (ET) nurse a week or so before your surgery. The nurse will counsel and educate you and your loved ones about life with a stoma. (A stoma is the name for the opening that is created during surgery between the skin's surface and an organ.) The nurse will usually mark your abdomen for the best location for the stoma. (See chapter 16 for more information.)

The preparation for elective major surgery for rectal cancer (radical proctectomy) is very similar to that described earlier in this chapter for elective radical surgery for colon cancer. Bowel cleansing is done, antibiotics are given, and, you will probably be admitted to the hospital on the day of surgery. You will meet the anesthesiologist and other members of the team in the preoperative area.

During the Surgery

After you are given general anesthesia, you will be positioned on the operating table so that the surgical team has simultaneous access to your abdomen and perineum (area of the anus and genitals). This is helpful when a low anastomosis or a combined removal of the rectum is necessary.

Because of the proximity of the rectum to the bladder and genitals, your surgeon may collaborate with a urologist—a doctor who specializes in diseases of the urinary tract and the male reproductive system—during your procedure. The urologist may place a stent in the ureters (the tubes that drain the urine from the kidneys to the bladder) to help the surgeon identify the ureters and avoid injury to them while removing the rectal cancer. The urologist inserts the stent by putting a lighted instrument called a cystoscope into the bladder and identifying the opening to the ureters while you are under anesthesia. This can be very helpful if the tumor is large and bulky or if there is a lot of inflammation present in the area of the cancer, which can make identification of the ureters difficult. A bladder catheter is also inserted to allow monitoring of your urinary output.

The incision, examination of the abdomen, and confirmation or change in the operative treatment plan are similar to the process used for colon surgery. The steps in radical proctectomy are: mobilize or free the rectum from its attachments in the pelvis, divide the blood vessels near their origin from the aorta (the main blood vessel from the heart that takes blood to the body, including the major organs), divide the rectum below the cancer with free margins, and do an anastomosis if possible or a total removal of the rectum and anal canal with construction of a colostomy if necessary.

Postoperative Recovery

Initial recovery from resection of the rectum is similar to recovery after a colon resection. One difference is that you may have drains in your pelvis to collect fluid for a few days after the operation. (A drain is a tube often inserted after surgery to help remove any fluid—blood, pus, etc.—that may collect after the closure of the incision.)

If a permanent colostomy was constructed after the rectal cancer was removed, you will have an incision in the perineum where the anus was removed in addition to the main abdominal incision. Some of your recovery time will be spent learning how to change the pouch and adjusting to the colostomy. Bowel function may not return as quickly or be as predictable after radical proctectomy and a low anastomosis as after colon resection. Your medications and diet may need to be altered to improve function. Your doctor will advise you about what to expect and how to manage any problems that arise.

Postoperative Treatments

Depending on the final pathologic stage (how extensive your cancer was found to be), additional therapy may be needed after your recovery from radical proctectomy. This may involve radiation to the pelvis, chemotherapy, or both. Your doctor will explain the purpose of the treatments and their potential side effects. (See chapters 11 and 12 for more information.)

You will also need to schedule periodic check-ups with your doctor to ensure a smooth recovery.

Overview of Rectal Surgery

The primary goal of surgery for the person with rectal cancer is cure. Other very important considerations include maintaining or restoring bowel, sexual, and urinary functions with a minimum number of complications.

Many rectal cancer treatments are currently available, spanning the spectrum from simple polypectomy to more complex resections. Many rectal cancer treatments involve radical surgery, radiation, and chemotherapy. This combination of treatments is called a multimodal approach.

Choosing the best treatment for rectal cancer is a complex process requiring the expertise of doctors from different disciplines. Even the most experienced surgeon requires other experts' input and technical expertise when treating rectal cancers.

The surgical management of rectal cancers differs from that of colon cancer in several important ways. Some rectal cancers are uniquely suited to treatment by local therapies because of their location in the last six inches of the large intestine. In these cases, rather than using a major incision in the abdomen to get at the rectal cancer, surgeons can gain access for treatment by working through the anus. Unfortunately, most rectal cancers are not suited to local approaches, so the surgeon performs a radical resection following the principles outlined earlier in this chapter. The resection of rectal cancer is considerably more challenging to the surgeon than radical resection of colon cancer.

One reason why is that the rectum is located deep in the pelvis, making it difficult to access. For the surgeon, reaching the pelvis is like working from a distance to remove an object firmly attached inside a small, rigid box. The adjacent mesentery containing the blood vessels that nourish the rectum and the lymph nodes draining the rectum must also be removed along with the rectal cancer. A second problem faced by the surgeon is that the pelvis is filled with other important structures, including major blood vessels to the legs; other organs, including the bladder, the vagina and uterus in women, and the prostate and seminal vesicles in men; as well as the nerves that control sexual and urinary functions. A third challenge is conducting radical resection of the rectal cancer in a way that provides the patient with good bowel function after the procedure is completed.

After radical resection of colon cancer, the connection of the two ends of the bowel (anastomosis) is relatively straightforward and ensures that bowel function will be close to normal. The same is true for rectal cancers located in the upper third of the rectum. However, this is not the case after radical resection of lower rectal cancers. In some cases of very low rectal cancer near the anus, there is no possibility of performing an anastomosis because the entire area—including the anal sphincter muscles—must be removed to cure the cancer. In such cases, a permanent colostomy is necessary.

In some cases, radical surgery is combined with radiation and chemotherapy treatments to shrink the tumor, thus making its removal less difficult and increasing the possibility of doing an anastomosis. In other cases, the surgeon can perform a radical resection of a low rectal cancer and leave a short stump of the lower rectum for an anastomosis. Doing a bowel connection deep in the pelvis is technically challenging, but new stapling devices have made this more manageable.

Even if the surgeon connects the bowel successfully, the resulting bowel function after low anastomoses may not be normal. Patients may experience a frequent and urgent need to evacuate stool and may even leak stool and gas. Fortunately, very poor function occurs in a minority of patients, and surgeons have developed new techniques to overcome many of these functional problems.

A final, important difference between colon and rectal cancer surgery is that the risk of recurrence of the cancer at the site of the surgery is much higher after surgery for rectal cancer than after colon cancer. To address this challenge, surgeons often combine radical surgery with radiation and chemotherapy treatments to decrease the risk of recurrence of rectal cancer.

Polypectomy

Rectal cancers usually develop from benign polyps growing from the lining of the rectal wall (mucosa). Snare polypectomy (see page 159) of a rectal polyp is most often done during colonoscopy examination of the entire colon with the assumption that the rectal polyp is benign. If the doctor is at all suspicious of cancer in a rectal polyp, the polypectomy site is marked and the precise level of the lesion is recorded.

Large polyps of the rectum that cannot be easily removed in one piece by snare polypectomy are generally best removed by a local excision as described below rather than using a piecemeal endoscopic snare excision technique (see page 159). This helps the pathologist identify the stage of the tumor.

Snare polypectomy alone is adequate to treat cancer in a rectal polyp if the growth is confined to the mucosa (Tis, in situ, or noninvasive cancer) or if the invasive cancer is confined to the head, neck, or stalk of a pedunculated polyp and the margins are free. If the margins are not clear or if the cancer extends into the submucosa of a polyp, additional anticancer treatment—such as transanal excision of the rectal wall, use of radiation and chemotherapy, or radical resection—will be necessary.

Local Therapies

The benefits of using local procedures to treat rectal cancer include minimal complications, preservation of bowel, bladder, and sexual function, and faster postoperative recovery.

In some cases, local therapy is the only alternative to permanent colostomy. The major risk of local procedures is that they put the person with rectal cancer at high risk of cancer recurrence.

Local therapy intended to fully cure the cancer may be used for treatment of rectal tumors that do not invade the anal sphincter (the ring of muscle that contracts to close the anus) and are confined to the rectal wall, providing they are small enough to be totally removed. If there is any spread to local lymph nodes or to distant organs, local therapy is ruled out.

Local therapy is also used as a compromise treatment for people with colorectal cancer in poor overall health who might not tolerate a radical procedure, or those who refuse a radical resection because of the potential for a permanent colostomy. Local therapy may be used along with chemoradiation (a treatment that combines chemotherapy with radiation treatments; this combination makes radiation more effective). In select cases, local therapy may be used as a palliative measure when the rectal cancer is incurable.

Local therapy procedures used to treat rectal cancer include excision, fulguration, and endocavitary radiation.

- Excision is the surgical removal of a rectal tumor.
- Fulguration uses a controlled electric current to destroy a rectal tumor.
- Endocavitary radiation therapy is a special technique that delivers radiation directly to a rectal cancer by using a radiation source that is passed through a special proctoscope inserted into the rectum through the anus. Because endocavitary radiation is aimed directly onto the rectal cancer, radiation does not pass through the skin and other tissues of the abdomen and only penetrates the rectal tissues for an inch or two. Complications are thus minimized.

These different local therapies provide varying amounts of information about the cancer that is present in the rectum. For example, excision techniques allow the pathologist to gather diagnostic information about the T stage, whereas endocavitary radiation and fulguration do not. This is because a local excision provides tissue for the pathologist to assess how widespread the cancer is, and thus to confirm or change the preoperative T stage. However, endocavitary radiation and fulguration destroy the cancerous tissue as part of the anticancer treatment, so no tissue is available to biopsy for the pathologist.

None of the local therapy techniques include removal of the lymph nodes, so it is impossible for the pathologist to provide information about the N stage (a measure of lymph node involvement) of the cancer in any of these circumstances.

Local Excision

The goal of local excision procedures is to resect a rectal cancer by cutting out a disc of the rectal wall containing both the primary rectal cancer and a clear margin of tissue. Local excision of rectal cancers is performed using one of two approaches: a transanal approach, in which the surgeon works through the anus without a skin incision, or a posterior approach, in which a skin incision is made in the low back area. If this incision is made next to the tailbone and sacrum (the area of the spine that consists of five fused vertebrae that is part of the pelvis) it is called a trans-sacral incision; if it is made through the anal sphincter, it is called a trans-sphincteric incision. Today, these posterior approaches are rarely necessary.

Figure 10.6 Transanal Excision of a Rectal Cancer

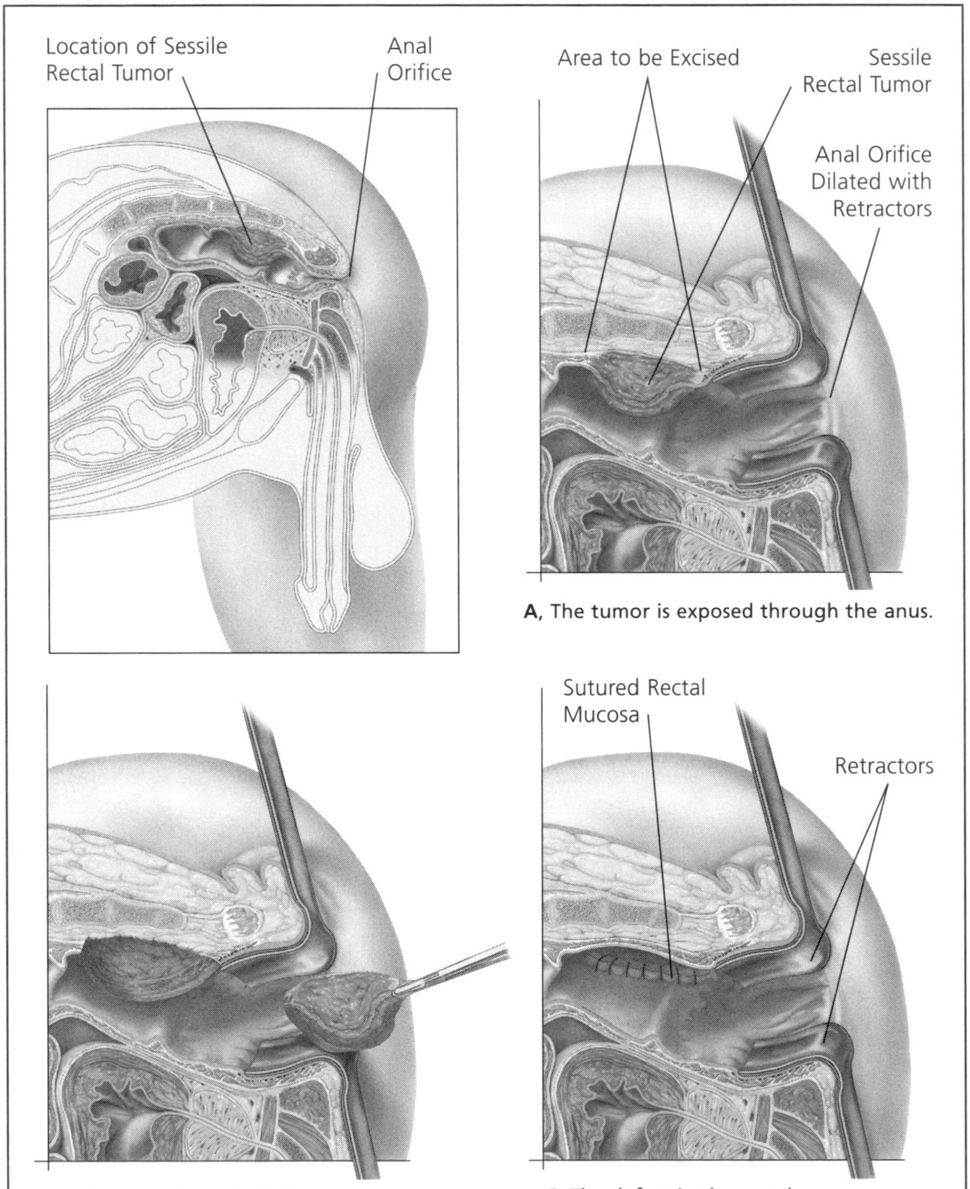

Location of Sessile Rectal Tumor

Anal Orifice

Area to be Excised

Sessile Rectal Tumor

Anal Orifice Dilated with Retractors

A, The tumor is exposed through the anus.

Sutured Rectal Mucosa

Retractors

B, The tumor is excised along with a disc of normal tissue.

C, The defect in the rectal wall is closed with sutures.

These are views of the right half of the body, as though we are seeing a front-to-back cross section. The shading in the main view indicates the area shown in illustrations A–C. Retractors hold back tissue so the surgeon has a clear view of the tumor and surrounding area.

With a transanal excision, the surgeon typically uses special retractors in the anus to provide a direct view of the cancer (see Figure 10.6). After cutting out the cancer, the surgeon closes the hole in the rectal wall. This technique is useful for small cancers located in the lower half of the rectum.

An alternative approach is called transanal endoscopic microsurgery (TEM). TEM is a specialized technique used in the local treatment of sessile polyps and T1 cancers of the middle to upper third of the rectum that lend themselves to this type of treatment. It requires special instruments and it is currently available at only a few cancer centers.

Endocavitary Radiation/Papillon Technique

Radiation to treat cancer is often delivered from a source located outside the body. Endocavitary radiation, also known as the Papillon technique, is different in that it delivers radiation delivered through a specially designed instrument called a proctoscope that is inserted into the rectum. This treatment works best on small growths located within a few inches of the anal verge (the junction between anal canal and anal skin) that do not extend around the entire circumference of the anus.

Endocavitary radiation has the distinct advantage of being an outpatient procedure done using local anesthesia with sedation. It is usually given over the course of two months. It requires special equipment and expertise; as a result, it is not widely available. (See chapter 11 for more information on using radiation to treat colorectal cancer.)

Fulguration/Electrocoagulation

Fulguration, also known as electrocoagulation, destroys a cancer by burning it with an electrode inserted into the tumor. The controlled electric current is applied and the buildup is scraped away until the cancer has been ablated (burned up) and only a margin of normal tissue remains.

Potential disadvantages of fulguration include postoperative fever, a need for repeated procedures, and the need, in a large number of patients, to convert to more radical procedures. As noted above, ablation also destroys any tissue that could have been used by a pathologist to provide staging information.

Fulguration is primarily used today to ease the discomfort of patients with bulky bleeding rectal cancers who are too ill for radical resection.

(continued on page 180)

Figure 10.7 Anterior Resection With Anastomosis

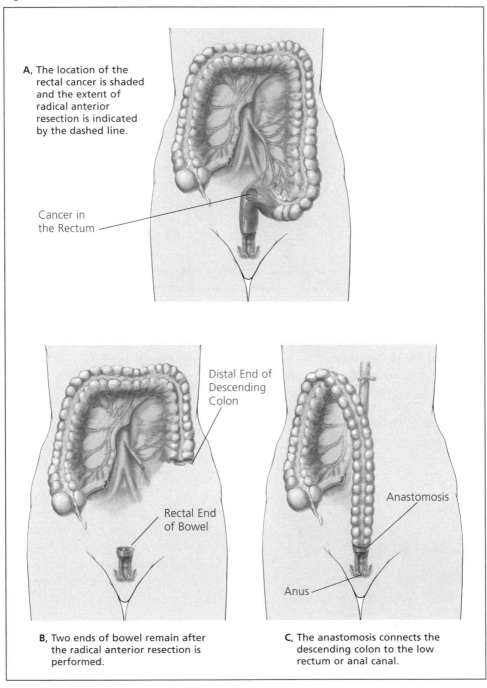

A, The location of the rectal cancer is shaded and the extent of radical anterior resection is indicated by the dashed line.

Cancer in the Rectum

Distal End of Descending Colon

Rectal End of Bowel

Anastomosis

Anus

B, Two ends of bowel remain after the radical anterior resection is performed.

C, The anastomosis connects the descending colon to the low rectum or anal canal.

Figure 10.8 Abdominoperineal Resection With Permanent Colostomy

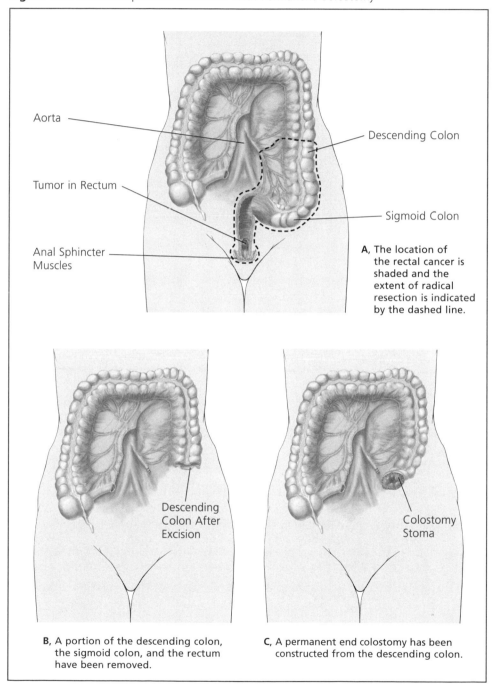

Aorta

Tumor in Rectum

Anal Sphincter Muscles

Descending Colon

Sigmoid Colon

A, The location of the rectal cancer is shaded and the extent of radical resection is indicated by the dashed line.

Descending Colon After Excision

Colostomy Stoma

B, A portion of the descending colon, the sigmoid colon, and the rectum have been removed.

C, A permanent end colostomy has been constructed from the descending colon.

Major Surgery

Most cancers of the rectum are removed through radical proctectomy. Radical surgery is a better choice than local procedures for cancers that have penetrated the wall of the rectum or that have spread to the lymph nodes.

The primary goal of radical resection is to remove the rectal cancer and adjacent mesentery with clear margins. A secondary goal is to preserve bowel function and do an anastomosis if feasible and safe. However, curing the rectal cancer is most important. Surgeons are usually able to preserve anal sphincter function unless the cancer is located very low in the rectum. If clinical staging shows the rectal cancer to be an advanced but potentially curable tumor, your doctor may suggest six weeks of radiation and chemotherapy before surgery. The radical proctectomy will be done four to twelve weeks later.

See page 162 for questions to ask your doctor about surgery.

Anterior Resection With Anastomosis

In an anterior resection with anastomosis procedure (see Figure 10.7 on page 178), the surgeon does a radical "sphincter-sparing" proctectomy. The sigmoid colon, rectum, and the associated mesentery are resected to a point at least one to three inches below the rectal cancer. After the proctectomy, the surgeon does an anastomosis between the colon and the stump of the rectum that may be hand-sewn or surgically stapled. Modern surgical stapling instruments make low anastomoses safer and more reliable.

Abdominoperineal Resection With Permanent Colostomy

In an abdominoperineal resection with permanent colostomy (see Figure 10.8 on page 179), the surgeon performs a "sphincter-sacrificing" proctectomy by removing a portion or all of the sigmoid colon, the entire rectum, the adjacent mesentery, and the anus. A permanent colostomy is constructed and the patient wears a pouch to collect stool and gas from the colon (see chapter 16).

Anterior Resection With Low Anastomosis and Temporary Proximal Diversion

Sometimes the surgeon is able to do a sphincter-sparing proctectomy (anterior resection) with a very low anastomosis deep in the pelvis but is concerned that the connection may not heal properly and that feces could leak from the anastomosis. In such cases, the surgeon may decide to do a temporary colostomy or ileostomy upstream from the low anastomosis. This temporary proximal diversion will temporarily divert feces into an ostomy pouch and prevent stool from going through the new connection. Once the anastomosis is totally healed after six to 12 weeks, a second operation is done to reverse the temporary colostomy or ileostomy. This staged approach is often used after especially low anastomoses and after pelvic radiation.

Extended Resections and Exenteration

Some patients have a rectal tumor that is invading nearby organs such as the bladder or the female reproductive organs or into nearby pelvic bone such as the sacrum. In general, the surgeon will still try to do a curative operation by removing all involved areas together. These extended operations may combine the removal of the tissues resected during an anterior or abdominoperineal resection with removal of the reproductive organs, bladder, or both by an operation called a pelvic exenteration. If necessary, the lower sacral vertebrae (the bones around the spinal cord at the base of the spine) can also be removed by an operation called a sacrectomy.

Adjuvant and Neoadjuvant Therapy

Although surgery is usually the primary treatment for colorectal cancer, sometimes doctors combine surgery with other treatments. These other treatments, such as radiation (discussed in chapter 11) and chemotherapy (discussed in chapter 12) are called adjuvant therapies. Adjuvant treatments can destroy cancerous cells left behind during an operation, delay the recurrence of cancer, and increase the chance that the primary treatment will result in a cure.

Adjuvant therapy given before the primary treatment (for example, radiation therapy to shrink a tumor before surgery) is called neoadjuvant therapy.

Surgery alone is usually all that is required to treat stage I cancer or stage II cancer with a low risk of local recurrence. People who have more advanced colorectal cancers—high-risk stage II, stage III (spread to lymph nodes), or stage IV (distant metastasis)—will probably be given neoadjuvant or adjuvant therapies.

Surgery for Metastatic Colorectal Cancer

Both colon and rectal cancer can metastasize (spread) to the liver, lungs, and other parts of the body. While no one wants to hear that cancer has spread, metastasis does not always mean that cure is not possible. Surgery to remove the metastasis is still the best hope for long-term cure and is possible in some patients.

Depending on the location of the metastasis, radiation with chemotherapy may be given before colorectal surgery to shrink the tumor and make it easier for the surgeon to remove the cancerous growth with clear margins.

Your doctor may discover metastases during the preoperative staging work-up or during follow up after the initial treatment (see chapter 18). When cancer spread is found before initial treatment, the surgeon will consider whether the metastasis can be removed during the same operation needed to remove the primary colorectal cancer. For example, a patient with a right colon cancer who also has a single metastasis to the liver may benefit from having both areas removed during the same operation. In some cases, though, this combined operation might be considered too stressful or dangerous for the patient, and a second surgery can be scheduled to deal with the metastasis.

If cancer has spread to an area outside the abdominal cavity—such as a single metastasis to the lung—the surgeon generally removes the colorectal primary tumor and allows the patient to recover for several months before a chest surgeon removes the lung metastasis. When surgery for metastasis is done in a separate operation, the diagnostic work-up is usually repeated to be sure additional metastases have not developed in the meantime. If the work-up shows that curative treatment is still possible, resection of the metastasis can move forward.

When doctors take a surgical approach to treating metastases, they consider several factors: the location of the metastases, their size, and their number. If a patient has a single metastasis, it is often possible to remove that spot surgically. If the surgery can be done with clear margins, the chances of long-term survival are approximately 30 percent. If there are several areas of metastases or if a single metastasis is very large, surgery may not be possible or useful.

As noted, sometimes the surgeon will combine techniques to control the cancer. For instance, a patient with multiple liver metastases may be treated by resecting the segment of liver that has most of the metastases, while other treatments are used to destroy the remaining spots of tumor. Most patients undergoing removal of a colorectal metastasis will also receive postoperative chemotherapy to prevent other metastases from developing.

If the cancer cannot be cured, chemotherapy in combination with radiation, surgical techniques, or both can be used to control the disease for many months or years. This type of palliative treatment has improved a great deal in recent years, and many patients now live comfortable and productive lives for a significant time even though their colorectal cancer has spread beyond the health care team's ability to cure it.

CHAPTER ELEVEN

RADIATION THERAPY

Christopher Crane, MD

For some people, radiation conjures up images of glow-in-the-dark swamp creatures from science fiction movies. But radiation is simply electromagnetic energy that is transmitted in the form of rays, waves, or particles. X-rays, ultraviolet light, visible light, near-infrared light, and heat (thermal) radiation are all different wavelengths of electromagnetic energy.

Radiation therapy is the medical use of this energy to treat diseases. Radiation therapy to treat cancer uses the same kind of X-rays that doctors commonly use to diagnose a broken bone or dentists use to take pictures of your teeth, but the X-rays used to treat cancer are more energetic and are delivered in higher doses. Special equipment is used during radiation therapy to deliver these high doses of radiation to cancerous cells, killing or damaging them so they cannot grow, multiply, or spread. In this chapter, we'll talk about how radiation therapy is used to treat colorectal cancer.

How Is External Beam Radiation Delivered?

When we talk about radiation therapy for colorectal cancer, we generally mean external beam radiation. This is the most common type of radiation therapy and involves delivering radiation from a source outside of the body to a precise location inside the body. There are also other delivery systems, which work differently and are used much less widely.

Before a patient can begin radiation treatment, the treatment must be planned or simulated using computer technology. During simulation, patients may be asked to drink contrast agents so that the doctor can visualize the intestine effectively. A metallic marker may also be placed on the anus as well so the radiation fields can be visualized and pointed away from the anal area to avoid painful skin reactions.

> *"I had rather a good time at radiation. Since the same people came at the same time five days a week, we all got to know each other. We never talked about our illnesses; instead we laughed a lot and had a good time with the gowns given to us to wear. We soon went out and bought our own house-coats. Laughter and fun made life easier."*
>
> —LAURA

Rather than using a single beam of radiation, doctors usually use three or four beams. The site where the beams intersect—the location of the cancerous tissue—receives an even distribution of radiation that is higher in dose than the separate radiation beams that enter the patient's body. Doctors may also take measures to try to ensure that other organs are out of the path of the radiation beams to minimize damage to normal tissue.

Specialized Radiation Techniques for Colorectal Cancer

So far, we've been talking about external beam radiation—radiation therapy that is delivered to a location within the body from a point outside of it. But doctors have other methods of delivering radiation to treat cancer. Two of these methods—brachytherapy and intraoperative radiation therapy—are used to treat colorectal cancer.

Brachytherapy

Brachytherapy, also known as internal radiation, is another way to deliver radiation therapy. Instead of aiming radiation beams from outside the body, radioactive seeds or pellets are placed directly into the tissue next to the cancer. Brachytherapy has the advantage of precisely delivering high doses of radiation directly to a tumor.

Figure 11.1 External Beam Radiation

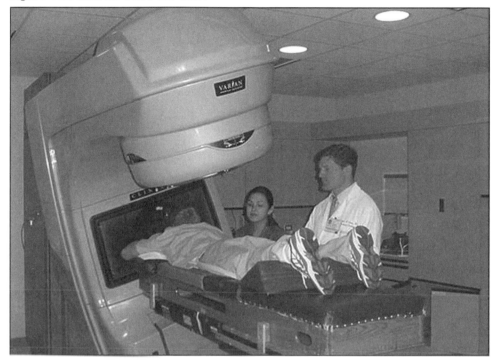

A typical external beam radiation treatment machine. This patient is being positioned for treatment of rectal cancer.

Source: Image courtesy of Andrew Lee.

Brachytherapy treatment has a very low risk of side effects but by itself does not usually treat all of the cells that are at risk. So, it is often used as a supplement after external beam radiation treatments.

Intraoperative Radiation Therapy

Either external beam radiation or brachytherapy can also be delivered during surgery. This is called intraoperative radiation therapy. After the tumor is removed, the normal organs can be moved and radiation can be delivered where the tumor grew to treat the cancer cells that the surgeon could not remove. This method of radiation delivery has a very low risk of side effects.

Who Delivers Radiation Therapy?

Many professionals participate in the treatment of people with colorectal cancer who receive radiation therapy. While the patient may only see the radiation therapist, nurse, and doctor, there are many others on the team who play important roles (such as developing the radiation plan, assuring quality, and actually delivering the treatment).

- The radiation oncologist is in charge of providing the information that a person uses to decide whether to receive radiation therapy. After discussion and collaboration with radiologists, pathologists, surgeons, and medical oncologists, the radiation oncologist decides which areas of the body need to be treated, and makes key decisions about the type, dose, and duration of therapy. The radiation oncologist does not administer the radiation treatment itself; that's done by the radiation therapist (see below). Therefore, during treatment, the patient will visit the radiation oncologist weekly to ensure the treatment is proceeding as planned and side effects are under control.
- Nurses who are knowledgeable about cancer care in general and radiation treatment in particular can educate people about side effects and help them navigate through the medical system of a cancer center.
- Radiation therapists run the radiation machines. They are trained to operate other types of X-ray equipment but specialize in the therapeutic application of radiation. Their role is to deliver the treatment exactly as the doctor planned.
- The dosimetrist creates radiation plans on a computer. Dosimetrists work with the doctor using specialized computer programs to create an exact representation of the best way to deliver a particular treatment plan for a particular person. They are also responsible for assuring the quality of the treatment that is given.
- Physicists who specialize in medical radiation delivery are also an integral part of the treatment team. Among other things, they calibrate the highly sophisticated radiation machines, check and double check the radiation output of the machines, and develop and maintain new equipment.

How Does Radiation Therapy Work?

Radiation in high doses kills cells or keeps them from growing and dividing. When this radiation deposits its energy in human tissue, the radiation causes chemical changes that destabilize DNA, the genetic material that directs a cell how to grow, reproduce, and die. Both normal and cancerous (malignant) cells are affected by radiation, but cancer cells divide more rapidly than most of the cells around them (making them especially susceptible to radiation). In addition, cancerous cells do not have the same ability as normal cells to repair DNA damage. Radiation oncologists take advantage of the fact that the normal tissues can heal better from radiation than the cancer can.

To protect normal cells, doctors carefully limit the doses of radiation and spread the treatment out over time. They also shield as much normal tissue as possible while they aim the radiation at the site of the cancer. (Damage to normal cells is one cause of radiation side effects; see page 189).

The dose of radiation that is prescribed depends on the goal of treatment and the organs surrounding the colon or rectum that need to be partially irradiated. To minimize damage to tissues, doctors deliver the lowest dose of radiation possible. However, this dose must still be high enough to effectively kill as many cancer cells as possible, because even when cancer is not visible on a CT scan or other imaging studies, it may still exist on a microscopic level. Because these small clusters of cancer cells are capable of growing into larger tumors and can spread to other parts of the body, the radiation dosage represents a delicate balance. The risk of tissue damage and side effects must be balanced with the possible advantage to the patient in terms of tumor control and cure.

Cancer that cannot be seen on a CT scan but still exists on the microscopic level can reliably be killed with five to six weeks of radiation treatments. Tumors that are large enough to be seen on a CT scan (larger than a half-inch) often need six to seven weeks of radiation to give the best chance for a positive outcome.

When Is Radiation Therapy Used?

Chapter 9 (pages 133–150) includes general information about the role of radiation therapy in treatment for colon and rectal cancers. As discussed, radiation therapy to treat colorectal cancer is most often given in combination with surgery, and sometimes also with chemotherapy as well. The reason that radiation alone cannot be used to treat most gastrointestinal cancers is that the surrounding organs cannot tolerate high doses of radiation without serious risk of complications.

Radiation therapy is a vital component of the treatment for many but not all people who have rectal cancer—especially those whose cancer has spread to their lymph nodes or those who are considered to have a high risk for cancer recurrence. In people with rectal cancer, radiation can also reduce the need for a colostomy.

Radiation therapy is given less often to people who have colon cancer, mostly in cases in which surgery alone is not likely to remove all of the cancer cells.

Why Radiation Is Used More Often for Rectal Cancer Than for Colon Cancer

Radiation often helps people with rectal cancer more than those who have colon cancer. This is because it is usually possible to surgically remove colon tumors without leaving many tumor cells behind. Surgeons can usually take out the growth itself as well as a comfortable margin of noncancerous tissue surrounding the tumor. There are no bones or structures in the abdominal cavity preventing the complete removal of the most common colon tumors.

Because of the anatomy of the affected areas, it is more difficult to completely remove a rectal tumor with surgery than a colon tumor. The difference is that the rectum—the last four inches of the large intestine—lies in the pelvis, which is a very confined space similar in shape to an ice cream cone. This space limitation makes it difficult for surgeons to maneuver. Because surgically removing rectal cancer is more of a challenge, doctors are more likely to combine surgery with radiation.

Radiation Therapy for Metastatic Cancer

Radiation therapy can also be used for palliation of the symptoms caused by the spread of cancer to bone or other tissues, such as the liver. Radiation can relieve pain, prevent obstruction, and stop bleeding by shrinking the tumors that are involving normal tissues.

Radiation and Surgery

When radiation therapy is used along with surgery, it is called an adjuvant therapy. (Adjuvant therapy is a "helper" therapy, a secondary treatment given to help boost the effectiveness of the primary treatment).

Radiation therapy is generally used to destroy tumor cells that might be left behind by the surgeon, regardless of how good the operation has been. The two treatment modalities can be combined to improve a patient's outcome, because radiation is most effective in destroying small volumes of tumor cells, while surgery does an excellent job of treating the bulk of the tumor (see chapter 10).

Radiation therapy given either before or after surgery is an effective way to kill the cancer cells that surround colon and rectal tumors or that have traveled to lymph nodes. Research shows that people with rectal cancer who receive radiation therapy before surgery tend to experience improved tumor control, less need for a colostomy, and fewer side effects than those who receive it postoperatively. Radiation can help control tumor regrowth and spread as well.

Radiation and Chemotherapy

Chemotherapy and radiation are two tools doctors can use to help control colorectal tumors. They are helpful when used singly, but because radiation and chemotherapy work in different ways to kill cells, doctors sometimes combine them for even greater effect. This is called chemoradiation.

Chemotherapy can also make the radiation more effective, a process known as radiosensitization. We'll talk more about chemotherapy in chapter 12.

Side Effects of Radiation Therapy

Before undertaking any course of cancer treatment, including radiation therapy, ask your doctor lots of questions about the process. You should be especially aware of the potential side effects you might experience. We'll cover both short-term (acute) side effects and longer term reactions (or late effects) in the following sections.

How Does Radiation Cause Side Effects?

Cells that are actively dividing are most sensitive to the effects of radiation because their DNA is more exposed to the damage that radiation causes. Cancer cells divide rapidly, making them especially vulnerable to radiation. But some healthy cells divide rapidly too, particularly the ones that need to constantly replenish themselves (such as cells of the blood, skin, and mucosal lining of organs). So, while radiation effectively targets cancer cells, rapidly dividing normal cells suffer too.

When these healthy cells are destroyed, the body can't function normally, and a person experiences side effects. For example, damage to the cells lining the gastrointestinal tract can cause diarrhea.

Types of Side Effects of Radiation Therapy

The side effects of radiation therapy are grouped into two categories: acute effects and late effects. Acute effects are temporary and occur while a person with colorectal cancer is receiving radiation therapy. Late effects of radiation, in contrast, may emerge many months after the treatment has been given. If they arise, they tend to be permanent. As noted earlier, the dose of radiation that doctors prescribe is based on minimizing the risk of these permanent complications.

Questions to Ask Your Medical Team About Radiation Therapy

- What is the purpose of the radiation therapy that is being recommended (for example, is it intended as adjuvant or palliative therapy)?
- What is the desired result of the radiation therapy that is being recommended? What are the chances that radiation therapy will achieve the result we want?
- Is my cancer at a high, intermediate, or low risk of recurring in the pelvis if I don't have radiation treatments?
- What will happen if the tumor comes back in the pelvis?
- How should I manage diarrhea if it occurs?
- How should I manage nausea if it occurs?
- How should I manage a skin reaction if it occurs?
- Will it be possible to spare my anal canal from the radiation beam?
- How long will the side effects last?

In the following sections, we'll provide an overview of side effects you might experience as a result of radiation therapy. We'll talk about how to manage these side effects in chapter 15.

Acute Side Effects

Generally, the blood cells, the lining of the gastrointestinal tract (mouth, esophagus, stomach, and intestine), and the skin are cells of the body are most sensitive to the acute effects of radiation. In the case of radiation treatment to the abdomen or pelvis, examples of acute side effects are diarrhea and weight loss, nausea, skin "burning," or low blood counts, which can cause weakness and fatigue. Hair loss could occur in areas of the body that are in the irradiated area and have hair.

Late Side Effects and Long-Term Risks of Radiation

Doctors think that the late effects of radiotherapy are caused by damage to the cells of the body that do not normally repopulate. Examples of late side effects include scar tissue in the skin or nerve injury resulting in pain. If a high enough dose of radiation were given, all patients would suffer these effects. On the other hand, these side effects may be avoided if a low enough dose of radiation is used. The dose of radiation that is prescribed to best treat cancer while minimizing side effects is based on experience gathered over the years.

> *"I found out it was very difficult to have intercourse because of the scarring and the burning in the female organs. So, I did go to my gynecologist and talk to him about that. He was surprised that the radiologist had not said anything to me about this being a possible side effect."*
>
> —CAROLE

SCAR TISSUE

Radiation can cause permanent damage to normal tissues, which may result in scarring. When radiation is delivered to the bowel to treat rectal cancer, scar tissue can cause bowel obstruction and rectal stricture (narrowing of the passageway). Fortunately, the risks of these side effects of radiation are very low. The risk is directly related to the amount of bowel that has to be irradiated to prevent cancer recurrence. Preoperative radiation has a lower risk of these complications because more of this normal tissue can be excluded from the radiation beam.

OTHER CANCERS

Radiation is a known carcinogen, which means it can cause cancer. Examples of other carcinogens are asbestos and tobacco smoke. Carcinogens do not cause cancer in every case or all the time. Substances classified as carcinogens may have different levels of cancer-causing potential. Some may cause cancer only after prolonged, high levels of exposure. And a person's risk of developing cancer will depend on many factors, including the length and intensity of exposure to the carcinogen and the person's genetic makeup.

It may seem odd to think that doctors would use something that can *cause* cancer as a way to *cure* cancer, but here's how it works: radiation damages DNA. It damages the DNA of cancer cells—which is a good thing—but it damages the DNA of normal cells too. The damaged DNA in normal cells can change how the normal cell's genes work. And these changes could eventually turn a normal cell into an abnormal cell, which can lead to cancer. However, getting cancer from medical radiation therapy is fairly rare and this process takes decades. So, because the risk of recurrence from a cancer that a person already has is much higher than the small risk of another cancer developing as a result of treatment, the benefits of radiation therapy far outweigh this risk.

PREGNANCY IN WOMEN AFTER RADIATION TO THE PELVIS

Radiation treatment to the pelvis can be a special concern to younger women who want to bear children. A fertile woman who receives radiation therapy to treat a colorectal cancer can lose the function of her ovaries and uterus.

If this is something that you are concerned about, tell your doctor. You may also want to explore other possibilities and assisted fertility methods, if needed, such as in-vitro fertilization and surrogate motherhood. An infertility specialist can provide specific recommendations regarding preservation of fertility after radiation therapy.

POTENCY IN MEN AFTER RADIATION TO THE PELVIS

If the testicles are directly irradiated, radiation can cause reduced sperm counts in male patients. Almost all men with rectal cancer can receive radiation to the areas at risk without direct irradiation of the testicles. However, whenever radiation therapy is given, a small amount of radiation scatters inside the body a short distance from the area. In male patients with rectal cancer, this rarely results in sterility, but often results in lowered sperm counts, which can affect fertility.

High-dose radiation—as is used for prostate cancer—can result in erectile dysfunction (impotence). However, there is no conclusive evidence that moderate dose radiotherapy—as is generally used for rectal cancer—results in impotence. (Patients should be aware that damage to the nerves during certain types of rectal surgery, however, might result in erectile dysfunction.)

Specialists can provide information and support services to help people deal with these potential challenges, including information about sperm banking. Talk to your doctor about any concerns and expected treatment outcomes.

CHAPTER TWELVE

CHEMOTHERAPY

Cathy Eng, MD

Chemotherapy is medicine that kills cancer cells. Like radiation therapy, chemotherapy affects both cancerous cells and normal cells. Unlike radiation therapy, chemotherapy is systemic. That is, it delivers medicine throughout the body. (Radiation therapy, in contrast, concentrates beams of electromagnetic energy on a specific body part.) Chemotherapy is provided intravenously (an injection by vein) or in a pill form. Regardless of the way it is given to you, it kills cancer cells by traveling through your bloodstream.

This chapter will provide a general overview of chemotherapy in the treatment of colorectal cancer and will help you to understand how chemotherapy may best fit in your treatment plan.

What Is the Purpose of Chemotherapy?

The purpose of chemotherapy depends on your unique medical situation, including your symptoms, your age, family history, and—most important—the stage of your cancer.

Chemotherapy in colorectal cancer is used commonly in the following scenarios:

- after colorectal surgery
- before colorectal surgery
- as palliative medicine
- with radiation

In the first scenario, your surgeon and/or oncologist may suggest additional chemotherapy despite complete surgical removal of the tumor to decrease your risk of cancer recurrence in the future. (Even when it appears that all cancer has been removed, microscopic cancer cells may still remain, either in the place that the tumor was removed or as micrometastases to other parts of the body.) This is known as adjuvant chemotherapy. Adjuvant chemotherapy may decrease your risk of recurrence by more than 30 percent.

The purpose of neoadjuvant chemotherapy—chemotherapy delivered before colorectal surgery—is to shrink the existing tumor so that surgery can be minimally invasive. Neoadjuvant chemotherapy can also prevent cancer cells from spreading.

Palliative chemotherapy is given if surgery is not a treatment option because of the extent of the cancer or if your surgeon has determined that surgery is too risky given your medical condition. Palliative chemotherapy can increase overall survival and may also temporarily shrink or stabilize a tumor, thus reducing symptoms, but will probably not cause cure or remission in patients with stage IV advanced disease.

In certain cases, chemotherapy may be used as a "booster" to enhance radiation and make more effective. This is called radiosensitization, because the chemotherapy medications make the cancer cells more sensitive and vulnerable to radiation. The majority of chemotherapy drugs (which we'll discuss later in this chapter) may be used this way. Usually, smaller-than-standard doses of chemotherapy are given for radiation sensitization so that the risk of side effects is reduced.

Misconceptions About Chemotherapy

Many people have preconceived notions and strong negative feelings about chemotherapy—they may assume that it always makes people bald, very weak, and nauseated. But chemotherapy is tailored to each person's unique medical situation and affects each person differently, resulting in different responses and side effects. Recent advances in the treatment of colorectal cancer have provided doctors with many excellent chemotherapy options.

Chemotherapy is a powerful tool doctors and patients have to combat the growth and spread of cancer. Don't let preconceived notions or misinformation about chemotherapy affect your decisions: get the facts. Talk candidly with your health care team about how specific chemotherapy agents (drugs) can help fight your cancer and what side effects they may cause. Your health care team should share with you their plan for dealing with side effects if they arise. Many potential symptoms can be controlled with other medicines (see chapter 15 for specific strategies for managing side effects).

You may also want your doctor to make clear what will happen if you *do not* take chemotherapy if it is part of your recommended therapy, so you clearly understand your options and potential outcomes.

What Are Your Other Options?

Discuss your options with your oncologist and other members of your health care team. In some instances, chemotherapy may not be the best option; for example, if your cancer is advanced and you are very sick, you may not be strong enough to tolerate the side effects of most chemotherapy agents. This is a decision that you should discuss fully with your health care team and your loved ones.

If at any point it appears that you are not tolerating your chemotherapy despite the use of other medicines to treat all side effects, or the side effects of chemotherapy are severe enough to negatively affect your quality of life, you should talk with your doctor about whether the benefits of chemotherapy outweigh the risks of further treatment. Sometimes it is simply a matter of educating your doctor about your side effects and trying other chemotherapy medications that might work more effectively for you.

> *"I asked [the doctor] to be frank with me. 'Tell me exactly,' I said. 'Don't try to hide anything. I want to know the real truth.' And he said, 'Well, it may extend your life 90 days.' When he told me all the bad things about chemo, I said, 'Hey, I'd rather have quality of life than quantity. No chemo.'"*
>
> —PETE

If your cancer does not respond to your prescribed chemotherapy treatment, your doctor will discuss other options with you, such as enrolling in a clinical study to receive a new treatment being investigated.

Chemotherapy and Herbal Treatments: Potential Interactions

People with cancer are becoming more interested in using herbal treatments in addition to standard medical therapies. *If you are taking or plan to take any herbal supplements, it is essential that you discuss this with your doctor.* Some herbal treatments may seem harmless but can interact with your chemotherapy medicines, undermine the effectiveness of your treatment, and/or cause you harm. See chapter 14 for more information on complementary and alternative approaches to cancer treatment.

When Is Chemotherapy Used?

Whether you receive chemotherapy depends mainly on the stage of your cancer. Sometimes chemotherapy is not appropriate at all. When deciding on the type of chemotherapy to use and how long to administer the medicine, doctors rely on evidence gathered from research and clinical studies on patients with medical profiles similar to yours. This evidence base can help you understand the expected results, benefits, risks, and side effects you may experience.

Chapter 9 (pages 133–150) includes general information about the role of chemotherapy in treatment for colon and rectal cancers. As discussed, chemotherapy is used in a variety of circumstances. Sometimes chemotherapy is offered before surgery, and in other cases, it is administered afterward. Chemotherapy can also enhance the effectiveness of radiation therapy.

How Is Chemotherapy Administered?

Your oncologist will determine which chemotherapy drug or combination of drugs is best for you given your specific medical condition. An oncology nurse will administer the chemotherapy to you.

Most chemotherapy drugs are administered intravenously through a needle, or a tiny plastic tube called a catheter, that is placed into a vein in your forearm or hand. This method is called intravenous, or IV. Intravenous drugs are given in the following ways:

- The drugs can be given quickly through IV tubing directly from a syringe over a few minutes, which is called an "IV push."
- An IV drip (infusion) can last 30 minutes to a few hours. A mixed drug solution flows from a plastic bag.
- Continuous infusions are sometimes necessary and usually last one to four days.

A bolus form of administration is a single injection of medicine; an infusional form is a prolonged intravenous injection given over several hours or days

The method of administration depends on the chemotherapy schedule and the chemotherapy agent itself. Some chemotherapies are provided through a semipermanent intravenous catheter connected to one of your major veins. This catheter will remain in your body for the entire length of treatment to minimize blood draws and eliminate the need to start a new IV line every time you receive a chemotherapy treatment. Some chemotherapy will only require a regular arm vein, making a semipermanent catheter unnecessary.

Occasionally, chemotherapy is provided in a pill form.

Location of Treatment

Where you get chemotherapy depends on the drugs you are getting, the dosages of each drug to be given, your hospital's policies, your wishes, and what your doctor recommends. You may be treated with chemotherapy at home, in your doctor's office, in a clinic, in your hospital's outpatient department, or you may be admitted to the hospital.

When you begin chemotherapy, you may need to stay in the hospital for a short time so that your doctor can watch you to see the medicine's effects and make any changes.

Duration and Frequency of Treatment

The selection of chemotherapy drug(s), method of administration, dose, and schedule for treatment is called a chemotherapy regimen. This regimen is developed by the health care team and is personalized based on your height, your weight, and the results of research on people like you with similar types of cancer.

"Following surgery for colon cancer in 1991, I faced one year of chemotherapy. When after the first weekly treatment was over and I commented. 'Only 51 more to go!' the nurse looked me straight in the eye and said, 'You're not going to do that, are you?' I smiled and nodded affirmatively! For me, looking ahead and remembering the adage, 'This too shall pass!' helped me cope with what seemed to be a long 12 months of treatment."

— SAN

How often you take chemotherapy drugs and how long your treatment lasts depends on:
- the kind of cancer you have, its stage, and grade
- the goals of the treatment
- the drugs that are used
- and how your body responds to them.

Physicians give chemotherapy in cycles of treatment. You may receive treatments daily, weekly, or monthly. Depending on the chemotherapy regimen, the duration of the cycle will vary. These breaks allow rest periods so that your body can build healthy new cells and you can regain your strength.

Adjuvant chemotherapy (chemotherapy given after colorectal surgery) is usually given for six months. Your doctor will monitor your health during the chemotherapy and after it is complete.

The duration of chemotherapy will depend on the stage of your cancer and your response to treatment. Periodic computed tomography (CT) scans or magnetic resonance imaging (MRI) will help doctors evaluate this.

Chemotherapy Options

New chemotherapy drugs introduced in the past few years have greatly altered the outcome for patients with both early and late stage colorectal cancer. For almost three decades, only one chemotherapy agent, called 5-fluorouracil (5-FU), was available to treat colorectal cancer. Now several new chemotherapy agents are available and may be combined or used alone.

Classes of Chemotherapy Agents

Chemotherapy drugs are divided into several categories or classes based on how they affect specific chemical substances within cancer cells, which cellular activities or processes the drug interferes with, and which specific phases of the cell cycle the drug affects. Knowing these effects helps oncologists decide which drugs are likely to work well together and, if more than one drug will be used, to plan exactly when each of the drugs should be given (in which order and how often).

Classes of chemotherapy agents used to treat colorectal cancer include antimetabolites, biomodulators, topoisomerase I inhibitors, and alkylating agents.

In addition to chemotherapy, other types of drugs may be used to treat colorectal cancer, such as monoclonal antibodies (see chapter 13 for more information on monoclonal antibodies and how they work).

Common Chemotherapy Drugs

5-Fluorouracil (5-FU, Adrucil, fluorouracil) is the drug most commonly used to treat colorectal cancer. Other frequently prescribed drugs include capecitabine (Xeloda), irinotecan (CPT-11, Camptosar), and oxaliplatin (Eloxatin).

Leucovorin (folinic acid) is given as part of some chemotherapy regimens to help boost the effectiveness of other drugs but is not technically a chemotherapy agent.

Cetuximab (Erbitux), and bevacizumab (Avastin) are monoclonal antibodies commonly given to treat colorectal cancer.

Each of these agents may be used alone or in combination but tend to be more effective when combined with each other in different regimens.

See Table 12.1 on pages 200–201 for an overview of common drugs used to treat colorectal cancer, how they work, and what precautions you should be aware of when taking them.

5-Fluorouracil

5-Fluorouracil (5-FU, Adrucil, fluorouracil) is the chemotherapy drug most commonly used to treat colorectal cancer. It is an antimetabolite, a drug that is very similar to natural chemicals in a normal biochemical reaction in cells but is different enough to interfere with the normal division and functions of cells. 5-Fluorouracil prevents cells from making DNA and RNA by interfering with the synthesis of nucleic acids, thus disrupting the growth of cancer cells.

Capecitabine

Capecitabine (Xeloda) is an oral form of the antimetabolite 5-fluorouracil that is usually used to treat colorectal cancers that have metastasized.

Leucovorin

Leucovorin (Citrovorum factor, folinic acid, FA) is a biomodulator, a biologic agent that mimics some of the natural signals that the body uses to regulate growth. Leucovorin calcium is a vitamin used as a "booster." Leucovorin helps drugs such as 5-fluorouracil work better and kill cancer cells more effectively than the 5-fluorouracil can alone.

Irinotecan

Irinotecan (CPT-11, Camptosar) is a type of chemotherapy drug called a topoisomerase I inhibitor. Topoisomerases are enzymes that help uncoil strands of DNA so that it can replicate itself. Irinotecan inhibits this ability, thus stopping the growth of cancer cells by preventing cell division and replication. Irinotecan is usually used to treat colorectal cancers that have metastasized—either alone or in combination with FU/leucovorin (or cetuximab, but only in previously treated patients).

Oxaliplatin

Oxaliplatin (Eloxatin) is an alkylating agent, a chemical agent that works directly on DNA during all phases of the cell cycle to prevent the cancer cell from reproducing. Oxaliplatin is used together with 5-fluorouracil and leucovorin to treat metastatic colorectal cancer.

Table 12.1 Common Chemotherapy Drugs Used for Colorectal Cancer

Class	Generic Drug Name (Trade Name)	How It Works
Antimetabolite	5-Fluorouracil (5-FU, Adrucil, Fluorouracil)	Prevents cells from making DNA and RNA by interfering with the synthesis of nucleic acids, thus disrupting the growth of cancer cells.
Antimetabolite	Capecitabine (Xeloda)	Prevents cells from making DNA and RNA by interfering with the synthesis of nucleic acids, thus disrupting the growth of cancer cells. Capecitabine is an oral form of 5-fluorouracil.
Biomodulator	Leucovorin (Citrovorum factor, folinic acid, FA)	Helps drugs such as 5-fluorouracil work better than the 5-fluorouracil can alone. This makes the 5-fluorouracil kill cancer cells more effectively.
Topoisomerase I inhibitor	Irinotecan (CPT-11, Camptosar)	Topoisomerases are enzymes that help uncoil strands of DNA so that it can replicate itself. Irinotecan inhibits this ability, thus stopping the growth of cancer cells by preventing cell division and replication.
Alkylating agents	Oxaliplatin (Eloxatin)	Alkylating agents work directly on DNA during all phases of the cell cycle to prevent the cancer cell from reproducing. Oxaliplatin stops the growth of cancer cells, which causes the cells to die.
Monoclonal antibody	Cetuximab (Erbitux)	Cetuximab fits, like a key in a lock, into receptors on the surface of the cancer cell, blocking an epidermal growth factor receptor (EGFR) from fitting into the receptor. The EGFR is unable to tell the cell to divide. This stops the growth of the cancer cell.
Monoclonal antibody	Bevacizumab (Avastin)	Bevacizumab prevents the growth of new blood vessels. Without new blood vessels, the tumor cannot grow.

Cetuximab

Cetuximab (Erbitux) is a monoclonal antibody, a special infection-fighting protein cloned in a laboratory and used to diagnose and treat some forms of cancer. In this case, cetuximab is used to treat colorectal cancer in certain people who are no longer responding to or cannot take the chemotherapy drug irinotecan.

Precautions	Notes
• Do not have any immunizations (vaccinations) without your doctor's okay. • May lower your blood counts (white blood cells, red blood cells, and platelets).	The chemotherapy drug most commonly used to treat colorectal cancer.
• Do not have any immunizations (vaccinations) without your doctor's okay. • May lower your may lower your blood counts (white blood cells, red blood cells, and platelets).	Usually used to treat colorectal cancers that have metastasized.
Side effects are rare.	Leucovorin calcium is a vitamin used as a "booster."
• Do not have any immunizations (vaccinations) without your doctor's okay. • May lower your blood counts (white blood cells, red blood cells, and platelets). • May cause nausea and vomiting. • May cause severe diarrhea.	Usually used to treat colorectal cancers that have metastasized. May be used by itself or in combination with FU/leucovorin or with cetuximab (only in previously treated patients). Not used as an adjuvant drug.
• Do not have any immunizations (vaccinations) without your doctor's okay • Can cause nausea and vomiting. • May cause numbness and tingling of fingertips or toes. • Be wary of cold temperatures.	Used together with 5-fluorouracil and leucovorin to treat metastatic colorectal cancer.
• Do not have any immunizations (vaccinations) without your doctor's okay. • May cause allergic reactions that manifest as fever, chills, shortness of breath, and swelling of the face or throat. • May cause rash	Used to treat colorectal cancer in certain people who are no longer responding to or cannot take the chemotherapy drug irinotecan.
• Do not have any immunizations (vaccinations) without your doctor's okay. • Rare side effects include: perforation of the intestines, bleeding, thrombosis, and high blood pressure.	Used to treat metastatic colorectal cancer.

Monoclonal antibodies represent an exciting new way of treating cancer. See chapter 13 for more information on monoclonal antibodies used to treat colorectal cancer and how they work.

Bevacizumab

Bevacizumab (Avastin) is also a monoclonal antibody. Bevacizumab is used to treat metastatic colorectal cancer. See chapter 13 for more information on monoclonal antibodies used to treat colorectal cancer and how they work.

Common Chemotherapy Regimens

Doctors have established common chemotherapy regimens to treat patients with specific shared characteristics. These regimens are described using acronyms that are based upon the chemotherapy drug combinations and the schedule for administration:

- IFL: irinotecan/bolus 5-FU/leucovorin
- FOLFIRI: irinotecan/infusional 5-FU/leucovorin
- FOLFOX: oxaliplatin/infusional 5-FU/leucovorin
- CAPEOX or XELOX: capecitabine/oxaliplatin
- CAPIRI or CAPEOX: capecitabine/irinotecan

A slash (/) means "in combination with." Recall that a bolus form of administration is a single injection of medicine, and an infusional form is a prolonged intravenous injection given over several hours or days.

Chemotherapy for Metastasis

Colorectal cancer, when it metastasizes, is most likely to spread to the liver, lungs, and abdomen. Doctors may suggest hepatic arterial infusion (HAI) for patients with liver metastases. HAI is a method by which chemotherapy is directly administered into the hepatic artery, the main blood supply of the liver. Direct injection of chemotherapy into the hepatic artery via a pump placed in the patient's abdomen aims to treat the liver metastases with little involvement of normal tissue. HAI is not commonly used, so your doctor may choose another method to treat liver metastasis, such as surgery or systemic chemotherapy. HAI is regional chemotherapy; as such, it will not treat areas of cancer outside the liver. HAI may or may not be combined with additional palliative chemotherapy.

Unfortunately, there is no regional chemotherapy treatment for the lungs or abdominal cavity that is not considered investigational. Currently, the best treatment available is chemotherapy alone.

What Are the Potential Side Effects?

Chemotherapy drugs are used to prevent cancer cells from dividing and growing, but they also affect normal cells to a lesser degree. When these normal cells are killed, side effects result. The symptoms you may experience depend on the chemotherapy agent(s), dose, and schedule that it is given. See Table 12.1 (page 200) for brief list of possible side effects linked to specific chemotherapy drugs and Table 15.2 (page 260) for a comparative look at common side effects of chemotherapy agents. A thorough inventory of treatment side effects and strategies for managing them can be found in chapter 15.

Side effects are commonly divided into two categories: short-term and long-term (or late) effects. Short-term effects occur during and shortly after treatment and tend to be reversible. Late effects may occur months or even years after treatment. Ask your doctor to be specific about what you can expect given your specific situation, but remember that everyone responds to chemotherapy medicines differently.

The most common short-term symptoms people experience because of chemotherapy include:

• Fatigue
• Nausea, vomiting, and loss of appetite
• Diarrhea
• Hair loss
• Swelling in the extremities
• Low blood counts—resulting in an increased chance of infection (because of a shortage of white blood cells), bleeding or bruising after minor injuries (because of a reduced number of platelets, which control blood clotting), and fatigue (because of low red blood cell counts)
• Changes to skin and nails, rashes, and mouth sores

These side effects are generally short term and reversible. There are many remedies for the temporary side effects of chemotherapy (such as antinausea and antianxiety medications), so if you have any unrelieved side effects, bring them up with your doctor. You may experience other, less common, symptoms (chest pain, headaches or migraines, etc.), so be sure to discuss all of your symptoms with your health care team on a regular basis.

Long-Term Side Effects

Most side effects from chemotherapy disappear once treatment stops. For example, if you lose your hair, it will grow back, although it might look different. However, you may experience long-term side effects. The following side effects may last longer than others.

- Nervous system: Damage to the nerves may result in a condition called sensory neuropathy, which is characterized by numbness and tingling in the hands and feet. This effect may not improve for weeks or months after the chemotherapy is discontinued. Effects on the nervous system may also result in insomnia, impaired memory, or a decreased attention span; these effects may resolve over weeks to months.

- Reproductive system: Regularity in menstrual cycle may not occur for a prolonged period after the chemotherapy is stopped. Fertility may temporarily impaired after the chemotherapy is discontinued. Regardless, an oral or barrier contraception method is recommended for at least 30 days after chemotherapy has been discontinued, because some chemotherapy medicines can cause birth defects.

- Organs: If the severity of the side effect potentially results in permanent organ damage, such as damage to the liver or lungs, the chemotherapy will be closely monitored and discontinued if damage is detected. However, permanent organ damage may not be evident until after the chemotherapy is discontinued.

How Will Chemotherapy Affect My Lifestyle?

The extent to which chemotherapy affects your lifestyle depends on your energy level and how well your body tolerates your chemotherapy treatment. You should be able to maintain your lifestyle, including going to work and continuing with regular exercise, unless your doctor suggests otherwise.

It may be wise for you to plan for additional rest and recovery time and arrange support at home and in the workplace. Talk to your doctor about any lifestyle changes you anticipate or experience—he or she may be able to recommend resources or strategies to help you adjust.

Which Chemotherapy Treatment Is the Best?

People with colorectal cancer considering chemotherapy often ask their health care team which treatment is best. There is no one superior choice—the best treatment is based on a number of factors: how well you tolerate the drug(s), what kind of side effects are produced, how effective the treatment is, and how it affects your survival. Your best response to chemotherapy will usually be with the first type of chemotherapy regimen that you receive.

When used as an adjuvant therapy, chemotherapy can decrease your risk of recurrence by approximately 40 percent and your risk of dying from colorectal cancer by one third. In the neoadjuvant or palliative setting, combination regimens are often more aggressive but may also result in a higher response rate and survival.

The IFL regimen has fallen out of favor in the treatment of metastatic disease because it less effective and produces more side effects. Both the FOLFOX and FOLFIRI regimens, with or without monoclonal antibodies, appear to be effective and to prolong survival. (The effectiveness of FOLFOX and FOLFIRI appear to be equivalent.) The role of adjuvant irinotecan remains unclear. Your oncologist may prescribe either oral capecitabine or 5-FU/leucovorin (recall that capecitabine is an oral form of 5-fluorouracil and that leucovorin is a "booster"). In addition, if appropriate, your doctor may choose to add a monoclonal antibody to your chemotherapy regimen, which may provide a greater response rate than to chemotherapy alone (see chapter 13).

Recurrence, Response, and Survival

For people with colorectal cancer whose cancer is stage I, II, or III, surgical removal of the cancer provides the greatest chance of cure. The expected survival rate at five years without adjuvant chemotherapy is 90 percent, but decreases if cancer has spread to the lymph nodes. Tumor recurrence is greatest usually within the first two years.

For patients with advanced metastatic disease (stage IV cancer), response and survival are the primary concerns. Response refers to a significant (usually 50 percent) shrinkage of the tumor being treated. Although capecitabine has a higher response rate than 5-FU/leucovorin (22 percent versus 13 percent) and causes fewer side effects, the overall survival of patients on these two medications is the same (approximately 13 months). Therefore, capecitabine has been determined to be equivalent to 5-FU/leucovorin, and most oncologists believe that they may be used interchangeably.

The chemotherapy drugs irinotecan, oxaliplatin, cetuximab, and bevacizumab have a clear positive effect on response rate and length of survival (see Figure 12.1 on page 200). The expected response rate for combination regimens ranges from 35 to 55 percent.

The best way to prolong your life as much as possible is by receiving all the chemotherapy regimens available to you as long as you are in good health and tolerating your treatment without difficulty.

Figure 12.1 Expected Median* Survival With Chemotherapy

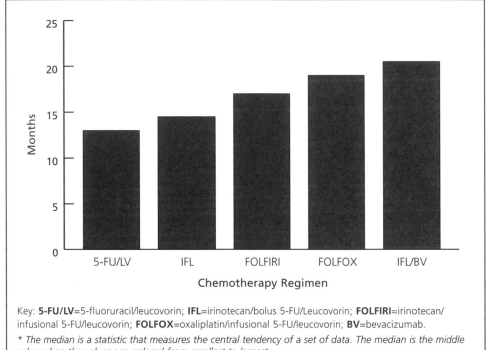

Key: **5-FU/LV**=5-fluoruracil/leucovorin; **IFL**=irinotecan/bolus 5-FU/Leucovorin; **FOLFIRI**=irinotecan/ infusional 5-FU/leucovorin; **FOLFOX**=oxaliplatin/infusional 5-FU/leucovorin; **BV**=bevacizumab.

The median is a statistic that measures the central tendency of a set of data. The median is the middle value when the values are ordered from smallest to largest.

Making Your Treatment Decisions

Whether to include chemotherapy in your colorectal cancer treatment plan is a matter you should consider carefully.

Keep in mind that the purpose of adjuvant therapy is to decrease your risk of recurrence; it is given for a finite time. Neoadjuvant and palliative chemotherapy aims to prolong your survival, shrink existing tumors, and/or improve your quality of life.

For patients with stage IV cancer seeking palliative chemotherapy, there are several exciting chemotherapy agents available that may help your quality of life and prolong your survival for an extended period. You always have the choice to refuse chemotherapy if you so desire.

Input from all of the health care professionals involved in your care will provide invaluable information, improve the quality of care your receive, and optimize an outcome, so it is important to communicate regularly with your health care team.

Questions to Ask Your Medical Team About Chemotherapy

- What stage is my cancer?
- Is chemotherapy recommended with this stage of colorectal cancer?
- What is the recommended regimen?
- What is the goal of the recommended regimen—adjuvant, neoadjuvant, or palliative?
- How soon after surgery should I start chemotherapy?
- What is my risk of recurrence or survival without and with chemotherapy?
- What is the duration of recommended chemotherapy?
- How often will I need to visit my doctor?
- How will the chemotherapy be given?
- What supportive medications do you recommend and how should I take them to treat any side effects?
- How often will I have to have my blood drawn?
- When will restaging be necessary?
- What side effects should I expect from this chemotherapy?
- Are there any clinical trials you would recommend for me?
- What symptoms would you be concerned about? Which ones should result in a phone call or emergency room evaluation?
- What kind of follow up do I need after adjuvant chemotherapy is over?

CHAPTER THIRTEEN

CLINICAL TRIALS AND EMERGING THERAPIES

Hanna Kelly, MD
Richard M. Goldberg, MD

Over the past few decades our knowledge of colorectal cancer has come a long way. We now understand many of the things that can cause normal cells to turn into cancerous ones. We can identify people at high risk of developing colorectal cancer. New treatments have emerged that improve survival and cure rates. As a result, the death rates for colorectal cancer have been declining since the 1970s.

However, even with these advances in our understanding of colorectal cancer, about 150,000 Americans a year are diagnosed with colorectal cancer and far too many people—more than 55,000—die every year from this disease. The more we know about how and why colorectal cancer develops, and what can be done to effectively treat it, the more these numbers will decline.

That's where cancer research comes into the picture. In this chapter, we'll discuss research studies (called "clinical trials" by people in the medical community) and experimental therapies, and how they can potentially help you and others who are diagnosed with colorectal cancer in the future.

What Is a Clinical Trial?

Scientists use research studies called clinical trials to try to answer questions that will help the medical community learn how to better prevent or treat a disease. Results from clinical trials advance our understanding of diseases and help doctors continually improve the care they provide, including cancer treatments.

Clinical trials are research studies in people. They take place after experiments on cells or animals suggest that a treatment or method of prevention is likely to be safe and effective in people. There are many types of clinical trials: those designed to answer questions about how to prevent disease, about how well a test works to diagnose disease, and about how well a new drug works to treat disease.

Most clinical trials in the field of cancer deal with new drugs or new combinations of drugs used to treat cancers. There are also clinical studies of new radiation therapy treatments, studies of the best ways to combine and sequence treatment modalities, and investigations of treatment to relieve side effects. These studies are designed to answer such questions as: Is this new treatment safe? Does it work more effectively than existing treatments? What side effects does it cause? Whom does it help?

Phases of Clinical Trials

Every new cancer treatment needs to go through three phases of study before it can become a standard treatment. A fourth phase is conducted after the new treatment has been approved by the Food and Drug Administration (FDA), a governmental agency that regulates the development, use, and safety of drugs, medical devices, food, cosmetics, and other related products.

Phase I Studies

Phase I studies ask: *Is this treatment safe? What dose can the patient tolerate?*

Phase I studies are designed to be sure the treatment being explored is safe in humans and to find the dose of the drug that balances the fewest side effects with the most effective result. Phase I studies are conducted only after a drug has proven successful in laboratory and animal studies.

Phase I studies are often offered to a small number of patients (perhaps only 10 to 20 people) whose cancer has not been cured by standard treatments and who want to try a promising investigational treatment.

Once a drug and a dose are deemed be safe in this small number of people, the treatment is tested in a phase II study.

Phase II Studies

Phase II studies ask: *Is this drug safe and effective?*

Phase II trials enroll a larger number of people (usually between 10 and 100). These studies continue to monitor the safety of the treatment in this larger group but are designed to learn whether the drug is effective as well.

Phase III Studies

Phase III studies ask: *Is the new treatment, either alone or combined with other treatments, better than the established standard therapy?*

To answer this question, larger numbers of patients are required, sometimes as many as several thousand people. Because phase III trials compare the outcomes of two or more interventions, patients are randomly assigned to receive one therapy or the other. Neither patients nor their doctors can choose which of the therapies is given or received.

Randomization prevents what is called selection bias in a study. For instance, if the doctors were allowed to decide which patients were to get the new drug X instead of giving the standard drug Y, they might all choose to give the new drug X to the sickest patients, thinking it was their best chance to be cured. However, if drug X and drug Y are equally effective, but all the sickest patients got drug X and the healthier patients got drug Y, patients on drug Y are likely to have better outcomes, even though the two drugs work equally well.

Often, the patients and doctors don't even know what drug they are getting until after the trial is over. This is called a blind study. This prevents a different bias, a reporting bias. If you know you are getting an experimental drug, you may be more likely to report strange or adverse effects than if you are getting the standard drug that has been used for decades.

Once a drug or intervention has been show to be safe, effective, and at least as good as the standard of care, the FDA may approve it for use in that setting.

Phase IV Studies

Phase IV studies ask: *What are the long-term effects of this drug or intervention?* Phase IV studies take place after a drug has received FDA approval. They continue to monitor patients who have received a given drug to be sure no serious long-term adverse effects result from its administration.

What Are the Benefits and Risks of Participating in a Clinical Trial?

Initially, the clearest benefit to enrolling in a clinical trial is to help advance the understanding of how to treat cancer. Some of our most powerful advances in cancer treatment have been made as a result of participation in clinical trials. For example, before 1990, only one drug (fluorouracil) was available to treat colorectal cancer. Now, as a result of clinical trials in the United States, five drugs are approved for use.

"I signed up for the protocol because there was really nothing else going on, and it looked good and it looked progressive and it looked futuristic. And, I thought, 'Well, if I can't help myself, this would obviously help a tremendous amount of other people.'"

—CARL

Another main benefit of clinical trials is that participation may give patients access to treatments that are not otherwise available. Participation in clinical trials is not limited to patients treated at a few nationally prominent cancer centers; many clinical trials are available in community cancer centers, and many oncology practices offer trials (especially phases III and IV) to patients they treat as outpatients.

Additional benefits include careful monitoring of your condition and the possibility of payment for part or all of the medical care received during the study by some study sponsors (this is not true for all clinical trials, so be sure you are aware of the costs of your participation).

Enrolling in a clinical trial is not without risk, however. Even though the federal government, granting agencies, universities and hospitals, and investigators take great care to ensure the cancer research protocols are as safe as possible, there are always uncertainties regarding the effectiveness and the side effects of these treatments.

This is especially true of earlier phase studies but is a factor for all clinical trials. This is why the study coordinators screen participants very carefully and require all participants to sign a waiver of informed consent.

In addition to the possible health risks that may be involved, there may be a financial burden if care provided during the study is not paid for. There is also the possibility that the patient may have to travel long distances to receive treatment.

Deciding to Enroll in a Clinical Trial

When you are discussing treatment options with your cancer team, your doctor may suggest that you consider participating in a clinical trial. Your health care team will answer your questions and help you get as much information as you need to make your decision. Ultimately, though, the choice is yours. If you do decide to participate in a clinical trial, it is important to thoroughly understand the goal of the study, the benefit can you might expect to receive from therapy, and the adverse effects you are at risk for.

Finally, if you do enroll, you may change your mind at any time. Participation in clinical trials is voluntary.

Where To Go To Learn More About Clinical Trials

To find out more about ongoing cancer clinical trials, ask your doctor. In addition, up-to-date information on clinical trials near you can be found at various sites on the Internet.

The American Cancer Society (ACS) offers a free clinical trial matching and referral service that provides patients with a list of clinical trials in which they are eligible to participate, based on information they provide about their medical situation, location, and preferences. For more information, visit the ACS clinical trials web site at http://www.clinicaltrials. cancer.org or call 800-ACS-2345/800-227-2345. You can also learn more from the National Cancer Institute (NCI) by calling 800-4-CANCER/800-422-6237 or visiting their web site at http://www. cancer.gov/clinicaltrials. The National Institutes of Health maintains a database of trials (http://www.clinicaltrials.gov), and the Coalition of National Cancer Cooperative Groups can also help (http://www.cancertrialshelp.org). If you do not have Internet access your local librarian should be able to help you gain access to these sites, or you can use the phone numbers listed.

> *"I'd recommend to somebody who's initially diagnosed to find out about every possible clinical trial they can.... I would look thoroughly, because there are new drugs out there and experimental trials that are certainly worth trying."*
>
> —MAX

Fewer than 5 percent of all cancer patients are offered and choose to participate in clinical trials, but an increase in this number could lead to the development of better options for the treatment of cancer and could speed up the amount of time it takes to evaluate new treatments, giving patients access to new treatments sooner.

New Approaches to an Old Problem

Surgery tackles cancer by removing cancerous cells. But sometimes cancerous cells have spread from the original site, or the surgeon does not remove all of the malignant tissue.

Traditional chemotherapy and radiation therapy kill cancer cells by taking advantage of distinctive characteristics of these malignant cells. As normal cells

Questions to Ask When Thinking About Participating in a Clinical Trial

- What is the aim of the trial?
- What benefit or response has been seen in previous studies using this drug or intervention? How does that apply to me?
- What side effects have been seen in previous studies with this drug? How are these side effects different from those in the standard approach?
- What are my options if I do not enroll in the trial?
- If I decide not to participate now, will I still be eligible for this and/or other clinical trials for my cancer in the future?
- Am I a candidate for any trials available elsewhere?
- How will my care be different if I am in the trial versus if I decline? Will I have to have more doctors' visits or extra tests?
- Will any of my medications interfere with the experimental drug?

change and become cancerous, they typically multiply more often and lose the ability to repair themselves when damaged. Chemotherapy and radiation therapy target these abnormalities by damaging cells while they are in the process of multiplying and by causing damage to cellular DNA and other structures critical to cell survival. In the best cases, this treatment is completely successful and kills off all of the cancer cells. (This happens more often in testicular cancer and Hodgkin's disease, but not often in patients with colorectal cancer.) Unfortunately, chemotherapy and radiation can damage normal cells too. And in most cases, chemotherapy causes colorectal cancers to shrink, or even disappear, but leaves residual cancer cells that can regrow once therapy stops.

As a result, scientists are considering new approaches treating for colorectal cancer. Instead of trying to destroy cancer cells by taking advantage of their rapid rate of division, the latest cancer therapies aim to reverse the molecular and/or genetic changes that cause a normal colon cell to become cancerous. To be successful in this approach, scientists need a better understanding of the molecular circuitry that governs the life of a cell and what goes wrong that causes a cell to turn cancerous.

These understandings can then be applied to new drug development. These new drugs target the specific defect in the circuitry and restore its normal function, ideally sparing normal organs from harmful effects in the process.

Emerging Therapies in Colorectal Cancer

A number of these new approaches and treatments for colorectal cancer have recently moved from the laboratory into clinical trials. The main categories of these emerging therapies are molecularly targeted drugs, immunotherapies, and gene therapies (see Table 13.1 on page 216). We'll try to provide simple explanations of the complex ways these new therapies work, along with a few specific examples of treatments designed to target colorectal cancer.

Molecularly Targeted Therapy

Cancer cells multiply without respect to the surrounding tissues, make new blood vessels to supply themselves with nutrients, and spread via the blood stream and lymphatic system. These are things that normal cells never do. The goal of molecularly targeted therapies is to disrupt one or more of these mechanisms to stop the cancer from growing.

The use of drugs that prevent cancer cells from growing by blocking tumor growth factors, one type of molecularly targeted therapy, has shown a great deal of promise.

Cetuximab and Bevacizumab

Researchers have discovered naturally occurring substances in the body that promote cell growth. These hormone-like substances are called growth factors. Growth factors activate cells by attaching to growth factor receptors, which are present on the outer surface of the cells. Once activated, these cancer cells may grow and replicate, form new blood supplies, metastasize (spread to other body parts), and override normal cell death processes (see Figure 13.1 on page 217).

One growth factor that has been linked to colorectal cancer is called epidermal growth factor (EGF). Twenty-five to seventy-five percent of colorectal cancer cells have abnormally high numbers of EGF receptors. One of these drugs, cetuximab (Erbitux), has been approved by the FDA for use against colorectal cancer.

Table 13.1 Emerging Therapies for Colorectal Cancer

Molecularly Targeted Therapy	Immunotherapy	Gene-Based Therapy
• Cetuximab (Erbitux) • Bevacizumab (Avastin)	• Interferon-α* (α-interferon, Actimmune, Alferon N, Avonex, IFN-α, Interferon-a 2α, Interferon-α 2b, Intron A, Roferon A) • Edrecolomab* • Cea-Vac	• p53 adenovirus • Onyx Virus

Interferon-α and Edrecolomab have proven unsuccessful in clinical trials and are no longer being pursued as colorectal cancer treatments.

Cetuximab is a monoclonal antibody (a special infection-fighting protein cloned in a laboratory) that fits, like a key into a lock, into epidermal growth factor receptors (EGFRs) on the surface of the cancer cell. When the cetuximab fills these receptors and acts as a placeholder, the epidermal growth factor has no place to attach. The EGFR is unable to activate the cell. This stops the cancer cell from growing.

Cetuximab (Erbitux), both alone and in combination with irinotecan (Camptosar, Camptothecan-11, CPT-11) has been repeatedly shown to shrink tumors in patients with advanced colorectal cancer after the cancer grew despite treatment with standard chemotherapy. Doctors don't know yet whether giving cetuximab to patients at an earlier stage in cancer care will improve survival.

Another growth factor, known as vascular endothelial growth factor (VEGF), helps tumors develop new blood vessels. Without building new vessels that tap into a new blood supply, the cancer has no way of getting nutrients or oxygen and dies. Several drugs are now in development to try to block VEGF in order to cut off the tumor's blood supply. Because the growth of new blood vessels is called angiogenesis, these drugs are known as antiangiogenesis drugs.

The most successful compound to prevent VEGF function in colorectal cancer has been bevacizumab (Avastin). Bevacizumab is a monoclonal antibody, similar to the ones our bodies make to fight infection, designed to specifically attach where VEGF normally does, thereby preventing VEGF from working.

A recent study showed that when combined, chemotherapy and bevacizumab may shrink tumor size and increase survival time of patients with advanced colorectal cancers. The next step in the testing of bevacizumab will be to see whether these antiangiogenesis drugs can prevent recurrence of colorectal cancer in patients who have had surgery for less advanced cancers.

Figure 13.1 Epidermal Growth Factor (EGF) and Cetuximab (Erbitux)

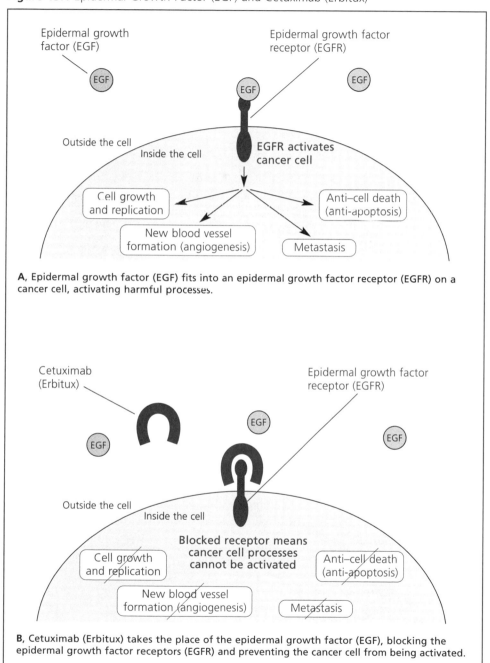

A, Epidermal growth factor (EGF) fits into an epidermal growth factor receptor (EGFR) on a cancer cell, activating harmful processes.

B, Cetuximab (Erbitux) takes the place of the epidermal growth factor (EGF), blocking the epidermal growth factor receptors (EGFR) and preventing the cancer cell from being activated.

Immunotherapy

The immune system defends the body against disease, infection, and foreign substances. The aim of immunotherapy is to find a way to help a person's immune system to recognize the cancer as a foreign invader that needs to be destroyed, just as it does bacteria, viruses, and other infections. To date, these methods have been extremely promising in laboratories but have not proven very effective when used in people with cancer.

Immune Stimulators: Interferon-α and Interleukin-2

The two most common substances used to boost the immune response to cancer are interferon-a (which goes by many trade names, including a-interferon, Actimmune, Alferon N, Avonex, IFN-a, Interferon-a 2a, Interferon-a 2b, Intron A, Roferon A, but is widely referred to as IFL) and interleukin-2 (sold as Aldesleukin or Proleukin; generally known as IL-2). Both IFN and IL-2 have been used to treat colorectal cancer.

Although some patients with metastatic colorectal cancer have shown a significant response to IFN therapy, on the whole the additional benefit of interferon has proven to be minimal. *Given the debilitating side effects and disappointing results, IFN is no longer being pursued as a treatment for colorectal cancer.*

Vaccine Therapy: Edrecolomab and Cea-Vac

To explain how cancer vaccines work, let's take the familiar example of a vaccine against the polio virus. The vaccine, the liquid actually in the shot, is made up of the polio virus that has been killed and so is not able to grow. Though harmless, it is still seen as a foreign invader, and the immune system generates its normal response to attack and kill this harmless virus. This powerful immune response creates cells and antibodies specifically primed to attack the polio virus. Once generated, the immune system remembers this response so that when infected with the real, harmful virus, the body is already prepared to isolate and kill it before it causes illness.

The idea of using vaccines to fight disease is not new, although scientists have only recently begun to explore the possibility of specific antitumor vaccines. One such antitumor vaccine is called edrecolomab; it is based on a molecule found on colorectal cancer cells, ep-cam, that works to keep cells attached to one another. When analyzed in blood samples from people with colorectal cancer, edrecolomab has repeatedly induced the desired type of immune reaction. *Unfortunately, clinical results have been disappointing, and further development of this vaccine has been abandoned.*

218

The second molecule to be targeted for vaccine-based immunotherapy is carcinoembryonic antigen (CEA), which is familiar to some as a colorectal cancer tumor marker. It is found on normal cells but appears more abundantly on many colorectal cancers. After immunization with a CEA-like molecule called Cea-Vac, an immune response has been repeatedly demonstrated in the lab, as with edrecolomab. Clinical trials with this therapy are still in the early stages.

Many other molecules could be used as targets for vaccine-based immune therapy in colorectal cancer. The trouble, however, does not seem to be in getting the body to produce an immune response from the vaccines, but rather in making the immune response have a meaningful affect on the outcome of cancer. Perhaps these therapies will end up being useful not in treatment but in prevention of cancer.

Gene-Based Therapies

Genes are sections of DNA that encode, or carry the blueprint, for a given trait. A change in the normal order of the basic units of the DNA, the genetic code, is called a mutation. When a gene becomes mutated it no longer carries the proper blueprint.

The goal of gene therapy is to give cancerous cells with mutated genes a healthy copy of the gene to restore normal balance and function. Scientists working with gene therapy take active viruses, render them harmless, and insert a copy of the gene they want restored into the virus. This new virus that carries a normal copy of a human gene is then injected into a person who has a gene mutation. If it all works, the virus infects the cells that are missing that gene and puts the new, normal copy into the person's DNA. The next time that gene is used to make a molecule, the normal blueprint has been restored, and the cell regains its normal function.

p53 Adenovirus and Onyx Virus

In colorectal cancer, a few genes are commonly mutated and, at least in part, cause cancer. One gene mutation found in about half of cancers, including colorectal cancer, is a mutation in the gene for the protein p53. Normally, when a cell's DNA is damaged, or any other critical imbalance happens, p53 keeps the cell from multiplying and growing until that damage can be repaired, or if the damage is too great, p53 sets cell death in motion. Cells that lack p53 continue to grow and multiply regardless of cell damage.

In this case, an adenovirus (a virus that causes respiratory tract and eye infections in humans and birds) is altered and used to replace the missing or defective p53 with functional p53. This has been successful enough in the laboratory to move into human trials.

Another novel approach to the absence of p53 in colorectal cancer is the Onyx virus. The Onyx virus may infect both normal cell and cancer cells, but it can multiply in cancer cells only. Once the virus replicates and makes new viruses within the cell it causes the cancer cell to die, while the normal cells remain unharmed. The Onyx virus has been deemed safe in early phase clinical trials and shows promise, although more study is needed.

Another way to take advantage of gene therapy techniques currently in early stages of testing is to use viruses to deliver genes that make a cancer susceptible to a drug that normally would be harmless. The goal is to provide a mechanism that takes a harmless substance and turns it into a chemotherapy drug, and to apply this mechanism only to cancer cells.

Given the high number of abnormal genes in cancer, many more exciting gene-based strategies are certain to emerge.

Lots of Progress, Still No Magic Bullet

We have moved into a new phase in the study of cancer treatments. These molecularly targeted, immune, and gene-based approaches tackle cancer therapy from a new angle, working more within the confines of the human body's delicate cellular balance to correct missing or damaged genes at the source of the cancer, rather than killing both cancerous and normal cells as traditional chemotherapy and radiation therapy do.

The success story of the newer drug imatinib (Gleevec), a drug that targets the exact gene defect in chronic myelogenous leukemia and puts most patients into remission, brought hope to all cancer patients that any one of these new targeted therapies could be the next magic bullet. Unfortunately, colorectal cancer and most other nonblood cancers result from not just one defect but multiple mutations and molecular imbalances acquired over a long time. For that reason, while the logic and laboratory successes behind many of these new therapies make it seem that any one of these could certainly cure cancer, in practice that has not been the case. With all of the mistakes that lead a cell to become cancerous, it is likely that scientists will need to use a number of different approaches in combination—including newer therapies and traditional surgery, chemotherapy, and radiation—to make a real impact on the course of cancer.

CHAPTER FOURTEEN

COMPLEMENTARY AND ALTERNATIVE MEDICINE

Barrie R. Cassileth, PhD

Andrew Vickers, PhD

K. Simon Yeung, MBA, MS, RPh, LAc

In recent years, American consumers have become more and more interested in complementary and alternative approaches to medical care. Complementary and alternative medicine (CAM) is a general term used to describe a wide variety of unrelated healing techniques outside the realm of conventional medicine generally practiced in the United States, everything from herbs to yoga, acupuncture to massage, special diets to oxygen therapy. Most people think of CAM as anything other than mainstream medical care.

Some of these treatments can help improve symptoms or side effects and others may have no discernable effect. However, some complementary and alternative treatments may interfere with standard cancer treatment and some can cause you serious harm. Because of this, you should *talk to your doctor about any CAM therapy you are considering*. In addition, you should know from the outset that *no complementary or alternative medicine slows or halts the growth or spread of cancer*.

> "My oncology team, they were so supportive [of my desire to use complementary therapies]. They were like, 'Well, you know, we don't have a lot of research that proves this to be a real big help. But if it makes you feel better, please, these specific therapies are not going to hurt you, go ahead and continue.'"
>
> —KIM

With that said, you may be interested in learning about complementary treatments that could help improve your symptoms or sense of well being, or you may be concerned about alternative medicines (such as dietary supplements advertised on the Internet or treatments administered at special clinics) that are falsely promoted as "miracle cures" for cancer in general or colorectal cancer specifically. This chapter will explain the difference between complementary and alternative treatments and give you a better understanding of which approaches might help and which are dangerous to your health.

What Is the Difference Between Complementary and Alternative Treatments?

The most important thing to ensure your safety is to understand the difference between *complementary* and *alternative* approaches. Complementary therapies, meant to be *used along with* traditional medicine, can effectively relieve many symptoms associated with cancer and cancer treatment. Alternative cancer treatments, promoted as a viable treatment option or for use *instead of* mainstream care, are *not* effective. They can cause side effects, and they tend to be extremely expensive while offering no benefit. In addition to these drawbacks, when patients forego conventional cancer treatment to try an alternative approach, they postpone the proven benefit of surgery, chemotherapy, and radiation therapy while their cancer continues to grow.

The body is a delicate machine and cancer is a complicated disease. *When considering the use of any complementary and alternative approaches to medical care, be sure to consult your health care team.*

What Are Complementary Treatments?

Complementary therapies are used in addition to standard medical treatment to reduce symptoms and improve quality of life. As the name suggests, they are designed to complement conventional methods. Examples of complementary therapies include acupuncture, hypnosis, imagery/visualization, massage, meditation, music therapy, relaxation, T'ai Chi, and yoga.

You may also hear the term integrative medicine. Hospitals and other health facilities that offer integrative medicine combine conventional medical treatments with complementary therapies that have been scientifically proven to be safe and effective.

Common and Effective Complementary Therapies

Research shows that complementary therapies can effectively decrease some of the symptoms and side effects of conventional cancer treatment (such as pain, anxiety and depression, and nausea and vomiting). Many complementary methods are safe, effective, and evidence-based. However, *complementary methods do not directly alter the growth or spread of cancer.*

If you are curious about any complementary therapy listed below, talk to your health care team. They can provide additional information and can refer you to qualified professionals who deliver these complementary treatments.

You should also investigate your insurance coverage before proceeding; many policies do not cover complementary therapies.

> *"Besides the usual treatment methods (surgery, chemotherapy and radiation), we now have other methods that can be used to complement the medical treatment you are receiving. Some of these include reflexology, massages, healing touch or other forms of energy work, guided imagery and meditation. There may be more, but these are the ones that I have tried and find are very relaxing and help me feel better."*
>
> —KRIS

Mind-Body Therapies

Mind-body therapies can relieve stress and enhance quality of life through relaxation. One popular relaxation technique, known as progressive muscle relaxation, involves tensing and relaxing of muscles. Another is meditation, which focuses on conscious attempts to calm the mind and body. Hypnosis is the induction of a deeply relaxed state followed by the use of suggestion. Visualization and imagery techniques involve the use of visual images, such as a mountain or peaceful beach scene, to enhance relaxation.

Patients can learn mind-body techniques to use during stressful situations, such as before surgery or to help reduce symptoms such as pain or nausea.

Acupuncture and Acupressure

Acupuncture is the insertion of tiny needles into the skin to help treat symptoms. Traditional Chinese medical theory is based in the Taoist concept of yin and yang and the flow of energy through the body, but today we understand acupuncture in terms of its effects on the nervous system. Acupuncture treatment is not painful; indeed, it is generally very relaxing, and is commonly used by patients with cancer to lessen symptoms such as pain and nausea.

Similar to the Chinese art of acupuncture, acupressure uses finger pressure applied in a massage-like fashion rather than needles to treat anxiety and stress, headaches, and nausea.

Therapeutic Massage

Massage is the manipulation of the soft tissue of whole or partial body areas to induce general improvements in health, such as relaxation or improved sleep, or specific physical benefits, such as relief of muscular aches and pains. Reflexology is a special type of massage given to the feet. Reiki is a form of light touch massage. Seek out a certified massage therapist who has experience working with patients with cancer. Research shows that light-touch massage is safe, pleasant, and beneficial for patients with cancer and relieves pain, fatigue, anxiety, and depression.

Music Therapy

Music therapy is the controlled use of music for clinical benefit. Although it is ideally provided live by trained therapists, music therapy often takes the form of recorded music. Music has been shown to be very effective for helping anxiety and depression.

Movement Therapies

Yoga is a philosophy and exercise system that combines movement and simple poses with deep breathing and meditation to promote relaxation and to reduce fatigue. T'ai Chi is an ancient Chinese practice in which sequences of movements are performed slowly, softly, and gracefully. The meditative nature of the exercises fosters relaxation and develops balance, alignment, fine-scale motor control, and rhythm of movement.

Complementary Treatments for Symptoms and Side Effects

Complementary techniques can help relieve a variety of symptoms and side effects caused by cancer or its treatments.

Complementary Treatments for Pain

The most common complementary therapies for cancer-related pain include mind-body techniques such as hypnosis and relaxation therapy, acupuncture, and therapeutic massage, and there is good evidence from clinical studies that all can be effective. Mind-body techniques are particularly useful because once they are learned, people with cancer can use the techniques themselves at any time.

Massage can have an immediate and dramatic effect on cancer-related pain, although it is not known how long the effects of treatment last, and many patients require regular treatment. Acupuncture, on the other hand, seems to have longer-lasting effects. Massage and acupuncture can be good treatment options when pain is not well managed by medication.

Complementary Treatments for Anxiety and Depression

Meditation has been shown to reduce anxiety and depression. Relaxation therapies have been shown to help both the short-term anxiety associated with treatment of cancer or a diagnostic procedure and the long-term anxiety common in many people with cancer. Clinical studies also show that massage reduces anxiety and depression, and that music therapy can dramatically improve mood. Acupressure can also help with stress and anxiety.

Complementary Treatments for Nausea and Vomiting

Although medicines to treat nausea and vomiting associated with chemotherapy have improved substantially in recent years, some patients still experience these distressing symptoms. Acupuncture is an effective treatment for nausea and vomiting. It can cut the rate of postoperative vomiting and may help with chemotherapy-related problems. Acupuncture appears to work best when given before chemotherapy; its effects seem to last about eight hours. Commercially available wrist bands that stimulate acupuncture points with a small electric current do not work well, but acupressure on the inner side of the forearm about an inch above the wrist may provide relief. Chemotherapy-related nausea and vomiting also can be relieved with self-hypnosis or other relaxation techniques.

Herbs and Supplements for the Treatment of Cancer

Herbs and supplements are used by many patients in the hope that they will either help conventional treatments to fight cancer or stave off its return. For example, someone who has undergone surgery and then a course of chemotherapy to treat colorectal cancer might start taking high-dose vitamins or an herb in the hope that this might prevent or delay a recurrence. In general, there is insufficient evidence to support the use of these supplements.

We do know, however, that herbs and supplements can sometimes interfere with chemotherapy, surgery, and radiation therapy. Because of these potentially dangerous interactions, *do not take any herb or supplement without first consulting your health care team, especially when you are actively receiving other cancer treatments.*

Dangers of Herbs and Other Supplements During Cancer Treatment

Herbs and other supplements can interfere with conventional treatments in several ways. Many botanicals may either induce or suppress the action of enzymes used to break down certain chemotherapy agents in the body. This may in turn decrease the cancer-killing effects or increase the toxicity of these drugs. For example, the popular herb St. John's wort has been shown to reduce the level of a chemotherapy drug in the blood by 40 percent.

The use of antioxidants is controversial. Antioxidants you may be familiar with include vitamins A, C, and E and supplements such as selenium. Many herbs, including garlic and gingko, also have antioxidant properties. Laboratory and clinical studies have had mixed results; some suggest that antioxidants can increase the effects of treatments such as radiation and chemotherapy. Other data suggest that antioxidants may actually be harmful. More study is needed in this area and research is ongoing.

Dietary supplements may also cause problems, especially during surgery. For example, garlic supplements and vitamin E have anticoagulant (blood-thinning) effects and can cause excessive bleeding during and after surgery. Botanicals that have stimulant effects (such as ma huang and guarana) or sedative effects (such as kava kava and St. John's wort) may potentially affect the action of anesthetic drugs. Some botanical supplements, including angelica, have been known to make the skin more sensitive to radiation, increasing the damage to healthy skin tissue during radiation therapy.

Here are some good basic guidelines to follow:

- Do not use herbs for children or if you are pregnant or breast-feeding unless your doctor tells you that they are safe.
- Stop all herbs one to two weeks before surgery, because they may interact with anesthesia or interfere with normal blood clotting.
- Avoid herbs if you are on chemotherapy because some have serious interactions with chemotherapy.
- Ask your radiation oncologist about any herbs you are taking before you begin radiation therapy. Some make the skin extra sensitive and may cause burns.

The following herbal products can have serious toxic effects and should be avoided:

- aloe
- cascara
- chaparral tea
- chaste tree berry
- chomper
- comfrey
- germanium
- kava
- pau d'arco
- pennyroyal
- licorice
- lobella
- ephedra (also called ma huang)
- plantain leaves
- St. John's wort (also called hypericum)
- yohimbe

Ask your health care team questions about other herbs and additional complementary and alternative therapies, or go to http://www.mskcc.org/AboutHerbs. Be sure to let your health care team know about all of the herbs, supplements, and over-the-counter medicines you are taking. They can help you incorporate the safe use of complementary therapies into your cancer treatment.

Common Herbs and Supplements

The use of herbs and supplements fall into the category of nutritional therapeutics and complex natural products. While it is true that many conventional cancer treatment drugs are derived from plant sources (such as paclitaxel, a chemotherapy agent based on a substance found in the Pacific yew tree), herbal medicines (or botanicals) differ from other pharmaceutical agents because they include whole plants or parts of the plant, rather than a single constituent, and because producers of these products are not required to prove safety and effectiveness.

The term dietary supplement is used to describe vitamins, minerals, animal products such as shark cartilage, and chemicals naturally found in the body, such as melatonin.

Some popular herbs and supplements are described here.

Beta-Glucans

Many mushrooms and fungi used widely in Asia contain chemicals called beta-glucans (also written as β-glucans). These have been studied for their effects on cancer. The largest study of beta-glucans used an extract of "polysaccharide Kureha" or PSK for short. Several good studies found that PSK given at the same time as chemotherapy improve survival in patients who have had surgery for colorectal cancer. PSK and other mushroom products are currently being studied, and they are widely available in the United States.

Carotenoids

Some epidemiology studies suggest that a diet high in beta-carotene (also written as β-carotene, a substance from which vitamin A is formed that is found in yellow and orange fruits, vegetables such as papaya and carrot, and green leafy vegetables) and lutein (a nutrient abundant in spinach that is also found in peaches, squash, kale, broccoli, and egg yolks) may help reduce the risk of colorectal cancer. However, no clinical data indicate that carotenoids can be used effectively as cancer treatment, and research suggests that beta-carotene supplements may produce negative effects.

Essiac

Essiac was originally developed in Canada and has been widely available for decades. It is also marketed as Flor-Essence and usually consumed as a tea. This product contains four herbs (burdock root, rhubarb, sorrel, and slippery elm) and has been promoted as a treatment for cancer and Acquired Immune Deficiency Syndrome (AIDS). However, no data or published clinical studies show efficacy for any claims made.

Green Tea

Interest in green tea as a cancer treatment agent originated from research showing lower rates of various cancers, particularly colorectal cancer, in Chinese and Japanese green tea drinkers. Green tea and some of its active components are under study as possible methods of preventing cancer, but it appears unlikely that green tea or its extracts can affect established disease.

High-Dose Vitamin C

In the 1970s and 1980s, Nobel prize winner Linus Pauling claimed that vitamin C in very high doses could help treat cancer. Because of intense public interest, clinical studies (including one that enrolled patients with advanced colorectal cancer) have compared high dose vitamin C with a placebo (an inactive substance containing no medicine), but there was no difference in survival.

Laetrile

Laetrile, a compound extracted from the pits of apricots and related plants, was an extremely popular alternative cancer treatment in the 1960s and 1970s. However, large studies showed no benefit, and a number of study participants experienced side effects related to the cyanide content of laetrile. *Laetrile is therefore not only ineffective but also toxic.* After the clinical trial, the sale of laetrile was banned in the United States and it fell out of use. However, this product has regained popularity in the last few years, at least partly because of active promotion by distributors. Often termed "vitamin B17" or sold as amygdalin, laetrile is available via the Internet and outside the United States.

Melatonin

Melatonin is a hormone naturally made by the body that regulates sleeping and waking. It is widely available as a dietary supplement and is used to treat insomnia and jet lag.

Because melatonin may affect cell growth, it has been suggested as a treatment for cancer. Several clinical studies have shown encouraging results for melatonin, but more study is needed before it should be used for cancer treatment.

Mistletoe

Mistletoe is a poisonous shrub with leathery leaves and white berries. Mistletoe extracts, widely known by the trade names Iscador, Helixor, and Eurixor, are popular cancer treatments in Europe and are used in some mainstream European cancer clinics. Laboratory and animal studies suggest mistletoe extract may stimulate the immune system to fight cancer. However, such effects cannot be duplicated in humans, and several clinical studies using an injectable form of mistletoe extract have produced disappointing results.

Shark Cartilage

Shark cartilage became popular as a treatment for patients with cancer after the publication of a book called *Sharks Don't Get Cancer*. Actually, sharks do get cancer. Some components in shark cartilage may inhibit the formation of new blood vessels that supply tumor growth; as a result, sharks do not appear to develop cancer as often as humans. Unrefined shark cartilage products typically found in health stores and on the Internet have not proved beneficial in a clinical trial. A pharmaceutical-grade extract showed promising results in clinical studies but will not be available to patients until completion of a current study.

What Are Alternative Treatments?

Unlike conventional medicine, which uses therapies that have been scientifically proven to be effective, *there is little or no evidence for the effectiveness of alternative methods*. In fact, many alternative treatments can be harmful and dangerous to your health.

Alternative therapies for cancer typically involve diets, vitamins, and unusual drugs; are often touted as "cures"; and are delivered at special clinics that may be located outside the United States to avoid usual regulations that govern the safety of drugs and the training of medical staff. Despite their ambitious claims, clinical studies have generally shown that these alternative therapies are ineffective.

Fraudulent Claims and Pseudoscience

Alternative therapies often involve unusual ideas. For example, one alternative cancer center's treatment is based on the claim that cancer is caused by a particular bacterium, an idea popular in the early 19th century. Not only is this idea inconsistent with current understanding of how cancer develops but also the bacterium in question is imaginary: it has not been described by anyone outside that clinic.

Another group of promoters of alternative therapies states that cancer is caused by the lack of a vitamin they term "B17." Yet, there is no such a vitamin; the name was an invention by promoters of the disproved and FDA-banned product called laetrile or amygdalin.

The Dangers of Alternative Treatments

Alternative methods often are used by people with cancer instead of conventional treatment. Conventional cancer treatments are potentially life-saving, so a decision to use alternative therapies in place of conventional care is literally a matter of life and death.

There is essentially no scientific evidence that alternative cancer treatments actually help patients. In fact, where studies have been conducted, alternative therapies have not been shown to have a positive effect on how long patients lived, and they often led to poorer quality of life. Nonetheless, alternative cancer "cures" are used worldwide.

Alternative Treatments: Buyer Beware!

Many patients are now discovering alternative cancer treatments via the Internet and are often attracted by the claim that cancer can be cured "naturally" or using techniques that are gentler than those used by doctors practicing conventional medicine. But buyer beware!

Avoid sources of information that also sell products, because they may make false or unsupported claims just to get your money. Stay with objective sources that can guide you best. The following resources provide reliable information on complementary and alternative treatments that is regularly updated:

- American Cancer Society (http://www.cancer.org/docroot/ETO/ETO_5.asp?sitearea=ETO)
- Memorial Sloan-Kettering Cancer Center "About Herbs" web site (http://www.mskcc.org/aboutherbs)
- National Center for Complementary and Alternative Medicine (http://nccam.nih.gov/)
- NIH Office of Dietary Supplements (http://dietary-supplements.info.nih.gov)
- Quackwatch (http://www.quackwatch.org/)
- University of Texas MD Anderson web site (http://www.mdanderson.org/departments/CIMER/)
- US Pharmacopeia (http://www.usp.org/USPVerified/dietarySupplements/)
- USDA Food and Nutrition Information Center (http://www.nal.usda.gov/fnic/)

When searching for information, it is important to consider its source. Avoid unknown sources and rely on those in which you have trust and confidence.

Avoid any treatment that involves the following:

- the treatment is promoted for use instead of conventional care
- using the therapy requires a change in mainstream cancer care
- there is a risk of serious toxicity without documented benefit
- using the treatment requires significant travel or financial cost

When in doubt, ask your doctor for guidance.

Toxicity

Not only are many of these alternative treatments not helpful but also they can cause serious harm. Though alternative cancer treatments are generally advertised as "gentle," "natural," and "safe," they can cause serious side effects. Some of these are exactly the same symptoms the patient may be trying to avoid from conventional treatment.

Side effects reported from alternative cancer treatments include nausea and vomiting, coma, headache, constipation, fatigue, confusion, sedation, heart problems, shortness of breath, and severe infections. Deaths have also been reported.

Cost

The treatments at alternative clinics can be very expensive. Costs of several thousand dollars per month running into tens of thousands of dollars per year are not unusual. Certain clinics charge a substantial fee at the start of treatment.

Health insurance does not cover alternative treatments.

Travel

Using alternative cancer treatment often means travelling great distances, which can be expensive. Treatment can lasts for weeks at a time, so food and lodging alone can become very expensive. In some cases, treatment requires follow-up visits every few weeks. This can add to the expense.

Lack of Supportive Care

People who travel great distances seeking care at alternative clinics must spend many weeks away from the love and support of family and friends.

In addition, patients who use alternative cancer clinics are not only delaying or forsaking proven cancer treatments, such as surgery, chemotherapy, and radiotherapy, but also a wide variety of supportive care services provided by cancer hospitals. For example, pain management is a common problem for patients with cancer. Cancer hospitals have specially trained doctors and other clinicians who are very experienced in treating cancer-related pain and in managing the side effects of pain medications. Such services are not generally available at alternative cancer clinics.

Some Higher Profile Alternative Cancer Therapies

Unfortunately, there are a wide variety of alternative therapies being falsely promoted as cancer cures to unsuspecting patients. Space limitations prevent us from including an exhaustive list in this chapter, but we'll look at a few of the most common ones in the next sections.

Burzynski and Antineoplastons

Stanislaw Burzynski, MD, is a doctor who treats cancer using what he terms "antineoplastons." These are mixtures of simple chemicals isolated from blood and urine that he claims promote the body's natural defenses against cancer. Burzynski has conducted his own research on antineoplastons, but his clinical studies do not meet the usual scientific criteria for such studies. Despite disappointing results from these studies, which were not sanctioned by the National Cancer Institute, the Burzynski Clinic's web site claims that the NCI has "replicated and expanded Dr. Burzynski's work." Great caution must be exercised in accepting such statements.

Electromagnetic Therapies

A variety of alternative cancer cures, including BioResonance Therapy, the Cell Com system, and the Rife machine, are based on the belief that cancer and other diseases are caused by disruptions of the body's electromagnetic fields. Proponents of electromagnetic therapies claim that these disruptions can be corrected using magnets or specific high-frequency electromagnetic waves, leading to cure. While there are no clinical studies of electromagnetic therapy for cancer, it appears highly unlikely that they could be effective: there is currently no good reason to believe that the devices used in these alternative clinics control cancer, and the basis for the therapy is fanciful and incorrect.

Metabolic Therapies

Metabolic therapies are based on the belief that cancer is a symptom of the accumulation of toxins. The aim of treatment is to "detoxify" using special diets, raw juices, enzymes and supplements. Treatment may also involve colonic irrigation and coffee enemas (cleaning the bowels by passing warm water or coffee into the large intestine through the rectum). Some higher-profile metabolic therapies are Gerson, Kelley/Gonzalez, and Livingston-Wheeler therapies. There have been several clinical studies of metabolic therapies, but their research designs have been flawed, and the reported positive results were incomplete and misleading. Nonetheless, a clinical trial funded by the National Institutes of Health is currently under way.

Oxygen Therapies

Proponents of oxygen therapy start from the science-based premise that tumors are often somewhat oxygen depleted. However, they go on to suggest that cancer cells cannot survive in an oxygen-rich environment and that unusual methods can be used to increase the amount of oxygen in the blood and thus kill cancer cells. These methods include injected oxygen directly into the blood; "ozone autohemotherapy," in which blood is removed, bubbled with ozone, and reinjected; and various types of "oxygenated" water, pills, and solutions.

There is no sound evidence that these techniques have an important effect on the amount of oxygen in the blood, let alone any effect on tumor cells. Nonetheless, they remain popular, despite reports of serious side effects, including death.

Hyperbaric oxygen therapy (a treatment in which the patient is enclosed in a pressure chamber, breathing oxygen at a pressure greater than one atmosphere) is a proven treatment for several conditions, including carbon monoxide poisoning and the "bends," a disorder sometimes suffered by deep-sea divers. It is being studied as a possible treatment for cancer in the belief that it can improve the effects of treatments such as radiotherapy. It is not a treatment for cancer on its own and should be avoided outside of a carefully conducted clinical trial.

The Purported Power of Positive Thinking

Many people, doctors and scientists included, believe that the health of the mind and body are linked. Although there is probably some truth in the cliché, "healthy body, healthy mind," or the importance of "keeping a positive attitude," some people have taken the extreme position that a person's state of mind can affect whether they live or die from cancer. Deepak Chopra, for example, who is a popular writer on complementary and alternative medicine, has written that patients with cancer can "control the course of the disease by using thoughts." Another popular figure is Bernie Siegel, who runs supports groups for "Exceptional Cancer Patients" in an attempt to strengthen their "will to live" and improve their rates of survival.

The idea that the mind can affect cancer is enormously appealing, because it gives us control over what is often a random, arbitrary, and terrifying disease. The best evidence, however, suggests that attitude does not have an important role in stopping or slowing the growth or spread of cancer. Not only is the idea that people can overcome cancer through the power of positive thinking unsupported, it advances a destructive "blame-the-victim" mentality, suggesting that is it is the patient's fault when cancer is diagnosed or when it advances. The health benefits of a positive outlook may include better mood, less pain, and improved quality of life (all important results), but a good attitude will not prevent or cure cancer.

Questions to Ask About Complementary and Alternative Treatments

When evaluating any complementary or alternative method, consider the following issues:

- What is my medical team's experience with complementary and alternative methods?
- What claims are made for the treatment? For example, does it reportedly cure the cancer, enable the conventional treatment to work better, or relieve symptoms or side effects?
- How does this treatment work and what does it involve?
- What are the credentials of those supporting the treatment? Are they recognized experts in cancer treatment? Have they published their findings in trustworthy medical journals?
- How is the method promoted? Is it promoted only on the Internet or in the mass media (books, magazines, TV, and radio talk shows) rather than in scientific journals?
- What are the costs of the therapy?
- Does my hospital or medical facility offer this method? Is the method widely available for use within the health care community, or is it controlled, with limited access to its use?
- Where can I go to find out more about this approach? Are there any books or videos about this method that my medical team can recommend?
- Will this technique help ease my pain or decrease my anxiety?
- How do I find a licensed or trained practitioner of this method?
- Which complementary and alternative methods should I avoid?
- Which method would my health care provider most highly recommend?
- Will my insurance cover this complementary or alternative method?

Do What's Best for Your Body

Some complementary treatments, such as acupuncture and acupressure, massage, and relaxation therapies, can help reduce symptoms, relieve side effects, and improve quality of life for people with cancer. However, complementary therapies do not prevent or cure cancer or even slow its growth. Many cancer centers now provide evidence-based complementary therapies along with mainstream cancer treatment.

Alternative cancer treatments promoted for use instead of mainstream cancer care are not effective and may be expensive, difficult to obtain, and/or dangerous. Their claims for efficacy by definition are anecdotal, fraudulent, or unproven by controlled scientific studies.

Pay special attention to the dangers associated with the use of herbs and other dietary supplements during cancer treatment, as they can interfere with chemotherapy, radiation therapy, and surgery.

The bottom line: *ask your doctor about any CAM therapy you want to know more about before proceeding.* Use the questions listed in the box on page 235 to help guide your conversation.

CHAPTER FIFTEEN

STRATEGIES FOR COPING WITH SYMPTOMS AND SIDE EFFECTS

Brenda K. Shelton, MS, RN, CCRN, AOCN

Cancer in the colon or rectum or its treatment can affect all aspects of your life, from your physical health to your emotional well being. This chapter will give you a broad overview of how to cope with these physical and emotional changes, but we encourage you to discuss your specific situation with your health care team. Many of these side effects can be effectively treated with small lifestyle adjustments and/or medication, so it is important to monitor your symptoms and report them to ensure you receive the best care possible. The more information you provide, the more helpful your doctor can be finding the best treatments.

Certain common symptoms and side effects are present in almost all people with cancer and those receiving cancer treatment. We'll discuss these most common symptoms first, looking at the differences in these symptoms after different kinds of therapy. Then we'll look at symptoms and side effects specifically associated with colorectal cancer. Finally, we'll discuss the potential side effects of

> *"Side effects will occur with your treatment. DO tell your doctor about them. Don't be a martyr (I tried this a couple times, figuring I could weather it out). They have medications that will help tame these side effects! It makes life much easier, even if it doesn't completely eliminate the side effects. I was able to control them most days and continue working."*
>
> —KRIS

Questions to Ask Your Health Care Team About Potential Side Effects of Your Cancer and Its Treatment

- What are the common side effects of this treatment?
- Is there anything I can do to lower my risk of getting these effects?
- When can I expect them to start, and when will they end?
- If these side effects occur, how will they be treated?
- What services or programs are available to help me cope with these side effects?
- Are there any unusual but serious side effects I should watch for?
- How severe should any side effect be for me to call the doctor's office?
- Which of these side effects help decide if I get my next treatment as planned?
- If my side effects are severe, what can we do to prevent or decrease them for the next therapy?

different treatment options, including effects of surgery, radiation therapy, chemotherapy, and biological therapy. Advanced cancer may cause additional complications, which we'll discuss at the end of this chapter.

In all cases, our focus is helping you understand these physical or emotional changes, and providing the practical information you need to effectively manage them. Again, work closely with your health care team—they can help reduce your discomfort and improve your quality of life.

Common Effects of Cancer or Cancer Therapies

Although everyone's experience with cancer is different, there are some common symptoms and side effects that many people experience. These can be the result of the cancer itself or can be caused by the therapy you receive to treat the cancer.

Knowing that these general effects occur in many people for different reasons will help you to understand the differences you feel in your body.

The most frequent symptoms described by people with cancer are fatigue, pain, depression, and problems sleeping. Most people with cancer—regardless of the type—will experience all of these general effects to some degree. You should consider how these physical changes might affect your normal activities and daily routine and, if you can, make plans to have extra help and support available. For example, you may need to request time off from work or flexible work hours or ask your partner or children to pitch in with household responsibilities while you recover from treatment.

Planning ahead and being aware of potential side effects may also help you catch them early and reduce their effect. For example, mild pain is much easier to manage than severe pain and is most easily treated if addressed before it becomes severe.

Knowing what to expect may also help you to cope. For example, if you are feeling depressed, it may help to know that many people with cancer experience depression, that depression as a result of cancer and its treatment is nothing to be ashamed of, and that your health care team has many resources, including medication and counseling, to help treat depression.

See page 238 for a list of questions to ask your doctor about potential side effects.

Fatigue

Fatigue is the most common symptom reported by people with cancer. Fatigue is a feeling of being overwhelmingly tired or drained of energy. It usually involves more than physical tiredness and extends to feeling exhausted mentally and emotionally as well. Fatigue can be present at the time when cancer is diagnosed, but it can also occur as a result of different cancer therapies. There are several theories of why fatigue occurs, but doctors haven't yet been able to pinpoint a specific cause for this generalized cancer fatigue, which can make it difficult to decide upon the best treatment.

Fatigue that occurs with surgery is usually the shortest, lasting until the body recovers from anesthesia and begins to heal. Chemotherapy-related fatigue may last up to about three weeks when the chemotherapy is given over just a few days, but persists longer when chemotherapy is given into the vein continuously. It may clear up sooner with

> *"The fatigue has been probably the worst for me. I have to stop what I'm doing and rest, and that bothers me. I've always been very active, very healthy. And just vacuuming one room, I have to stop, sit down, rest. I've had to take one or two naps each day, just to get through the day, and then sleep at night. It's much more than I normally would sleep."*
> —JACY

chemotherapy medications that do not reduce blood counts. Fatigue caused by radiation therapy begins in about the third week and lasts until several weeks after it ends. Biologic therapy is notable for the development of fatigue that begins early in treatment and lasts for weeks to months after it ends.

When you feel fatigued, almost all other parts of your life are affected. Unlike the fatigue that people normally experience, rest or sleep does not relieve the fatigue of cancer and cancer treatment. You may find yourself sleeping more, or sleeping during the day, and still not feeling rested upon waking. The feeling of tiredness interferes with your concentration, your ability to make decisions, and coping in general. Factors that can worsen fatigue include anemia, emotional distress, inadequate nutrition or hydration, infection, medications, pain, prolonged low activity level, and sleeplessness.

Managing Fatigue

Feeling fatigued may be unavoidable, but there are things you can do to decrease its impact on your life. First are things to actually reduce your amount or severity of fatigue. Think of these as the things you do to counteract the effect before or as it occurs.

- Talk to your health care team about the possible causes of your fatigue and how long it will last.
- Talk to your health care team about medications that may help reduce fatigue.
- Eat a nutritious, well-balanced diet.
- Avoid excessive sugar or caffeine if possible. Their effects on your energy level are often short-lived and make you feel more tired when they wear off.
- Drink plenty of fluids. Do not allow yourself to become dehydrated; not having enough fluids and electrolytes (or minerals) will worsen your fatigue.
- Plan quiet, distracting, and entertaining activities such as reading, coloring, painting, or listening to calming music or tapes or CDs designed for relaxation.
- Some people believe that certain aromas can enhance energy levels. Aromatherapy with oils or candles smelling like peppermint, citrus, or other energizing substances may be helpful. (All complementary therapies should first be reviewed by your doctor to make certain they will not interfere with your treatment. See chapter 14.)

Second are activities that conserve energy so that you are not too fatigued to do the things you enjoy and value the most.

- List your usual activities and prioritize the ones that are most important that you do.
  - Give away some activities to other people.

240

- Consider asking friends and family to help with errands or assisting with meals.
  - Consider hiring assistance for heavier duties like household chores or yard work if no family or friends are available.
- Be creative with your problem solving. For example, keeping a cooler full of chilled drinks and nutritious snacks beside the bed or couch can reduce your number of trips to the kitchen.
- Plan rest periods and ask the support of family members to hold these times sacred.
- Maintain a level of light activity on a daily basis to avoid fatigue from inactivity.
- Plan ways to ensure you can get enough rest and sleep. Several shorter rest periods are better than one long rest time.

Pain

Pain is an unpleasant sensation caused by tissue injury or pressure on the nerves. It is one of the most feared and dreaded symptoms associated with cancer. Fortunately, there are many treatment options to reduce and eliminate pain.

For many people with colorectal cancer, pain is one of their symptoms at the time of diagnosis (doctors call this a presenting symptom). As pain recurs, people may be concerned that their disease has come back, although pain has a wide variety of causes. The degree to which a person feels pain or is distressed by it is very individual. Because pain has so many different causes and features, your health care team will ask you to provide a detailed description of the pain and its level of intensity. You should be prepared to offer the following information about your pain:

- What is the severity of your pain on a scale of zero to ten, where "zero" is no pain at all and "ten" is the worst pain imaginable?
- Where is the pain located?
- When did the pain begin?
- How long does the pain last?
- What does the pain feel like? Is it sharp or dull? Is it on the surface, or deep inside the body?
- Does the pain move or "radiate" from one place in the body to another? If so, under what circumstances?
- Do other symptoms occur along with the pain (such as nausea or sweating)?
- What makes the pain better?
- What makes the pain worse?
- How upsetting is the pain?
- How does the pain affect your life?

Ask the health care team questions about what kind of pain to expect, and what solutions will be included in the treatment plan. They should be able to tell you if pain medications will be needed, and suggest other therapies for pain. They can also call upon the services of a pain specialist. It is also important to discuss the level of pain relief that is expected, what you consider an acceptable level of pain, and when to notify the health care team.

Types of Pain

Pain can be described as short-term or long-term depending upon whether it is new or persistent. We know that some types of pain will resolve as the body heals, but other kinds of pain cause permanent changes and last for life. Health care professionals also classify pain by the parts of the body involved: pain in the organs is visceral pain, pain experienced in the skin and soft tissues is somatic pain, and nerve pressure or injury is neuropathic pain. The severity and type of pain will help determine the treatment plan.

Factors That Increase Pain

Pain is a subjective experience that cannot be measured by tests. Because the experience of pain involves personal interpretation of physical sensations, a person must always think of pain as it relates to other symptoms. Pain may be considered tolerable when it is the only symptom a person experiences, but it may be more distressing if a person is also suffering from loss of sleep. Factors that are known to increase people's pain or distress related to the pain include: anxiety, depression, fatigue, fear, hunger, and sleeplessness. Having a lot of concerns and worries such as unpaid bills or childcare problems can increase a person's feelings of pain too.

Try to control the other factors that can contribute to the pain by making sure you eat well, seek help and support if you are depressed or anxious, and rest when necessary.

Managing Pain

The goal of pain management is to prevent, stop, or limit pain symptoms to a level that is acceptable to the person experiencing the pain.

If you are having pain, try to define as many specific features of the pain as you can, including activities that improve or worsen the pain. The doctor will consider your descriptions and perform a physical examination and diagnostic tests to better define factors that may be causing or affecting the pain.

Pain medications (sometimes called analgesics) are prescribed in most instances. Complementary pain management strategies can also help. If pain is related to damage to body tissues or tumors pressing on parts of the body, surgical correction will be considered.

PAIN MEDICATIONS

Medications are used to treat pain in a large number of cases and can be very effective in controlling pain. The choice of pain medication and method of taking it is determined by the cause of the pain, its location, and its severity. Pain medications work in lots of different ways: they can reduce inflammation or swelling, numb affected nerves, alter the brain's interpretation of the pain, and boost the effectiveness of other pain medications. An overview of some common pain medications and cautions are included in Table 15.1 on page 244.

Many people mistakenly believe that they can become addicted to pain medicine if they take it throughout the day and night to relieve their pain. Not all pain medications create physical dependence with continued use. In addition, studies show that people who take the medication they need to relieve pain do not become dependent, and their usage decreases as their pain goes away.

If you are prescribed pain medication, you can ensure it is most effective by following some specific guidelines:

- If pain is ongoing, make sure you take the medication around the clock to prevent pain before it becomes severe. Check with your health care team if you think the medication schedule should be changed. Pain medication is only taken as needed when the pain is reducing or going away.
- Take your pain medication with you on trips and errands so that if you are delayed you can still take the medication on time.
- Keep at least one week's worth of pain medication on hand. This provides extra if you need to have the dose increased, or if something prevents you from getting to the pharmacy.
- Be physically active as much as the pain will permit. Sometimes activity eases pain and sometimes it worsens it. Adjust your activity as needed, but avoid excessive inactivity if possible.
- Ask the health care team for medications to control side effects of pain relievers, such as nausea or constipation, if they occur.
- Rate your pain on a number scale at least once a day to help the health care team determine whether the medication plan is adequate. Also, rate your pain after taking medications ordered for breakthrough pain. This will help the health care team decide how to adjust both the around-the-clock dose and the dose for breakthrough pain.
- Never stop taking pain medication suddenly. Instead, reduce the medication dose gradually under the supervision of your doctor.

Table 15.1 Types of Pain Medication

Type of Pain Medication	Type of Pain	Examples Generic name (Trade names)	Common Side Effects
Nonsteroidal anti-inflammatory medications	Bone pain Mild to moderate discomfort	• naproxen (Aleve) • indomethacin (Indocin, Indocin SR, Indotech) • ketorolac tromethamine (Toradol)	• kidney failure with prolonged use • stomach upset and bleeding
Moderate strength opioids	Moderate to severe discomfort	• oxycodone (Endodan, OxyContin, Percocet, Percodan, Roxiprin)	• constipation
Severe pain opioids	Severe discomfort	• morphine (Astramorph, Duramorph, Infumorph, Kadian Morphine Sulfate Sustained Release, MS Contin, MSIR, Oramorph, Roxanol) • hydromorphone (Dilaudid) • fentanyl (Actiq)	• constipation • nausea • itching
Local anesthetic agents	Local nerve pain	• lidocaine (Xylocaine) • bupivacaine (Marcaine, Sensorcaine)	• itching, tingling, or burning sensation in skin • altered physical sensation and risk for injury
Adjuvants	Neuropathic pain	• Antidepressants, such as amitriptyline hydrochloride (Elavil)	• hypertension
		• Anticonvulsants, such as diphenylhydantoin (Dilantin), carbamazepine (Tegretol), and gabapentin (Neurontin)	• hypotension
	Increase effectiveness of other pain medications	• Dexamethasone (Decadron, Deronil, Dexasone, Dexone, Hexadrol, Mymethasone)	• mood changes • increased appetite • fluid retention • increased blood sugar

Call the health care team if:
- you experience any new or sudden change in pain
- you are unable to take your pain medication or keep it down without vomiting
- the pain is not relieved long enough by the pain medication using the plan prescribed
- you have constipation, nausea, are unable to urinate, have excessive sleepiness, or have confusion

COMPLEMENTARY MANAGEMENT OF PAIN

Complementary nondrug treatments are now widely used to help manage cancer pain. There are many techniques that are used alone or along with medicine. These methods include: relaxation, biofeedback, imagery, distraction, hypnosis, skin stimulation, transcutaneous electric nerve stimulation (TENS), acupuncture, exercise or physical therapy, and emotional support and counseling. You may need the help of health professionals—social workers, physical therapists, psychologists, nurses, or others—to access or learn these techniques. See chapter 14 for more information on complementary therapies.

Depression

After being diagnosed with cancer you may feel that others cannot possibly understand what you are going through, you may feel alone, or you may have concerns that you will be a burden to others. Depression is the feeling of extreme sadness and loss of enjoyment in normally rewarding activities. Depression can interfere with appetite and sleep and can make other symptoms worse.

As many as one in four people with cancer have feelings of depression. These feelings may be related to physical symptoms or they may be a result of dealing with bad news and tough situations. Many people with depression have a specific chemical imbalance causing the symptom, so do not assume that all feelings of depression are psychological or emotional.

It is normal to have short periods of unhappiness, disappointment, and frustration, but when they become frequent, persist over several weeks, or interfere with your ability to take care of yourself, you should seek help from your health care team. If these sad feelings are accompanied by a sense of helplessness, despair, or worthlessness, it may signal serious depression. *If you experience thoughts of death or suicide, or you begin to think about hurting yourself, contact your health care team immediately.*

Managing Depression

Insomnia, excessive sleep, decreased appetite, the inability to enjoy normal activities, erratic changes in temper, or frequent crying spells are early signs of depression. Serious signs of depression may include harming yourself or others. There are many medications and counseling treatments that can help you cope with feelings of depression. Almost all are reimbursed on common medical insurance plans. Here are some strategies to help you manage the effects of depression:
- Discuss the possible benefits of counseling with your health care provider.
- Discuss the potential benefits and risks of antidepressant medications with your health care provider.

- Remember that it is okay to feel sad and frustrated.
- Share your feelings and concerns with someone you trust rather than keeping them inside.
- Be patient with feelings of depression. Allow time for physical symptoms to improve; this may decrease depressive feelings.
- Consider seeking emotional support through internal thoughts that provide you with feelings of peace. This may include prayer, meditation, positive self-talk, or self-hypnosis.
- Engage in calming activities such as massage, deep breathing, and relaxation techniques.
- Explore available support groups and online chat forums.

Problems Sleeping

People with cancer or those undergoing cancer therapy often require more sleep than usual and have trouble finding the right balance of sleep and activity. At the same time, extreme fatigue may lead to daytime sleeping and nighttime wakefulness, worsening sleep problems. For people with colorectal cancer, this may be worsened by the side effects of therapy that interrupt sleep (such as diarrhea), or an infusion device that must remain connected 24 hours a day. Other factors that may interfere with sleep include anxiety, depression, nausea, and pain. Sleep may also be disrupted by certain stimulating medications such as corticosteroids, antinausea medications, or medications used to treat blood pressure, diarrhea, urinary incontinence, and wheezing.

Managing Sleep Disturbance

The following strategies may help reduce the problem of sleeplessness:
- Try to exercise at least once every day.
- During the nighttime, sleep as long as your body wants.
- Avoid stimulants such as coffee, tea, caffeinated sodas, and chocolate for at least 6 hours before bedtime. If sleeplessness persists, you may have to eliminate these items from your diet.
- Drink warm, decaffeinated drinks before bedtime.
- Some suggest the aromas of lavender and vanilla enhance relaxation and aid sleep.
- Some people will tell you that taking melatonin will assist in resetting the sleep-wake cycle, but there is very little research to support its use as a sleep aid, particularly in people receiving cancer treatment. So, if you are considering using melatonin, talk it over with your health care team.

- Take action to ensure you do not have pain at or near bedtime.
- Consider taking a warm bath immediately before bed.
- Have someone rub your feet or back with warm oil or lotion just before bed.
- Try to establish routine bedtimes.
- Take sleeping medications at a regular time before bed as prescribed.
- Make sure the bed is conducive to comfort and sleep. For example, use heating pads or blankets as needed, and have comfortable pillows and clean, wrinkle-free sheets.
- Use white noise (for example, ocean sounds, rain sounds, the whirr of a fan) to block distracting noises that may prevent sleep.
- Darken the room as much as possible to prolong sleep.

Nausea and Vomiting

Nausea (upset stomach or feeling of queasiness) or vomiting (regurgitation or throwing up) can be caused by cancer, cancer treatments, or other general health problems. The problem of nausea or vomiting will vary with certain therapies and will even be different among people getting the same therapy. If you consider your past experiences with the flu or other "stomach upsets" such as pregnancy, or after eating a meal that does not agree with you, it may reveal how you will respond to the symptom when it occurs with your cancer.

When considering the severity of nausea or vomiting, your doctor will usually add up the amount of times or hours a day you have the symptom and also consider how much distress it causes you to feel.

Managing Nausea and Vomiting

There are a variety of effective treatments that can help people with cancer manage nausea and vomiting. In some cases, symptoms can be totally eliminated.

Medicines for nausea and vomiting are usually given before the expected nausea is due to start and continue until nausea and vomiting should be gone. It is important not to wait until the nausea or vomiting is distressing before taking medication, because then some people will develop a feeling of nausea or begin to vomit before even receiving the therapy (called anticipatory nausea and vomiting), and this is much more difficult to treat.

People receiving chemotherapy generally receive a dose of medication before treatment, and then take medications on a regular schedule or as needed for a number of days after the treatment. For nausea and vomiting related to radiation therapy, daily long-acting medications may be given along with a prescription for medicine to control additional nausea.

It is extremely important that you share with the health care team any feelings of nausea you have, any vomiting you experience, and how bothersome these symptoms are to your everyday life. Many people will need several medications to control their nausea; in fact, more than half of people receive at least two medications.

If you are prescribed corticosteroids such as dexamethasone or prednisone for treatment of nausea and vomiting, be certain you never stop taking the medication abruptly. With corticosteroids, the dose may have to be reduced gradually over a period of time.

Complementary therapies such as acupressure, aromatherapy, and relaxation with imagery have proven effective for some people. Specially designed wrist bands (one brand name is Sea Bands) may help nausea related to motion sickness, but early studies have not shown them to be effective in controlling nausea related to cancer treatment. More information about complementary therapies is included in chapter 14.

Loss of Appetite

Cancer and its treatment causes decreased appetite and desire for food. Appetite loss has several possible causes:

- upset stomach or nausea
- taste changes affect a person's desire for specific foods
- motivation to eat can be affected by fatigue, anxiety, or depression

In addition, colorectal cancer may disrupt the digestive system and cause unpleasant effects (for example, a tumor can block the passage of food through the large intestine), which may in turn affect your desire to eat. Treating the cancer (such as surgically removing the tumor or shrinking it with radiation) can reverse this effect.

Managing Appetite Loss

If your lack of appetite is a result of nausea, talk with your doctor above the variety of antinausea medicines that are available (see the previous section). Once you do not feel queasy or sick to the stomach, you may be more eager to eat.

Some therapies affect your desire for certain tastes such as salt or sugar. Avoid foods that don't appeal to you and stick with foods that sound appetizing. Begin with foods that are bland like crackers or toast. Progress to more varied foods you like, keeping the portions small and eating often.

If fatigue interferes with your ability to prepare your own meals, ask family and friends to prepare food for you, or talk to your health care team about a "Meals on Wheels" type of program in your community. Have someone pack your favorite foods and drinks and keep them close by your resting place to avoid having to move to a different room to eat. If you are too fatigued to eat, try to eat very small amounts of nutritious foods as often as you can manage, and avoid consuming empty calories such as unsweetened drinks, celery, or lettuce.

The key to eating adequately when you simply do not enjoy eating is to "graze" (consume small portions frequently) rather than forcing yourself to consume a large meal. Be careful not to drink too much of anything before or during the time you are eating or you will feel too full to eat. Many people find that drinking a small amount of wine before eating helps stimulate their appetite, but alcohol can interfere with the effects of some medications, so talk with your doctor first.

If you cannot maintain a healthful weight because of appetite loss, a dietitian may recommend you drink specially formulated milkshakes or take supplements that can help boost your intake of calories and nutrients. There are also medications that help improve appetite, although a doctor will generally prescribe these medicines only when other approaches have failed.

Symptoms and Effects Related to Cancer in the Colon or Rectum and Its Treatment

Diarrhea and constipation are common for people with cancer of the colon or rectum. Colorectal cancer and its treatments can also affect self-image and sexual function. These symptoms are described together and are not presented in each treatment-related section.

Diarrhea

Diarrhea is an abnormal increase in the frequency and liquidity of your stools. Diarrhea may also come before or with abdominal pain or cramping, sweating, or nausea. Since people's bowel habits vary widely, it is important to think about the frequency and liquidity of your stools in relation to your own normal bowel activity. If you have a tendency for diarrhea caused by other conditions (such as previous gall bladder removal), you may be at higher risk for this symptom. If you have a disease that make you more prone to constipation (such as irritable bowel syndrome), you may have fewer problems with diarrhea.

Diarrhea is a common symptom of people with colorectal cancer. You can expect at least intermittent diarrhea throughout the disease continuum, and some patients experience it constantly.

There are many reasons diarrhea can occur. It is commonly related to surgery, radiation, and chemotherapy. For example, one of the most important jobs of the large bowel is to reabsorb water; if a large section of the bowel has been surgically removed, this can result in loose stool. Radiation treatments can cause local inflammation in the area that is treated, resulting in diarrhea. And unfortunately, the chemotherapy agents that are most active against cancer in the colon or rectum also happen to cause significant diarrhea. Diarrhea can be caused by factors other than cancer treatments as well. For instance, infections in the bowel can cause diarrhea, and injury to the liver or pancreas or the growth of a tumor in the pancreas can cause diarrhea as a result of lack of normal enzymes. Some people's bowel habits are affected by specific foods or emotions like stress. Your doctor will consider the likeliest cause(s) of your diarrhea and use this information to create your treatment plan.

> *"There are about eight or nine what they call possible side effects. After my first round of chemo I decided to get all of them, from hair loss, diarrhea, vomiting, mouth sores, blisters on my fingers and toes, sore skin, the whole gamut. We had to wind up reducing my chemo for the next round and then we reduced it one more time. The two that I've had the most trouble with have been the diarrhea and the fatigue. And that's lasted through the whole six months of treatment."*
>
> —JACY

You should take notice of certain characteristics of the diarrhea to help the health care team decide on the best treatment for it. Consider your answers to the following questions:

- Is diarrhea constant or intermittent?
- When did it start?
- Has the severity changed?
- What brings it on? Does it occur shortly after eating? Are there certain foods you notice it with more than others (for example, sugary, greasy, fatty, or milk-based products)? After drinking? At night? Without a pattern?
- Do you have other symptoms with the diarrhea such as cramping pain in the abdomen? Sweating? Nausea? Headache?
- What does the bowel movement look like? Watery, partly formed, soft, thin and ribbon-like? What color is it (light clay, yellow, bright green, black, or tarry)?
- Does the bowel movement have a stronger or different smell than usual?
- Do you have control over when you go or is it uncontrolled?

When you have diarrhea, this material moves quickly through your bowel, decreasing the amount of time your body has to absorb important nutrients from the food you have eaten. Diarrhea may be very watery, and the longer and more severe the diarrhea, the more water is passed. This can quickly cause dehydration if you do not replace your fluids, and some people with severe diarrhea may need to be admitted to the hospital to receive fluids intravenously.

Managing Diarrhea

Diarrhea can be particularly distressing because the overactive bowel response causes little physical warning signs before the diarrhea occurs, making it uncontrollable in timing. Fortunately, eating and drinking cautiously can reduce the risk of this happening, and medications can help too.

Medications given to treat diarrhea slow down the bowel's activity. Some examples of medications used to treat diarrhea include loperamide (Imodium), attapulgite (Kaopectate), and diphenoxylate with atropine (Lomotil). Report any side effects from the medications, such as headaches, drowsiness, shortness of breath, or an increased heart rate, to your doctor.

Here are some other tips for reducing or managing your diarrhea symptoms:

- Make sure you replenish your body's fluids, but drink fluids slowly and avoid hot liquids if possible.
- Avoid foods or drinks that may increase your bowel activity. Some people experience increased bowel activity when they eat sugary foods, fatty foods, spicy foods, warm drinks, or milk products.
- Foods served at room temperature are least likely to cause diarrhea.
- Switch your diet to clear liquids when diarrhea is expected to begin. Clear liquids include apple juice, clear broth, gelatin, peach or pear nectar, popsicles, sports drinks, and decaffeinated tea.
- When diarrhea has slowed, introduce foods low in fiber and residue such as applesauce, bananas, dry toast or saltine crackers, lowfat cottage cheese, mashed potatoes, and rice.
- Proteins are the easiest foods to digest, and some people have more diarrhea when they eat fatty, sugary foods, or vegetables than when they eat meat or cheese.
- Eat foods to replace potassium that is lost with diarrhea (apricots, bananas, citrus fruits and juices, green leafy vegetables, potatoes).
- Take vitamins as advised by the health care team. Nutrients are not well absorbed with diarrhea, but a multivitamin may help supplement your intake of needed vitamins or minerals.

- If you have diarrhea without an increased risk of infection, such as during chemotherapy, you may find "probiotics" (normal bacteria that grow in the bowel) a helpful supplement to obtain regular stools.
- Take special care of the skin around the anus. Clean and dry it after every bowel movement and apply water-repellent cream (such as diaper cream or ointment).
- Pain at the rectum may also be relieved by a warm sitz bath that involves seating the buttocks in warm water.

Constipation

While less common than diarrhea in people with colorectal cancer, constipation (hard, dry stools that are difficult to pass in a bowel movement) can occur. Constipation in patients with colorectal cancer is most likely a result of excessive amounts of medicines for diarrhea or pain, or a tumor blocking the bowel that prevents you from having a bowel movement.

Managing Constipation

The cause of constipation is an important part of planning the treatment. If the bowel is blocked, it is important *not* to give medicines that increase the contractions of the bowel. If you have constipation because of excessive medicines for diarrhea or pain, you may benefit from the following:
- Increase your intake of fluids, especially warm fluids.
- Increase the amount of fiber in your diet (fiber holds water, which softens stool).
- Increase your activity level if possible.
- Do not take any prescribed or over-the-counter medications to treat constipation unless your doctor is aware and approves of your plans.

If you experience any of the following symptoms, call your doctor: severe pain after eating, vomiting shortly after eating, swollen or enlarged abdomen, constant fever and cramping in the abdomen, or severe pain when you press down or let up on your abdomen. If you have pain along with dizziness, feeling of fuzziness or confusion, or low urine, you should go to the nearest emergency room.

Altered Self-Image

It is not unusual to feel that cancer and its treatment changes your view of yourself both physically and psychologically.

Treatment for colorectal cancer can alter your physical appearance, such as hair loss due to chemotherapy or the placement of a colostomy. Such changes can make you feel self-conscious and can be a reminder of your illness.

Cancer can also affect your psychological sense of yourself. If you formerly viewed yourself as strong, able, and vital, you may now be feeling frightened, frail, and no longer invincible.

Coping With Changes in Your Self-Image

Feelings of loss and sadness about the changes in your body and self-image are normal reactions. Talk to others about your feelings and concerns, and be as involved as possible in managing your own care. Engage in hobbies or activities that reaffirm your talents and assets and spend time with people who can comfort and reassure you. Support groups and web site chat rooms may also provide you with positive feedback about yourself and can strengthen your ability to cope with changes in your body and lifestyle. Some people find spiritual support helps them grow accustomed to the changes cancer and its treatment have caused.

Looking attractive enhances your general feeling of well being. Do not let your appearance run down. Continue your routine grooming activities as much as possible (shaving or wearing make-up, brushing your teeth, styling your hair), even if you are confined to bed.

Sexuality and Altered Sexual Function

Sexuality includes all the feelings and actions associated with loving someone. It includes holding hands, special looks, hugging, and kissing. It is not just the act of sexual intercourse. A person's sexuality and the specific ability to function sexually involve a variety of factors that cancer and its treatment can affect.

You may experience physical changes affecting your ability for normal sexual function. For example, colorectal cancer can affect the blood flow or nerves in the pelvis, which may affect your ability to physically perform or enjoy usual sexual activities. Men may experience impotence or erectile dysfunction. Radiation delivered to the lower part of the abdomen to treat colorectal cancer can involve your sexual organs, potentially causing irritation, swelling, dryness, and pain that may temporarily interfere with your ability to have sex. Surgery—especially removal of the rectum—can change the shape of a woman's vagina. Cancer- or treatment-related fatigue, pain, or other distressing symptoms may also interfere with your sexual function.

Emotional or psychological changes can affect your usual sexual or intimate activities too. Altered self-image (see above), depression, and anxiety or stress can change the way you experience desire, intimacy, and pleasure.

Other factors may also interrupt your normal intimate relationships and activities. These include hospitalization, visiting family members, or the presence of caregivers in the home.

Ask your health care team whether you should expect to experience changes to your normal sexual function as a result of your cancer or its treatment. Based on your condition and the treatment options you have chosen, your doctor should be able to tell you what to expect in terms of changes to your sexual function, the physical causes of these changes, and how long these disruptions to your normal sexual activities should last. Some changes are temporary, while others may be permanent.

Coping With Altered Sexual Function

During this time, it is essential that you communicate your questions and feelings to your doctor or nurse, and most importantly, to your partner.

Whenever possible, try to develop a pattern of normal personal time with your loved ones. Preserving the time and relaxing atmosphere for your loved ones may offer opportunities to talk about feelings as well as explore new methods of intimacy. Don't push yourself to engage in sexual activity if you are not ready. Remember, warmth, caring, physical closeness, and emotional intimacy are as necessary and rewarding as any other kind of human interaction.

Cancer, chemotherapy, and radiation are not communicable—that is, you cannot pass them on to your partner. Although you may choose to refrain from sexual activity during this time, you may be able to comfortably participate if you use lubricants. Ask your health care team about medications, lubricants, hormones, surgery, or medical implements that may help you. The American Cancer Society offers helpful education booklets on this topic.

Genitourinary Problems and Fertility Cautions

Depending on the type of treatment and dose, women having chemotherapy or radiation therapy in the pelvic area may stop menstruating, have irregular menstrual cycles, and have other symptoms of menopause (such as hot flashes). Treatment also can result in vaginal itching and burning and painful intercourse. Report these symptoms to your doctor so you can learn about options for relieving these side effects. Use a lubricant such as K-Y Jelly to help with dryness.

For men and women older than 50 years—the population colorectal cancer most frequently affects—infertility is generally not a concern. But for younger men and women planning families, chemotherapy and radiation therapy have some important effects on fertility. Women should ask their doctors about birth control options and how treatments may affect fertility. It is not a good idea to become pregnant during cancer therapy because radiation and chemotherapy may harm the fetus and result in birth defects. If you are pregnant, let your health care team know before beginning treatment.

For men, chemotherapy or radiation therapy to an area that includes the testes can reduce both the number of sperm and their ability to function. This does not mean conception cannot occur, however. If you want to father a child and are concerned about reduced fertility, talk to your doctor. One option is to bank your sperm before starting treatment.

Signs and Symptoms Related to Surgery

Surgery is the preferred treatment for colorectal cancer if the cancer is limited in size and location. The most common surgeries involve removing a portion of the bowel and either reconnecting it or creating a colostomy, an artificial opening from the colon through the abdominal wall. See chapter 16 for more information about types of ostomies, coping with a colostomy, and colostomy care and management. Palliative surgeries—operations that can help control discomfort but are not intended to cure the cancer—are also performed.

Effects of Anesthesia

Surgical procedures use anesthesia (medication to reduce sensation, especially pain), which generally slows down all body processes. Common anesthesia-related symptoms after surgery include nausea and vomiting, dizziness, muscle weakness, trouble urinating, and slowed bowel function or no bowel movements. These effects are temporary and go away after the anesthetic wears off and leaves your system.

Wound Management and Preventing Infection

Bowel surgery will always include at least one incision in the abdomen. (Laparoscopic surgery, discussed on page 154, may result in a several smaller incisions rather than one larger cut).

Most surgeons use surgical staples or sutures to close the wound; these are removed five to ten days after the surgery.

As the wound heals, you will be expected to keep the area clean and dry to prevent infection. The moist skin around a wound is prone to infection, so you must frequently change cotton dressings on draining wounds to reduce skin breakdown and infection. Small, isolated wound infections may have redness, swelling, or pain at the incision site. A change in the drainage amount, color, or odor may also signal an infection.

If you have these symptoms, alert the health care team immediately. Early treatment can prevent the infection from spreading. Your health care team will perform a wound culture to determine whether the wound is infected, and they may draw blood to make sure the infection has not spread. A fever is the most likely symptom of an infection that has spread beyond the wound.

If there is also swelling or severe pain on touching the wound site, there may be an abscess under the skin. This is a little more likely with surgeries of the bowel because of the bacteria that normally live inside the bowel.

A colostomy is designed to heal "open" rather than closed and requires specific wound management strategies; see chapter 16 for more information.

Adhesions With Bowel Narrowing

In one of every three surgeries involving the bowel, scar tissue will form where the bowel is reconnected. Sometimes, these tissues grow together in an abnormal way; these areas are called adhesions. Adhesions may develop as early as a few months after surgery or many years later.

Adhesions can narrow the inside of the bowel, slowing the movement of contents through it. Adhesions can also obstruct or block the bowel.

Symptoms signaling possible bowel obstruction include severe, constant abdominal pain, vomiting with all food or drink, fever, and a swollen abdomen. Report these symptoms immediately—if your doctor cannot see you right away, you may need to go to an emergency room for tests to determine whether an obstruction is present. Partial bowel obstruction may be managed by medications that help speed the bowel contents along the tract, but surgery is also a good and potentially successful treatment. Some patients are temporarily admitted to the hospital so they can be treated and observed until surgery is performed.

Signs and Symptoms Related to Radiation Therapy

Radiation therapy is a local treatment, which means it directly acts upon the cells in the part of the body where the cancer is or was located. The radiation beam is usually directed through the skin, so skin or other tissue immediately surrounding the area being radiated will be affected. Most side effects are limited to the area that is radiated.

Radiation used to treat colorectal cancer is most likely to cause skin reactions, gastrointestinal upset (see the sections on nausea, diarrhea, and constipation earlier in this chapter), urinary bladder problems, and pelvic genitourinary symptoms, including altered sexual function (see section earlier in this chapter) and fertility issues.

Topical (Skin Surface) Reactions

One of the most common reactions to radiation is skin redness and irritation where the radiation beam goes through the skin. This is similar to an intense sunburn. Most skin reactions should go away a few weeks after treatment is finished. In some cases, though, the treated skin will remain darker than it was before. Be gentle with your skin. Suggestions include:

- Use only lukewarm water and mild soap. Just let water run over the treated area. Do not rub.
- Do not wear tight clothing over the treatment area.
- Try not to rub, scrub, or scratch any sensitive spots.
- Avoid putting anything that is hot or cold, such as heating pads or ice packs, on your treated skin, unless advised by your doctor.
- Do not use powders, creams, perfumes, deodorants, body oils, ointments, lotions, or home remedies in the treatment area while you are being treated and for several weeks afterward, unless approved by your doctor or nurse. Many skin products can leave a coating on the skin that may cause irritation, and some can interfere with penetration of radiation into the body.
- Avoid exposing the area to the sun during treatment and for at least one year after your treatment is completed.

Radiation that involves the rectum may be particularly problematic because the area around the anus is already prone to irritation, and it is not easy for you to check. You should have someone help you look at this area every day for the signs of skin redness, irritation, abrasions, or signs of infection. Normal creams used with hemorrhoid irritation are not recommended for use in this situation. You can create your own soothing sitz bath by sitting in a warm bath and running a continuous flow of warm water over the area by a shower attachment or squirt bottle or pouring cups of warm water over the area while sitting on a commode. If you have irritation in the rectal area, use baby wipes for cleaning after every bowel movement. You can also cover the area with baby oil after cleaning to prevent stool from sticking and reduce the effort to remove it with wiping. Your health care team can provide recommendations about products to use.

Infection in the rectal area is not uncommon. Signs that an infection may be present include: severe and continuous pain, increased pain when you press on the site, fever, or chills. An infection in this area should be treated immediately since it can quickly spread to the bloodstream and cause serious complications.

Bladder Irritation

The radiation beam may penetrate body organs near the colon or lymph nodes that are being radiated. One of the most commonly affected areas is the urinary bladder. Radiation therapy can cause irritation and bleeding of the inside of the bladder. This may result in pain in the lower abdomen or back, pain when urinating, frequent feeling of needing to urinate, or bloody or cloudy urine. Bladder irritation symptom is usually related to the location of your tumor, the area being radiated, and the dose of radiation. You may reduce the risk of this complication by drinking a lot of fluid (aim for a gallon a day) to keep urine constantly flowing through the bladder. People with a higher risk of infection or who have symptoms of an irritated bladder may be prescribed antibiotics to prevent infection, and may need to be hospitalized to have a catheter and fluid rinses of the bladder until the mucous membranes heal.

Signs and Symptoms Related to Chemotherapy

Chemotherapy is a common treatment offered to patients with colorectal cancer that is advanced and cannot be completely removed. It is also used to treat people who have undergone surgical removal of a tumor but who still have positive lymph nodes or at high risk for recurrence.

Chemotherapy drugs are made to kill fast-growing cells, but because these drugs travel throughout the entire body, they can affect normal, healthy cells. Damage to healthy tissue is the cause of side effects. The most common side effects of chemotherapy agents used to treat colorectal cancer are described in Table 15.2 on page 260. We'll discuss common chemotherapy side effects we haven't yet covered in the following sections. (See the earlier portion of this chapter for tips on coping with nausea, vomiting, diarrhea, fatigue, etc.)

Hair Loss

The normal scalp contains approximately 100,000 hairs. They are constantly growing, and old hairs fall out and are replaced by new ones. As chemotherapy drugs travel throughout the body to kill cancer cells, some hair follicles may be damaged in the process, causing the hair to fall out. In addition to the hair on your head, facial hair (eyebrows, eyelashes, beard or mustache), arm and leg hair, underarm hair, and pubic hair all may be affected.

Hair loss or thinning usually begins about two to four weeks after the start of chemotherapy and persists for several months, but the extent and length of time for hair loss is very individual. Hair loss is highly variable. Some people experience it and others do not, even when they are taking the same drug.

People being treated for cancer have differing feelings about the impact of hair loss. If the thought of losing your hair is distressing to you, visit a wig shop before hair loss so you can match your normal hair color and texture. (Ask your doctor for a prescription—a wig may be covered by insurance.) You can also experiment with scarves and hats.

In the meantime, treat your remaining hair gently. Use mild shampoos and gentle brushes, and avoid the use of heated implements (curling or straightening irons, hot rollers, hair dryers on high heat), harsh styling products, or hair dye. Also be careful with your new balding head—it will be very prone to sunburn, and can be a source of heat loss in cold weather.

> *"My big thing was I used to have very, very, very long hair. I didn't care about having a colostomy. I didn't care about having my body cut up. I didn't care about any of that stuff, but my hair was like this really big thing for me. But my hair has all grown back in and it's short and it's curly. I've gotten more compliments about my hair now than I ever did when my hair was long. So I call it 'my cancer hairdo.'"*
>
> —DONNA

Your hair may begin to grow back even before your chemotherapy ends. When your hair grows back, you may be surprised—it may be more curly, or even a different color.

Skin Reactions

You may have minor skin reactions to chemotherapy, including redness, itching, peeling, and dryness, especially if you are receiving 5-fluorouracil (5-FU, Adrucil, Fluorouracil). Of these skin reactions, the most severe is a blistering rash, most common of the palms of the hands or soles of the feet. The rash is painful and may cause tingling as well. This symptom seems to be related to higher doses of the drug or to slow detoxification of the drug (caused by kidney or liver problems). This severe reaction usually occurs early in the course of therapy and may limit the amount of drug you will be able to receive. Less severe skin reactions can include an overall pink and itchy rash or swelling from higher doses or longer times on treatment. It is also possible to develop darker skin tone, especially along

Table 15.2 Common Side Effects of Chemotherapy Agents

Chemotherapy Agent*	Common Side Effects†												
	Difficulty breathing	Abdominal pain or cramping	Fatigue or weakness	Loss of appetite	Brittle or discolored nails	Diarrhea	Hair loss	Low blood counts	Mouth sores	Nausea and vomiting	Neuropathies (numbness or tingling in extremeties)	High blood pressure	Skin irritation, sensitivity, or rash
5-Fluorouracil (5-FU, Adrucil, Fluorouracil)					X	X	X	X	X	X			X
Capecitabine (Xeloda)						X		X	X	X	X		X
Leucovorin‡ (Folinic acid)													
Irinotecan (CPT-11, Camptosar)		X	X			X		X		X			
Oxaliplatin (Eloxatin)	X		X			X			X	X	X		
Cetuximab (Erbitux)			X										X
Bevacizumab (Avastin)			X	X		X			X			X	

** Generic drug names are listed first, followed by trade names in parentheses.*
† Not all patients will develop all side effects. Those listed here are the most commonly experienced by patients receiving these chemotherapy drugs. Other side effects not listed above can also occur in some patients. Tell your doctor or nurse if you develop any problems.
‡ Side effects related to the use of leucovorin, a water-soluble vitamin given to boost the effectiveness of 5-fluorouracil, are rare.

the veins where chemotherapy medicines have been infused. Use of cetuximab (Erbitux) can cause acne-like skin rashes on your face, neck, and torso.

The treatment for these severe skin reactions is to stop taking the medication, and treat the symptoms until the skin reaction is completely healed. Skin symptoms can occur anytime during treatment, but usually improve significantly within five to seven days after stopping the medication.

The following strategies may help relieve your discomfort and lessen further irritation:

- Use only lukewarm water and mild soap when washing.
- Do not wear tight clothing over the irritated area.
- Try not to rub, scrub, or scratch any sensitive spots.
- Avoid putting anything that is hot or cold, such as heating pads or ice packs, on your skin, unless advised by your doctor.
- Do not use powders, creams, perfumes, deodorants, body oils, ointments, lotions, or home remedies unless approved by your doctor or nurse. Many skin products can cause additional irritation.
- If you expect to be in the sun for more than a few minutes, wear protective clothing (such as a hat with a broad brim and shirt with long sleeves) and use a sunscreen. Ask your doctor or nurse about using sunscreen lotions.

Some people may also experience nail changes such as bluish or darker coloring, lines across them, or even loss of nails. These changes are not usually painful, but can cause you to feel self-conscious. Since there is not a specific treatment for these nail changes, you may want to cover your nails with polish to hide the effect.

Low Blood Counts

Most chemotherapy drugs used to treat colorectal cancer also block growth of the rapidly dividing cells inside the bone marrow. This lowers the number of white blood cells (which fight infection), platelets (which aid in blood clotting), and red blood cells (which carry oxygen). As a result, your body's ability to carry out these tasks is impaired. We'll talk specifically about how to prevent infection and manage bleeding and anemia in the next section.

Low blood counts usually begin seven to ten days after the start of chemotherapy and rebound to normal in a few days. Low blood counts caused by chemotherapy can not be prevented, but there are medications called growth factors or colony-stimulating factors that can shorten the time in which they are decreased, or prevent them from going as low as they would have normally. These growth factors can reduce the symptoms of infection, bleeding, and anemia for people receiving chemotherapy but are costly and may not be covered by insurance. Ask your healthcare team whether growth factors could assist in your treatment and recovery.

Infection

Your body's white blood cells help fight infection. Because they only live a short amount of time (hours to days), their levels drop most quickly after chemotherapy is given. Doctors call this low white blood cell count neutropenia. When there are fewer cells available to protect the body against disease, the chance that a bacterium or virus can cause an infection is much higher.

People whose number of white blood cells remains low for seven days or more are at an increased risk of infection, as are people whose counts are below 1000/mm^3. When the count is lower than 500/mm^3, the risk for infection is deemed very high and requires special protective actions to prevent an infection.

Here are some measures you can take to help protect yourself from an infection during this time:

- Stay away from crowds, small children outside of your own family, construction, soil disruption, and animal excrement.
- Consider wearing a mask in areas of possible infection risk (for example, when shopping, using public restrooms, or walking through areas of construction).
- Make sure any children you are exposed to are fully immunized and have limited exposure to childhood illnesses.
- Maintain good personal hygiene. Bathe and change clothes daily, brush your teeth after every meal, and wash your hands frequently—especially after going to the bathroom.
- Take special infection prevention precautions with pets. Keep them clean, wash your hands after handling them, try to keep their bedding separate, and do not handle their excrement.
- Consider potential risks for infection at home. You may want to consider using bottled water, washing all clothes and dishes in hot water, and using separate eating utensils from other family members.
- Monitor the food you eat and avoid potential contaminants such as blue cheese, cultured yogurt, nonpasteurized products, raw food such as sushi, and store-bought sandwiches or salads with eggs or mayonnaise.
- Wear loose-fitting, comfortable clothes. Choose white cotton underwear and socks.
- Clip nails with care and avoid the use of false fingernails.

Most patients will not have severe neutropenia or it will be present for only a few days. During this time, watch carefully for any signs of infection:

- Take your temperature twice a day and report a fever above 100.5°F or 38.5°C to your doctor.
- Examine your body every day, paying close attention to any areas of redness, swelling, or pain.
- Look for changes in the color or odor of your urine, bowel movements, or discharge from any sore or opening.
- Report any abnormal feelings (headaches, dizziness, muscle ache, etc.) to the health care team so they can evaluate whether an infection is present.

262

If you develop an infection, your doctor will prescribe antibiotics. If you are in good general health, and the white blood cells are not low for a long period, the healthcare team may allow you to remain at home and take antibiotic pills. Most of the time, you can expect to be admitted to the hospital and receive intravenous antibiotics for about seven to ten days.

Bleeding

Platelets are small cell fragments that are essential for blood clotting or coagulation. When your platelet count falls, your body may not be able to stop the bleeding if you are injured. During this time, you'll need to be extra careful. If minor bleeding occurs, firm pressure and elevation of the body part can usually stop the bleeding. On rare occasions these measures do not work, and medications to prevent or stop bleeding may be prescribed, or special ointments and treatments can be applied to the skin.

The following precautions can help you avoid problems with bleeding.

- Maintain a safe environment in your home. Avoid clutter or open corners on which you can injure yourself.
- Discontinue hobbies, activities, or sports that put you are risk of injury during this time.
- Always wear feet coverings.
- Use only an electric razor.
- Maintain good dental hygiene to prevent your gums from bleeding.
- Be attentive to changes in the color and odor of your urine and bowel movements; such changes can signal hidden bleeding.

BLOOD CLOTS

Receiving chemotherapy and having cancer also places you at risk for developing blood clots. Blood clots may occur in your calves, lungs, or in your intravenous catheter. Common symptoms (which should be reported to your health care team right away) include pain, swelling, warmth in your calf, shortness of breath, or inability to withdraw blood from your intravenous catheter site.

Anemia

Anemia occurs when the blood has too little hemoglobin, the part of the red blood cell that carries oxygen throughout your body. Symptoms of anemia will begin to appear as your level of hemoglobin decreases; these can include shortness of breath, difficulty breathing on exertion, and fatigue. These symptoms occur because your body tissues aren't receiving enough oxygen.

The red blood cells live longer than any other cells in the bone marrow, and therefore they are the last to become low after chemotherapy. In fact, most people develop anemia later in treatment, not in the early stages. Because anemia is slow to develop, it may also take low red blood cell counts a while to return to normal.

You can manage anemia by addressing the source of the problem or managing the symptoms it causes, such as fatigue (see page 239.)

One way to address the source of the problem, the lack of hemoglobin, is to boost your body's red blood cells. To do this, doctors may administer a medicine called an erythrocyte growth factor (erythropoietin or epoetin). This substance, which is normally produced by the kidneys, helps the body make its own new red blood cells. Erythrocyte growth factor requires two to four weeks until its best effect is realized, but its continued administration makes the symptoms stay away.

A transfusion of red blood cells also may be given to treat anemia, especially in cases where the hemoglobin level needs to be raised quickly, but the positive effects from a transfusion wear off in a few weeks. Transfusions carry the added risk of infection or reactions.

You can also address anemia by eating nutrient-rich foods, taking iron and folic acid supplements, and stopping bleeding.

Mouth and Throat Sores

Many chemotherapy agents kill rapidly dividing cells in addition to the tumor cells. The skin and mucous membranes that line the digestive tract are among the most rapidly dividing cells in the body. As the mucous membrane dies and falls off, raw, new tissue is exposed, and painful sores can develop. Mouth and throat sores may be small and isolated or continuous on the lips and throughout the mouth, throat, and area used for swallowing. They can vary in severity, from small, red irritations and blisters to open, bleeding sores. The presence of mouth sores is called mucositis, and the condition usually develops about five to seven days after chemotherapy is started and lasts until the cells regrow (about twelve to sixteen days after chemotherapy).

Although this side effect can't always be prevented, studies have shown that frequent rinsing with any comfortable fluid helps wash away bacteria that worsen the mucositis. Most people find cold fluids most soothing, although warm salt water or a baking soda and water solution may also be helpful. Numbing solutions containing lidocaine or liquid diphenhydramine may also be soothing. Avoid using mouthwashes, since most of them contain alcohol, which will sting open sores. Maintain good oral hygiene including regular brushing with a soft nylon toothbrush.

When eating, choose chilled foods and fluids (popsicles, frozen yogurt, sherbet, smoothies, and ice cream) and avoid citrus fruits, such as oranges, lemons, limes, and tomatoes. Avoid hard or coarse foods such as crusty breads, crackers, raw vegetables, potato chips, or pretzels, and do not eat hot, spicy foods such as pepper, curry powder, or horseradish. Drink at least two to three quarts of fluids daily with approval from your doctor, but avoid citrus juices, carbonated beverages, and alcohol, which will irritate your mouth sores. Instead, try warm tea or apricot, pear, or peach juice.

In rare circumstances, you may need to request pain medications until your symptoms resolve. Persistent or severe mouth sores may lead the health care team to change your chemotherapy schedule or dose.

Peripheral Neuropathy

Some chemotherapy drugs used to treat colorectal cancer may cause temporary damage to the nerves, resulting in decreased feeling starting in the fingers and toes and extending up into arms and legs. This decreased sensation, called peripheral neuropathy, can be accompanied by tingling or shooting pains. This lack of feeling will affect your ability to sense things that can cause injury, such as extreme temperatures and sharp objects. People with neuropathies are at risk for burns or cuts that they do not even notice because of the lack of feeling. It may also cause difficulty doing small, fine, movements requiring sensation such as buttoning clothes or attaching jewelry clasps.

Oxaliplatin is the chemotherapy agent that is most commonly associated with peripheral neuropathy. At this time, scientists believe that this symptom is related to high doses or long-term use of the drug, and will go away when the chemotherapy is discontinued. Unlike other medicines with these effects, oxaliplatin does not seem to produce any permanent nerve damage, and it does not affect the nerves deeper in the body that control activities like the speed of the heart or activities of the bowels. If you are having trouble with the feeling in your fingertips, or toes, notify the healthcare team so they can perform a more thorough examination. Any other unusual symptoms such as a racing heart, or sudden severe cramping in the abdomen should also be reported.

Reduced Memory and Concentration Ability

Chemotherapy is known to affect your memory and ability to work on complex mental tasks, but the exact way it does this is unknown. While the chemotherapy medication itself may play a primary role, there are probably multiple factors that cause difficulty with mental abilities; symptoms such as fatigue, pain, loss of appetite, sleep problems, infection and anemia have all been verified as contributing to difficulty with thinking. If you believe you are experiencing problems remembering, concentrating, or focusing on a task, talk to your healthcare provider. Some of the contributing symptoms may be manageable, and tests can be performed to assess the cause.

Knowing this is a problem for some people can also help you to prepare and reduce this effect. Develop the habit of creating lists or voice messages for remembering important things. Some find it useful to keep all their thoughts and lists in a journal so they know it is all in one place. Organize the notes in a predictable way, and develop habits of following the same routines. For instance, you may want to establish a place to always store your keys or obtain a weekly medication storage bin to ensure to do not miss any doses. Allow longer times to perform mind-challenging tasks such as balancing a checkbook, or delegate tasks to others who are close to you and want to help. Some careers will be difficult to return to, while others simply need some changes in the work environment or workload. Write down directions to all activities whenever possible.

Most important, if you feel that you are experiencing changes in memory, concentration, or calculating ability, discuss it with others so they understand your difficulties and can help you mobilize resources to compensate.

Other Symptoms

Chemotherapy affects every person differently. In addition to the most common symptoms listed above, you may also experience other symptoms, including a runny nose or temporary nasal congestion, headaches or migraines, an allergic rash, and/or chest pain. Report all symptoms to your health care team.

Signs and Symptoms Related to Biological Therapy

There are few biologic agents used in treatment of colorectal cancer, and all are currently given in conjunction with chemotherapy agents. Therefore, it can be difficult to separate the symptoms of chemotherapy and biological therapy.

The growth factors used to prevent bone marrow suppression are classified as biological therapy. For most people, they cause only mild symptoms. White blood cell colony-stimulating factors cause rapid bone marrow growth of white blood cells, resulting in mild to moderate bone pain. Some people also experience mild fevers and aches in their joints of muscles. Platelet colony-stimulating factor is more likely to cause swelling and excess fluid. Erythrocyte colony-stimulating factor increases production of red blood cells, thickening the blood, causing adverse effects such as high blood pressure or blood clots.

There are also other biological agents used for treatment of colorectal cancer. Most biological agents cause fever, chills, aches, malaise, and other vague and general symptoms that are similar to those of the flu or colds. Most people find that taking mild pain and cold medicines effectively relieve these symptoms. Each agent also has a specific set of adverse effects.

Leucovorin (folinic acid) is used in conjunction with chemotherapy agents and can cause fatigue and body aches for a small number of people. On very rare occasions, medicines have been unable to relieve these flu symptoms, and patients take a short break from their therapy.

Cetuximab (Erbitux) is an antibody directed at a special molecule on the tumor cells of some patients. Allergic reactions have been reported, but otherwise, the most common effect is acne-like skin eruptions.

Bevacixumab (Avastin) blocks the creation of new blood vessels in the tumor. Because of some rare cases of wound incisions reopening, patients are not pre-scribed this agent within 28 days of surgery. While there are usually almost no adverse effects, some other patients with colorectal cancer have experienced high blood pressure or bowel rupture. If you receive this agent, you can expect frequent blood pressure monitoring and visits to your healthcare professionals to monitor the status of any surgical wounds, and for an abdominal assessment. If you are receiving bevacixumab, be certain to call your healthcare provider with any new changes in your symptoms, especially if they are in your abdomen, or are symptoms of high blood pressure such as headache, blurred vision, or dizziness.

Signs and Symptoms Related to Advanced Cancer

One of the most difficult and challenging aspects of life after cancer treatment is the fear of recurrence. Healthcare professionals do not want you to fixate with worry over this possibility; instead, you should simply be informed of symptoms that may indicate a return of disease. This way, recurrence can be caught at its earliest and most treatable point. See chapter 18 for more information about recurrence.

General Nonspecific Physical Symptoms Related to Cancer Recurrence

Vague symptoms that may signal return of your cancer include fatigue, anorexia, and weight loss. These occur because the cancer cells are stealing important nutrients and calories needed by the body. These are similar to those experienced with therapy, but may be a little more pronounced or resistant to normal treatment.

Another problem that is connected to the presence of cancer cells in the body is a tendency to clot (see page 263). Sometimes the clot lodges in a vein in the leg or abdomen, although clots can occur anywhere in the body. These clots are usually recognized because they cause pain, redness, and swelling. If the clot becomes dislodged, it can travel to the heart and cause shortness of breath. When someone has a known risk for clotting, blood thinners (anticoagulants) are usually prescribed. Once you have had a clotting episode, you can expect to receive the blood thinners for the rest of your life. Taking blood thinners requires that you take precautions to prevent bleeding (see page 263).

Blockage (Obstruction) of the Bowel

One of the more common locations for colorectal cancer to recur is in the area where it was originally located or another place along the gastrointestinal tract. This area is usually already damaged and narrower than other parts of the bowel because of the surgery itself or scar tissue from the surgery (called adhesions) or other treatments.

When cancer recurs in this area, there is a high possibility that the bowel will become blocked. Bowel blockage causes backup of the normal bowel contents and slowing of all digestive processes. Even when only partly blocked, people describe feeling nauseated, vomiting, lacking appetite, having a bad taste in their mouth, feeling bloated, or actually having a swollen abdomen. Some also experience abdominal pain that is more severe and cramp-like after eating or drinking. Most symptoms are more extreme if the obstruction is higher in the bowel, although pain is more prominent in lower bowel obstructions. Early on, excessive gas and fluid causes somewhat severe symptoms. As the bowel slows down, constipation occurs, and there is less feeling of gas, but instead there is a progressive feeling of fullness. If the bowel totally closes and treatments are not effective, it will eventually rupture. Abdominal pain is a common symptom, but it will often decrease as the condition worsens; after total blockage, sleepiness and low blood pressure are the most common symptoms. An X-ray of the abdomen may be unable to verify a bowel blockage, so most people must have a CT scan to determine whether this is a problem.

If detected when only partially closed, medications to increase the movement of gastrointestinal activity may be prescribed, such as erythromycin (E-mycin, ERYC, Erythrocin, Illotycin), tegaserod (Zelnorm), and octreotide (Sandostatin). If the obstruction becomes more severe, a person is usually admitted to the hospital and a tube is inserted to drain the stomach. When the tumor can be safely removed by surgery, that is the preferred treatment. Some chemotherapy and radiation therapy may also be used to shrink the tumor and relieve these symptoms

Spread to Other Organs

Since the gastrointestinal tract has a large blood supply, the liver is the most common location for spread of colorectal cancer. The liver accepts all the blood draining from the gastrointestinal system. Other places where the tumor may spread include the lung or urinary system.

Spread to the Liver

Symptoms of spread to the liver include nausea, vomiting, lack of appetite, bloated abdomen, diarrhea, yellow discoloration of the skin and eyes, and itching. The early symptoms relate to the body wastes beginning to collect in the blood. As the liver becomes more dysfunctional and tumors grow inside, it will enlarge and leak fluid, causing swelling of the abdomen. This abdominal swelling can become very extreme, causing some difficulty moving, lying down, and breathing. Fluid can be removed to relieve the pressure and size of the abdomen. Later, waste products cannot be removed by the liver, and as the amount in the blood increases, a yellowish skin or eye discoloration called jaundice occurs. Jaundice comes from the bilirubin that is usually removed by the liver. High levels of bilirubin cause itching and dry skin. Continued liver failure will cause extreme sleepiness. Spread to the liver is diagnosed through blood studies that are routinely monitored in patients with a history of colorectal cancer. Although they can detect changes fairly early, many people describe symptoms before the presence of laboratory abnormalities. A CT scan of the abdomen will detect abnormalities early if intravenous contrast is used for the scan.

On rare occasions, when a single, isolated tumor has spread from the colon to the liver, surgery can be performed. Most other cases of cancer spread to the liver are managed with treatments for the uncomfortable symptoms. Sometimes jaundice can be relieved by placing a catheter inside the gallbladder duct inside the liver. Skin cream and anti-itch medicines may also be prescribed.

Spread to the Lungs

After gastrointestinal recurrence and liver spread, the lung is the next most common site for colorectal cancer to spread. Many people with tumors in their lungs have no symptoms at all. At other times, difficulty catching their breath is the symptom most reported. This "shortness of breath" can occur only with activity or may be present all of the time. It will depend upon the amount of lung that is involved and other body mechanisms needed to compensate. As breathlessness increases, people will become sleepy and not able to feel the symptom so much.

The presence of lung tumors that have spread from the colon is often detected during routine follow-up scans, even before symptoms or laboratory abnormalities occur. If there is extra fluid in the lungs, medications to aid urination are prescribed, and if fluid is in the layer outside the lung (pleural effusion), a needle can remove the excess fluid. Oxygen therapy, breathing treatments (such as those given to people with asthma), and some pain medications all help relieve the breathlessness associated with these lung tumors.

Spread to the Urinary System

Although not common, colorectal cancer can spread to the urinary system. The tubes reaching from the kidneys, located above the hips, to the bladder, located in the lowest part of the abdomen, are called ureters. There is one on each side of the body. These are the most likely to be compressed as tumors in the abdomen grow. If the ureters become obstructed, people feel hip and back pain (often only on one side) and have less urination. They may also show signs of infection as the urine is trapped inside the kidney.

Ureteral obstruction is detected by a scan of the kidney, ureters, and bladder. An ultrasound may also show the enlarged kidney from urine back-up. When possible, doctors prefer to place a plastic pipe into the ureter (called a stent) to hold it open. More often, this is not possible, and so the more common treatment is to place a catheter into the kidney to allow outside urine drainage. These drains produce minimal discomfort, and are not difficult to learn to manage. They are attached to a drainage bag that is emptied periodically, and covered with a simple dressing. Specific care of these "nephrostomy tubes" varies from one institution to another, so information about them is best obtained from your health care provider. On some occasions, the tube can be placed internally and connected to the bladder.

CHAPTER SIXTEEN

LIVING WITH A COLOSTOMY

Brenda K. Shelton MS, RN, CCRN, AOCN
with the United Ostomy Association

Ostomies are far more common than most people realize. The next time you're in a large public place—an airport, a sports event, or a concert—look around you. Although you probably couldn't pick them out in a crowd, one in 500 people has some type of an ostomy.

On the other hand, improvements in surgical techniques for colorectal cancer mean that fewer and fewer colostomies are being done, and many that are done are temporary. For patients with colorectal cancer, a permanent colostomy is rarely needed. Most patients who have a colostomy need it only until the colon or rectum heals from surgery. Approximately one in eight people with rectal cancer require a permanent colostomy.

It is estimated that a little more than half of the people who have ostomies have them as a result of colorectal cancer. Others may be a result of other illnesses, injuries, or birth defects.

Although many people are frightened or dismayed when faced with the possibility of having ostomy surgery, the procedure can be a lifesaving one, and people with ostomies can enjoy a full range of life experiences, including traveling, physical activities, intimate relations, and work.

Preconceived notions about ostomies should not influence your decisions about treatment. This chapter will provide you with the facts about colostomies and will give you a realistic sense of what it is like to live with a colostomy so that you can make educated, informed treatment decisions.

What Is an Ostomy?

An ostomy is a type of surgery required when a person does not have the normal function of the bladder or bowel because of birth defects, disease, injury, or other disorders. Types of ostomies include colostomies, ileostomies, and urostomies. A colostomy—the surgical option for most people treated for colorectal cancer—is created when a portion of the large intestine (colon) is removed or bypassed. The end of the remaining portion of the functioning colon is brought through the abdominal wall, creating a stoma. This results in a change of normal body function to allow elimination of bowel contents.

> "I have run into people who would have elected to die rather than have that. But I didn't have a whole lot of options, and I was just glad to be alive. A colostomy was just a minor thing in order to survive."
>
> —DREW

An ileostomy is a surgically created opening in the small intestine, usually at the end of the ileum. A urostomy is a general term for a surgical procedure that diverts urine away from a diseased or defective bladder. Because colostomies are the type of ostomy most frequently associated with colorectal cancer, this chapter focuses on colostomies. However, many of the tips, strategies, and resources discussed in this chapter are relevant to all types of ostomies.

Ostomy surgery allows normal body wastes to be expelled through a new surgical opening on the abdominal wall called a stoma (see Figure 16.1). Most people with an ostomy must wear a special pouch over the stoma.

Colostomies may be temporary or permanent. A temporary colostomy is performed when a portion of the colon has been removed, and the colon needs time to heal. To prevent stool from reaching this part of colon, the temporary colostomy diverts the stool so it can be eliminated through the stoma. The usual time for a temporary colostomy to be in place is two to three months, though healing can take up to a year. Eventually the temporary colostomy is reversed and normal bowel elimination is restored. Temporary colostomies are more common when colorectal cancer affects the ascending or transverse colon and cancer is not widespread.

When cancer invades the descending or sigmoid portion of the colon or the rectum, the diseased portion must be totally removed or permanently bypassed, sometimes requiring a permanent colostomy. This provides a permanent alternate

Figure 16.1 Colostomy and Stoma

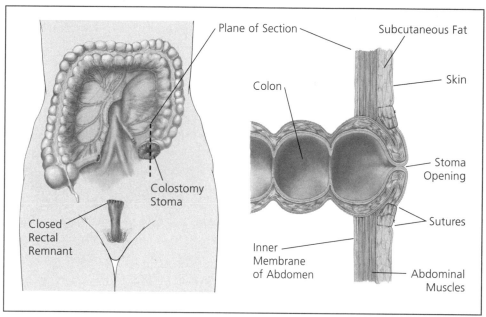

The right view shows a side (cutaway) view of the stoma and surrounding area.

exit for stool. A permanent colostomy may also be recommended if a patient's other health problems make it unwise for the doctor to perform additional surgery.

The Stoma

An ostomy refers to the surgically created opening in the body for the discharge of wastes. A stoma is the actual end of the bowel that can be seen protruding through the abdominal wall. When you look at a stoma, you are actually looking at the lining (the mucosa) of the intestine. It is warm and moist and secretes small quantities of mucus. Stomas are rose to brick red in color, with a shiny wet appearance. Unlike the anus, the stoma has no valve or shut-off muscle. For this reason, willful control of the passage of stool is not possible.

There are several different types of stoma openings that vary depending upon the part of the bowel involved and whether the doctor hopes to reconnect the bowel at a later time. The three types of stomas are end stoma, loop stoma, and double-barrel stoma. (A double-barrel stoma and an end stoma are illustrated in Figures 16.2 and 16.3, respectively, on pages 275 and 276).

An end stoma brings the bowel out onto the skin surface. This is usually a permanent stoma, and the rest of the bowel has either been removed or has been sewn shut inside the abdomen. To create a loop stoma, a loop of intestine is brought through a small opening in the abdominal wall and a plastic rod is placed under the loop for support. The loop is slit and it is turned back upon itself. This produces a stoma with two openings: one opening will discharge fecal matter while the other opening will emit mucus. A double-barrel stoma brings both ends of a separated bowel onto the surface of the skin to form two separate stomas. The top one is functioning, and the bottom one is for mucus drainage.

The appearance of the stoma depends on the type of colostomy and on individual differences in the human body. While the stoma may be quite large at first, it will shrink gradually and attain its final size in six to eight weeks after the surgery. There may be some swelling of the edges for two to three weeks after surgery or a small amount of bleeding from the stoma at first, and at times mucus may come out of it. The consistency and type of stool drainage will depend upon the location of the ostomy.

Positioning the Stoma

The location of the colostomy on the abdomen depends on which part of the colon is used to create it. The ostomy nurse or surgeon will determine the correct location for the stoma. The preferred site lies near the midline of the rectus abdominus muscle (more commonly called "the six-pack"), which is located between the ribs and the pubic bone in front of the pelvis. The nurse or surgeon will also take into account factors such as the contours of a person's abdomen, skin folds, and areas of possible irritation, such as where a belt or waistband might rub.

Types of Colostomies

Different types of colostomies are named by their location in the bowel:
- Ascending colostomy: a relatively rare procedure that results in an opening in the ascending portion of the colon. It is located on the right side of the abdomen.
- Transverse colostomy: the surgical opening created in the transverse colon, resulting in one or two openings. It is located in the upper abdomen, in the front or on the right side.
- Sigmoid or descending colostomy: the most common type of ostomy surgery, in which the end of the descending or sigmoid colon is brought to the surface of the abdomen. It is usually located on the lower left side of the abdomen.

Figure 16.2 Transverse Colostomy with Double-Barrel Stoma

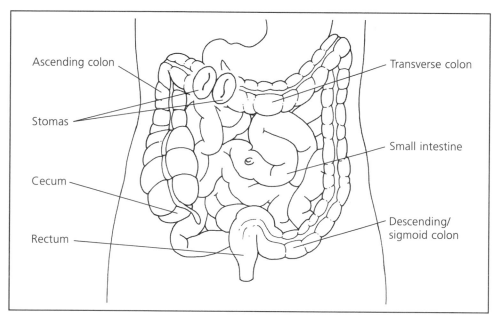

Source: Copyright © 2004. United Ostomy Association. Colostomy Guide, Rev. ed. Irvine, CA: United Ostomy Association; 2004:4.

Ascending Colostomy

The ascending colostomy is located on the right side of the abdomen. When a colostomy is located in the right half of the colon, only a short portion of colon remains. As a result, the discharge through the stoma is liquid. This type of stoma is rarely used since an ileostomy is the best option when the discharge is liquid. A drainable pouch is worn for colostomies of this type.

Transverse Colostomy

The transverse colostomy is in the upper abdomen, either in the middle or toward the right side of the body. This type of colostomy allows the stool to exit from the colon before it reaches the descending colon. The transverse colostomy will either be a loop procedure or a double-barrel colostomy.

The discharge from the transverse colostomy is semisolid, unpredictable, and contains some digestive enzymes. A person who has a transverse colostomy usually wears a drainable pouch, although a closed-end (nondrainable pouch) can be used for convenience during special activities.

Figure 16.3 Descending or Sigmoid Colostomy with End Stoma

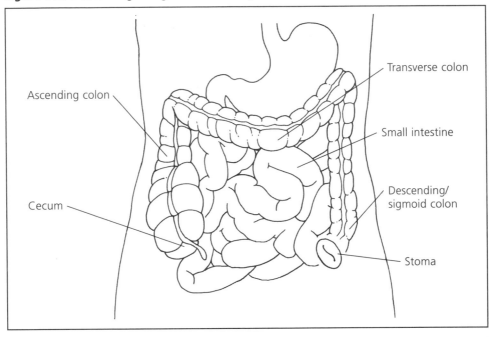

Transverse colon

Ascending colon

Small intestine

Descending/
sigmoid colon

Cecum

Stoma

Source: Copyright © 2004. United Ostomy Association. Colostomy Guide, Rev. ed. Irvine, CA: United Ostomy Association; 2004:6.

Descending or Sigmoid Colostomy

Located on the lower left side of the abdomen, the sigmoid colostomy is the most frequently performed type of colostomy. See Figure 16.3.

Because the stoma is at the end of the gastrointestinal tract, the discharge is generally firm, resembles normal bowel movements, and does not contain caustic digestive enzymes. People who have a descending or sigmoid colostomy may return to a predictable bowel movement pattern and may be able to pass stool easily, which is then collected in a lightweight, disposable pouch.

Irrigating (via an enema through the stoma) to assist with regulated bowel movements is another option. A nurse specialist called a wound, ostomy, and continence nurse (WOCN), or simply an ostomy nurse, will help you set up and perform irrigations through a special colostomy cone. The bowel movement occurs after the stoma is irrigated (and thereby stimulated) once a day or every other day. Working with an ostomy nurse will help you understand how to perform the irrigation and teach you how to fix problems that may occur.

Ostomy Management and Care

The first step in caring for an ostomy will always involve covering it with a clear drainage pouch. This allows the health care team to easily see the stoma, drainage, and condition of the skin in the area around the stoma. Since most problems occur soon after the ostomy is first created, this early observation is important.

A nurse in the hospital will help you to find and fit a skin barrier faceplate or flange around the stoma. This protects the skin in the area, and is where the pouch attaches. The pouches are changed as they become soiled and stained, but the faceplate or flange remains in place as long as it sticks well to the skin and does not leak. Immediately after surgery, colostomies will drain liquid and mucus. If it is a closed loop colostomy, it will not drain until opened. If your colostomy is placed in the descending or sigmoid colon, you may be able to choose to regulate it so that you have a bowel movement on a regular schedule. If you do not want to regulate it, you can keep a pouch over it.

If your surgeon determines that you will need a temporary or permanent colostomy, an ostomy nurse or wound, ostomy, and continence nurse (WOCN) will join your health care team. He or she will educate you about your colostomy and will help you learn how to manage your ostomy, to obtain and use supplies correctly, and to adapt your lifestyle to accommodate the colostomy.

Complications

You may experience complications related to your ostomy. The most common problem after colostomy surgery is the development of a hernia around the stoma site. This takes the form of a bulge in the skin around the stoma and causes difficulty irrigating and partial obstruction of the stoma.

A less serious complication is skin irritation in the area near the stoma. A colostomy that discharges firm stool usually causes few, if any, skin problems. But if the stool is loose and contains caustic digestive enzymes, as is often the case with transverse colostomies, it can irritate the skin. To prevent skin problems, keep the area clean and dry and change the pouch regularly. Call the doctor immediately if any of the following symptoms develop:

- severe cramps lasting more than two to three hours
- unusual odor lasting more than a week
- unusual change in stoma size and appearance
- obstruction at the stoma
- prolapse of the stoma (when the bowel protrudes through the opening)
- excessive bleeding from the stoma opening or a moderate amount of blood in several emptyings of the pouch

277

- severe injury or cut to the stoma
- continuous bleeding at the junction between stoma and skin
- watery discharge lasting more than five to six hours
- chronic skin irritation
- stenosis (narrowing) of the stoma

Ostomy Supplies

Always keep a comfortable quantity of supplies on hand to ensure that you don't run out. However, ostomy supplies do have a shelf life and can be affected by heat, so don't purchase too many at once. You can order ostomy supplies from pharmacies, medical supply distributors, and on the Internet. Check the yellow pages under "Ostomy Supplies," "Surgical Supplies," or "Hospital Supplies." The United Ostomy Association (http://www.uoa.org) is also an excellent resource.

Pouches

Many people with colostomies wear a pouch. Pouches collect stool that may expel expectedly or unexpectedly. Pouching systems may include a one- or two-piece system. Both kinds include a faceplate, or flange (also called a wafer because of its thin, disc-like shape), and a collection pouch. The pouch attaches to the abdomen by the faceplate or flange and is fitted over and around the stoma to collect the diverted stool. The barrier is designed to protect the skin from the stoma output and to be as neutral to the skin as possible.

Pouches come in a variety of styles and sizes that do not show under clothing (see Figure 16.4). Some are open at the bottom for easy emptying. Others are closed and are removed for emptying when they become filled. Others allow the adhesive face plate or flange to remain on the body while the pouch is detached, emptied, or replaced. Everyone, including those who irrigate, needs some type of stoma pouch on hand, if only for emergency purposes.

Cotton pouch covers fit over the pouch and are designed for comfort and to protect the skin. They can also be used to cover the pouch during intimate occasions.

Stoma Covers and Caps

If your colostomy is regulated, a gauze-type covering can be placed over the stoma and held in place with waterproof tape, or you may be able to use a stoma cap.

Other Supplies

Depending on your unique situation, you may also use some other supplies:

Figure 16.4 Types of Colostomy Pouches

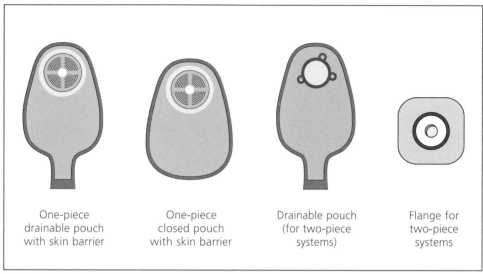

| One-piece drainable pouch with skin barrier | One-piece closed pouch with skin barrier | Drainable pouch (for two-piece systems) | Flange for two-piece systems |

Source: Copyright © 2003 O'Reilly Associates. From Kalibjian C. Straight from the Gut: Living with Crohn's Disease and Ulcerative Colitis Sebastopol, CA: O'Reilly; 2003. Reprinted with the permission of O'Reilly Media, Inc.

- Various skin barrier products, such as liquids, wipes, or powders, can help protect the skin under the faceplate and around the stoma from irritation caused by digestive products or adhesives. They also aid in adhesion of the faceplate.
- Tapes are sometimes used to help support the flange or faceplate and for waterproofing. They are available in a wide range of materials to meet the needs of different skin sensitivities.
- Ostomy belts wrap around the abdomen and attach to the loops found on certain pouches. Belts can also be used to help support the pouch or as an alternative to adhesives if skin problems develop.

Insurance Coverage for Supplies

For all consumers, but especially for people with permanent ostomies who will need supplies indefinitely, the selection of insurance is critical. Both the cost and coverage of ostomy supplies are important factors to consider.

Most individual health insurance plans typically will pay you 80 percent of the "reasonable and customary" costs after the deductible is met, but you need to investigate exactly what is covered. Sometimes everything is covered. Other plans will cover pouches but not tape, may pay only for a certain type of pouch, or may limit where you can buy supplies. If your claim is denied, learn how to appeal.

When changing insurance carriers, you should also investigate whether having a colostomy constitutes a pre-existing condition, which might render you ineligible for benefits.

Medicare Part B covers ostomy equipment, but only allows a predetermined maximum quantity each month.

Coping With a Colostomy

Living with a colostomy—that is, managing the everyday tasks associated with changing and emptying a pouch and maintaining good colostomy hygiene—is different from *coping* with a colostomy. Coping with a colostomy is about psychologically learning to live with a colostomy and accepting the changes it may require in your lifestyle.

> "I find that having a permanent colostomy doesn't stop me. I go to the pool in the morning, and I'm very, very active. You live with a permanent colostomy. You do realize you have it, that's not anything you can forget. You take a little bit of extra care when you apply it, make sure that you're not going to have an accident later on. I'm not embarrassed or afraid of it anymore, but I was at the beginning."
> —LUCY

There are times after surgery when you may feel discouraged. You may feel alone and isolated. Because the whole experience is so new to you, you may feel awkward, frustrated, and uncertain. You may feel uncomfortable dealing with your personal bodily functions, and you may worry about repulsing others or may yourself feel some initial revulsion emptying your pouch or irrigating your stoma. These feelings and reactions are normal. You might cry, be hostile or angry, and react in ways that are unusual for you.

Talking to your partner, a trusted friend, or a member of the clergy can help. The members of your health care team (especially an ostomy nurse, social workers, and counselors), and other people with ostomies may help you work through these feelings. Many people say that they worried about not being able to see themselves in the same way again and wondered whether they would be able to regain and maintain their normal lifestyle. There will certainly be some changes as you adjust to a colostomy, but many people can attest to the fact that most aspects of your life can proceed as before an ostomy.

You will find as you talk to people that ostomies are more common than you realize. A variety of medical conditions may require ileostomy or colostomy, including cancer, diverticulitis, bowel obstruction, injury, and birth defects. Many people live with their ostomies for years.

Finding Support

Your doctor, an ostomy nurse, and other health care professionals on your team are important sources of information and support. Because one of the most difficult aspects of having an ostomy can be the initial reaction to seeing the stoma and pouch on your abdomen, your health care team will help you change and empty your pouch and will teach you how to manage and adjust to this change in the days and weeks immediately after the surgery.

The United Ostomy Association (UOA) web site has information about ostomies and supplies. Emotional support is available through local chapters. You can locate a chapter near you by calling the American Cancer Society at 1-800-ACS-2345, or visiting the UOA web site at http://www.uoa.org.

Taking part in an ostomy support group or participating in an online "chat room" may also help. A support group allows you to share your feelings and ask questions. It also allows you to share your successful adjustment with others who may need the benefit of your experience.

> "I am 46 years old. I have a colostomy, and I just want you to know, that it's not the end of the world. And you know what? Nobody even knows that you have it. There's no red light over my head that goes and says, 'Oh, gee whiz, this lady poops in a bag.' ...And this surgery saved my life. Yes, it does take a little bit of maintenance. Yes, it's kind of a pain in the neck, I will grant you that. But there's nothing wrong with it, and it functions just as normally in every aspect, every aspect. And that means personally, sexually, all those kinds of things. ...Nobody would ever know unless you tell them."
>
> —DONNA

The Wound, Ostomy, and Continence Nurses Society (800-224-9626 or http://www.wocn.org/) also supplies information and can give local referrals for ostomy nurse specialists.

Telling Others About Your Surgery

You might be worried about how others will accept you and how you will explain your surgery. You can tell your friends and relatives as much as you want them to know. If you have children, answer their questions simply and truthfully. If you take a matter-of-fact approach, they are likely to adopt it too. If you are considering entering into a serious or intimate relationship, discussions with your partner about life with a colostomy will help to alleviate misconceptions.

Resuming and Maintaining Your Lifestyle

People with colostomies can do everything they did before their surgery—dine out, wear stylish clothes, go to work, take a bath, play sports, and have sex. You may have to take a few extra precautions depending on your situation, but an ostomy should not prevent you from leading an active, healthy, happy life.

Clothing and Appearance

Because colostomy pouches are fairly flat and inconspicuous, you shouldn't be concerned about special clothing. The pressure of undergarments with elastic will not harm the stoma or prevent the bowel from functioning; however, avoid tight waistbands directly on the stoma. Women may find that knit underwear or pantyhose gives added support and security. Men can wear either boxer or brief-style underwear.

Eating and Digestion

In the first weeks and months after your surgery, you may be asked to follow a low-residue diet of foods that are bland and easy to digest.

After healing is complete and the ostomy is functioning normally, most people with colostomies can return to a regular diet. Introduce foods back into your diet a little at a time and monitor the effect of each food on the function of your ostomy. Some less digestible or high-roughage foods are more likely to create blockage problems (for example, corn, coconut, mushrooms, nuts, raw fruits, and raw vegetables). You may also want to choose your foods more carefully to minimize gas and odor and to avoid diarrhea and constipation (see Table 16.1).

Managing Intestinal Gas

During the first weeks and months after surgery, you may experience excessive intestinal gas. This will lessen after the bowel has had time to heal and you have resumed a regular diet.

To help prevent excessive gas, eat at a leisurely pace in a relaxed atmosphere with your mouth closed, and chew well. Avoid the food listed in Table 16.1. Constipation or unsatisfactory irrigation may also cause gas.

Table 16.1 How Foods May Affect an Ostomy

Foods That Can Cause Odor	Foods That Can Cause Gas	Foods That Can Cause Diarrhea	Foods That Can Cause Constipation
Alcohol	Beans	Alcohol	Cheese
Asparagus	Beer	Beer	Chocolate
Cruciferous vegetables	Carbonated drinks	Coffee	Eggs
(broccoli, Brussels sprouts,	Cheese	Fresh, unpeeled fruit	High-fiber foods
cabbage, cauliflower)	Chewing gum	Vegetables	
Eggs	Cruciferous vegetables	Spicy foods	
Fish	(broccoli, Brussels sprouts,	Whole grains	
Garlic	cabbage, cauliflower)		
Onions	Cucumbers		
	Onions		
	Soy		
	Sprouts		

If intestinal gas is a continuing problem for you, write down what you eat and how it is prepared. These notes can help you learn what causes the problem.

Controlling Odor

Certain foods tend to produce more odor than others (see Table 16.1). Some medicines such as vitamins and antibiotics also cause stools to have odor. Some options for odor management include oral products (such as bismuth subgallate) and deodorant drops in the pouch. These products are more effective with transverse colostomies.

Coping With Constipation and Diarrhea

Constipation is often the result of an unbalanced diet, not enough food or liquids, or certain medications. If you had constipation problems before surgery, remember how you solved them and try the same methods. However, *do not use laxatives without asking your doctor first.*

Diarrhea must be distinguished from loose bowel movements, which are common in transverse colostomies because of the shortened length of the colon. Loose bowel movements in and of themselves are not a sign of sickness or disease. However, if you experience an increase in frequency of stools compared with normal, or bowel movements that are looser than usual, report those changes to your doctor.

See Table 16.1 for a list of foods that can contribute to diarrhea and constipation. If you have persistent diarrhea or constipation, talk with your doctor or ostomy nurse. They may be able to prescribe medication to help you manage these symptoms. Also, see pages 251 and 252 for tips on coping with diarrhea and constipation.

Colostomy Quick Tips

- If you feel self-conscious, as though everyone can see your pouch even though it is hidden by your clothing, keep these questions in mind: Did you know what a colostomy was, or where a stoma was located, or what it looked like, before you had surgery?
- If you find your pouch filling with gas and bulging under your clothing, a quick trip to the restroom can take care of this problem.
- To muffle noisy discharges of gas, put your hand discreetly over the stoma.
- If you are worried about your pouch filling up immediately after eating at a social event, remember, people without colostomies often need to go to the restroom after eating and nobody will think it unusual if you do the same.
- Check the pouch occasionally to see whether it needs emptying before it gets too full and causes a leakage problem. Always empty before going out of the house and away from a convenient toilet.
- To empty the pouch, sit on the toilet with the pouch between your legs. Hold the bottom of the pouch up and remove the clamp. Slowly unroll the tail of the pouch and empty contents into the toilet. Clean the outside and inside of the pouch tail with toilet paper. Replace the clamp.
- Keep an ample supply of supplies on hand to avoid accidents.

Returning to Work

As your strength returns, you can go back to work. Persons with colostomies can do most jobs; however, heavy lifting may cause a stoma to herniate or prolapse. Check with your doctor about your type of work.

If you feel you are being discriminated against on the job because of your cancer or your colostomy, contact the Equal Employment Opportunity Commission (EEOC) at http://www.eeoc.gov/ or 800-669-4000.

Intimacy and Sexuality

Sexual relationships and intimacy are important aspects of your life that can and should continue after ostomy surgery. Your attitude is a key factor in re-establishing sexual expression and intimacy, although a period of adjustment after surgery is to be expected.

The creation of a colostomy usually does not physically affect sexual function. Body contact during sexual activities will usually not harm the stoma or loosen the pouch from the abdomen. The colostomy itself should not interfere with normal sexual activity or pregnancy. If there is a problem, it is almost always related to the removal of the rectum. Changes to your emotional state (depression), your physical health (pain), and the effects of other cancer treatments, such as radiation and chemotherapy, all may play a role.

After surgery, while you are recovering and learning to manage your ostomy, you may not experience sexual feelings for days, weeks, or even months. You may fear rejection or suffer changes in your body image and self-esteem. On the other hand, you may begin to focus on sexual feelings while still in the hospital. You need to let your partner know what to expect from you about intimacy and sex.

Partners of people with ostomies may feel anger and resentment toward a sick mate or may express concern about hurting the stoma during intimate encounters. Such feelings and fears are natural. Try to discuss sexuality concerns openly and honestly. Seeking the support and advice of a professional counselor can be a great help.

You may also need to surmount some physical and psychological barriers. Illness and medical treatments often lower sexual desire, as do pain, medication, and fatigue. See page 254 for more on coping with symptoms and side effects related to sexual function.

As you engage in sexual activity, you may have to adjust your routine somewhat. Here are some tips on preparing for sex and making love:

> *"What I would be embarrassed about was my thought of going back to work with a permanent colostomy, thinking that I might have an accident. I wasn't embarrassed as much as I was afraid of having an accident. And then I found the people that I work with saying, 'Listen, we love you. We don't worry about you having an accident, we're just so happy that you're here.'"*
>
> —LUCY

> *"It could have been a problem but my wife was a rock; she was very, very, very understanding. Intimacy was not a problem with my wife because she did not mind the pouch."*
>
> —JOHN

- Good ostomy hygiene is always important, but it is especially important before sex. The colostomy covering or pouch for your ostomy should be clean and neat. Unless sex is absolutely spontaneous, the pouch should be emptied beforehand. Pouches should be odor free and fastened securely.

> "There is love and caring and sex after the ostomy. These things need to be talked about, because so many men think if their wife is going to have an ostomy, ileostomy, or colostomy, that their sex life is gone. And it certainly is not. We've been married 54 years, and I've had the ostomy for 29 of those years. As far as my husband goes, we're in love. I think love conquers all, and that's the way we feel about it."
>
> —NINA

- Pouches should be opaque, or covered with a pouch cover. You might also try wearing a sexy cover-up, such as a negligee or short robe.
- Experiment with different positions if the pouch or other stoma covering seems to be in the way during intercourse.
- There is much more to a loving, intimate, physically satisfying relationship than sexual intercourse. Cuddling, manual stimulation, or otherwise pleasuring each other can be delightful.

Participating in Physical Activities

An ostomy should not prevent you from leading an active lifestyle or participating in sports. People with ostomies participate in most types of physical activities, including running, skiing, and swimming. However, you may want to avoid contact sports and heavy weight lifting (a severe blow could injure the stoma and heavy weight lifting could result in a hernia at the stoma). If you are unsure, ask your doctor before undertaking any physical activities.

Bathing

You may bathe with or without your pouching system in place. If you wish to take a shower or bath with your pouch off, you can do so. You can also leave your pouch on. Normal exposure to air or contact with soap and water will not harm the stoma and water will not enter the ostomy opening.

Travel

Don't avoid road trips, camping, cruises, and air travel because of your colostomy. There is no reason you can't travel, as long as you take a few extra precautions. For example, leave home fully prepared and take along enough supplies to last the entire trip plus some extras in case your return is delayed. If you are taking a plane flight, carry an extra pouching system and other supplies on the plane with you in case your checked luggage gets lost.

CHAPTER SEVENTEEN

TAKING CARE OF PRACTICAL MATTERS:
Work, Insurance, and Money

Maureen Coyle, MSW, LCSW-C
Eden Stotsky

Given the many physical and emotional challenges that come with cancer, it may be difficult for you to focus on daily tasks such as keeping records and paying bills. Yet, if you are willing to spend a little bit of time thinking about these issues, you may come across some useful information that can make your experience with colorectal cancer a little easier.

In this chapter, we'll explore what you need to know to stay informed about your job, insurance, and financial situation as you undergo treatment for your colorectal cancer.

Employment and Workplace Issues

Facing a cancer diagnosis often brings with it an increased sense of the importance of work in a person's life. For many people, work is an important part of their identity. Professional accomplishments can boost your self-esteem. Fulfilling your work duties can remind you that there is more to who you are than your cancer. Work can also preserve your daily routine and sense of normalcy, and it can distract you from cancer treatment. In addition, cancer can be extremely isolating, and being around people at work can be a great comfort. For most people, work is also a very important part of their financial well being.

Figure 17.1 Work Schedule Chart

Day	Schedule
Sunday	
Monday	
Tuesday	
Wednesday	
Thursday	
Friday	
Saturday	

Preparing for Time Away From Work

Your return to work will be easier if you have done a little planning before your absence. This isn't always possible, but if it is, you may want to make logs of your usual work schedule and responsibilities and refer to them when organizing any flextime, shifted responsibilities, or time off. It may help to fill out a Work Schedule Calendar and Work Responsibilities Log (see Figure 17.1 and Figure 17.2 on page 290). These tools can help your coworkers handle situations while you are away.

To better prepare for your time away from work, you'll need to have a detailed understanding of what your treatment involves, including how long you'll need to be away from the office, how long your recovery will take, and how your cancer or its treatment might affect your energy level or ability to function. Some specific questions to ask your health care team are listed in on page 291.

Telling Your Employer and Your Coworkers

A diagnosis of colorectal cancer is particularly difficult because it's a type of cancer that few people want to talk about, and it affects parts of the body that people generally aren't comfortable discussing. How open you are with your employer and coworkers about your cancer is a personal decision. Many people bring it up soon after diagnosis to give supervisors ample time to adjust to work schedules or personal assignments. Other people wait until they begin treatment, when they are more mentally prepared to discuss their cancer.

A few even choose to go it alone without workplace support. Although this is certainly an option, it is the most difficult. Keep in mind that if you do not tell your employer about your illness and you have difficulty performing at work or fulfilling your job duties, you will not be protected by federal laws that prevent employers from discriminating against people with chronic illnesses or disabilities (see page 292). Discuss with your family and health care team what is best for you.

In some environments, it won't benefit you to share details. It might help to first decide who is most likely to understand your situation. You can then confide in that person or those people and ask for help in developing the best plan for telling others and for requesting time off.

In some work settings, people may react to your cancer diagnosis and absences due to treatment with understanding and helpfulness. Some people will be very supportive. It is likely that many supervisors and coworkers have had people close to them who have had cancer. Think about what approach will work best for you at work. You may want to talk with your employer about options such as flextime, job sharing, or telecommuting if it would help you fulfill your job responsibilities.

Figure 17.2 Work Responsibility Log

Current Projects	Scheduled Meetings	Important Dates/Deadlines	Responsibilities to Be Shifted	Person to Do Them

Questions to Ask Your Health Care Team About Work and Cancer Treatment

- Will I be able to work throughout my treatment?
- If I have to stay home to recover from surgery or other treatment, how long will I be away from my job?
- Will I be able to return to work after treatment?
- If I do return to work, do I need to have a different work schedule?
- Will any of my abilities to perform my job be impaired as a result of treatment?
- How will I know if I am overdoing it at my job?
- Do I need to give my place of employment any special forms or other documentation from my doctor before taking time off from work? (You can also ask this question of your employer.)

Your cancer may cause coworkers to feel uncomfortable around you. Employers and coworkers may react awkwardly from a vague fear or uneasiness about cancer, thinking of cancer as something that is contagious or dangerous. Many people are bothered by it as an unpleasant reminder of their own mortality. Coworkers may ask intrusive or odd questions about your health or may avoid you. Your coworkers may also take on extra responsibilities because of your absences; they may resent having to do this or they may do it willingly.

Worries About Discrimination

Even though attitudes toward understanding cancer are generally improving, some prejudices and preconceived notions remain, and these can sometimes result in workplace discrimination.

It is a good idea to keep records of your contacts with your employer's human resources department, including the names of the people with whom you spoke about your cancer, the date and place you spoke, and the information you discussed.

It's also a good idea to keep documentation of your job performance evaluations. If you are a member of a union, union officials are also good sources of information about illnesses and the workplace.

> "Because I was self-employed, I did not experience any of the job discrimination that has been part of other cancer stories I've heard. I did learn that the playing field was no longer level when I attempted to buy life insurance. I would have to wait five years to be insured at standard rates."
>
> —DICK

If you have cancer, an employer should not discriminate against you because of your diagnosis. In fact, there are laws to protect you from such discrimination. In many cases, you would be covered by the Americans with Disabilities Act (ADA). (Although you may not think of yourself as disabled, you are "disabled" within the definition of the law if your health condition substantially limits one or more major life activities.)

The ADA makes it unlawful to discriminate in employment practices such as recruitment, job application and hiring, training, job assignments, tenure, promotions, pay, benefits, leave, firing, and all other employment-related activities. For additional information, including information about filing a complaint, call 800-514-0301 or 800-514-0383 (TTY) or visit the ADA web site at http://www.ada.gov.

Employers are not required to lower standards for a disabled employee. However, an employer must make a change or adjustment to a job that allows an employee with a disability to perform the "essential functions" of the job or to enjoy the benefits and privileges of employment equal to those enjoyed by employees without disabilities. If you need time off for treatments, a reasonable accommodation may be a part-time or flexible work schedule. Speak with your employer to clarify the benefits to which you may be entitled. To find out more about job accommodations that may work for you, contact the Job Accommodation Network at 800-526-7234 or http://www.jan.wvu.edu.

If you think you have been discriminated against in employment on the basis of disability, you can file a complaint with the US Equal Employment Opportunity Commission (EEOC) within 180 days of the alleged discrimination (according to some state or local laws, you can take up to 300 days). For more specific information about ADA requirements affecting employment, contact the EEOC at 800-669-4000 or 800-669-6820 (TTY) or visit their web site at http://www.eeoc.gov. You may also want to consider consulting an employment discrimination attorney.

The Family and Medical Leave Act

The Family and Medical Leave Act (FMLA) requires that employers of more than 50 people provide 12 weeks of *unpaid* leave on account of medical reasons. This applies to an employee's own medical condition or those who are caring for an immediate family member (spouse, children, or parents) with a serious health condition. Many employers require that accrued paid vacation or sick time be used first. The 12 weeks of leave may be used continuously or intermittently within a 12-month period.

To be eligible, the employee must have been employed there for at least 12 months and have worked 1250 hours during that time. You will need to provide to your employer medical documentation that a serious health condition exists. By law, people must be returned to the same or an equivalent position, including pay and benefits. Your employer is required to maintain your group health insurance; however, you may be responsible for your share of the premium.

You may also be entitled to similar time off from a smaller employer depending on your state's laws.

If you feel that you have been treated unfairly under this act, you can file a complaint with the US Department of Labor. Call 866-4-USA-DOL/866-487-2365 or visit http://www.dol.gov/esa/whd/fmla/ for more information about the FMLA.

> *"There was one medication for nausea that my new oncologist gave me a prescription for. So, I got the prescription, and it was $10, and usually I don't look at the full retail price of the prescription, I just file away the receipt. And I happened to glance at it, and 20 antinausea pills were almost $400! I think you've got to know about your plan, and you need to know what's covered and how it works."*
> —EDDIE

Insurance

Your insurance is important to assure you receive appropriate treatment for your cancer. There are many types of insurance, including health insurance, disability insurance, and life insurance. These policies may have been made available to you through your work, or you may have purchased them separately.

> *"I had absolutely no problem with my insurance. I was just really blessed with that, because that's one hassle that you just don't need on top of everything else."*
> —JACY

Health Insurance

If you have health insurance, it is important to know how your coverage works and what it covers. For example, if you have a type of managed-care coverage, it may be that insurance company approval is needed before you can see a doctor, receive treatment, or purchase medicine. Even then, you may be limited to the doctor or treatment center that

Questions to Ask About Your Health Insurance

- What is the best number to use to contact my insurance company with questions about my coverage?
- Does my policy have a monetary cap on benefits?
- What treatments for colorectal cancer are covered by my policy?
- What is my coverage for inpatient hospital visits?
- What is my coverage for outpatient chemotherapy and/or radiation?
- If my doctor prescribes an oral chemotherapy agent, will this be covered by my prescription plan?
- Do I need to have procedures preauthorized and, if so, whom do I contact?
- Do I have to see a doctor who is in-network? If I go outside of the network, what is my coverage?
- If I am eligible for a clinical trial, will this be covered by my insurance?
- What is my coverage for ostomy supplies, and do I need to order them from a specific supplier?
- Am I eligible for case management services, which may offer me additional benefits?
- For what out-of-pocket expense will I be responsible?
- Am I eligible for transportation services to/from treatments and/or doctor visits?

the insurance company chooses. Or you may have the kind of policy under which you see whatever doctor you choose and then submit the bill.

The key is to learn how your coverage works and figure out what the plan really covers, especially in the case of an illness like cancer. If the description from your employer or insurance company isn't clear, ask for clarification in the benefits department of the hospital or doctor's office or call the insurance company. The questions above can help you learn more about the specifics of your health care coverage.

Claim Disputes

It is important that you keep your medical bills organized and submit them as soon as they are received. If any of your claims are denied, ask the billing department at your doctor's office or hospital for assistance.

Sometimes the insurance company will deny claims based on specific language in the policy, or by the incorrect use of codes by the billing department. Contact your insurance company to find out how you can appeal the denial. Keep track of the people with whom you have spoken, including the date and time, and make copies of all written correspondence. If further intervention in necessary, contact your state insurance commissioner by looking in your local phone book or by visiting the National Association of Insurance Commissioners web site at http://www.naic.org.

Health Care Resources

Many health care and insurance-related resources exist to help you with insurance issues and related services. We'll share some of the most common resources; your hospital's social worker can also connect you with resources and organizations who can help.

MEDICARE

Medicare is a federal program that pays for medical care for those who are 65 or older, have been on Social Security Disability Insurance (see page 298) for over 24 months, or have end-tage renal disease. Medicare is made up of two parts, A and B. Medicare part A covers inpatient hospital care, skilled nursing facilities, hospice, and home health care. Medicare part A is free if you or your spouse has paid Medicare taxes while working. Medicare part B covers doctor's services, outpatient services, diagnostic tests, X-rays and laboratory tests, and home durable medical equipment. In 2004, part B was $66.60 per month. It can be automatically deducted from your Social Security check.

> *"All of my treatments, my radiation, my chemo, my surgery, were all covered, but we did go through battles, because while I was taking my chemotherapy, my oncologist would submit a bill for the pump and the chemotherapy. One month or one week the insurance company would pay it without a problem and the next week they would send us back a statement that said I'd gone out of network, or I was doing something that wasn't covered, and it was the very same procedure we had done the week before with the chemotherapy. So, we had to go back in and, in fact, I have a bill today still sitting in my desk that we are still trying to get the codes corrected so that the insurance company will pay for the things that they paid for during different time periods of my treatment."*
>
> —PATTI

295

Medicare benefits are subject to change, so to ensure that you have the most accurate and current information about Medicare, call 800-MEDICARE/ 800-633-4223 or visit http://www.medicare.gov.

MEDIGAP

If you receive Medicare benefits, you may be able to add more coverage with a Medigap policy or a Medicare HMO to provide for things not covered by Medicare (co-pays, deductibles, and prescription costs, for example). There are 10 Medigap policies issued by private companies, which are identified by letters A through J. Medigap policies require underwriting, which means that a person with a serious disease like cancer may not be eligible. Under the Medicare Modernization Act of 2003, Medigap policies will be changing, so contact Medicare at 800-MEDICARE/800-633-4223 or check online at http://www.medicare.gov for the most updated information.

MEDICAID

Medicaid is a government program that covers the cost of medical care for those with limited incomes and resources. Check with your local Medicaid office to find out what the financial limits are in your state. You may qualify if you are pregnant, disabled, blind, elderly, or part of a low-income family with children. If you are receiving Medicare with limited resources, you may also be eligible for Medicaid to help with deductibles and co-payments, part B premiums, and some pharmacy coverage.

VETERANS' BENEFITS

If you are a veteran, you may qualify for health, income, or other benefits from the government, administered by the Department of Veterans Affairs. To find out if you are eligible, contact them at 800-827-1000 to speak with a benefits counselor, or visit http://www.va.gov.

HILL-BURTON PROGRAM

Under the Hill-Burton Program, hospitals and other health facilities that have received federal funds for construction, renovation, or expansion must provide a specific amount of free or reduced-cost medical care each year to those who are unable to pay. Each facility chooses which services it will provide free or at lowered cost. Eligibility for Hill-Burton funds is based upon family size and income. For more information about this program, or to locate the nearest Hill-Burton facility, call 800-638-0742 or visit http://www.hrsa.dhhs.gov/osp. The admissions or business office of the medical center where you are receiving your treatment can tell you how to apply for assistance.

THE HEALTH INSURANCE PORTABILITY AND ACCOUNTABILITY ACT

The Health Insurance Portability and Accountability Act (HIPAA) provides nationwide standards and a guarantee of access to health insurance coverage in the individual market. This legislation protects people from discrimination based on pre-existing medical conditions. Because of HIPAA, many employees may not lose their insurance when they change jobs.

Although HIPAA is a national protection, some criteria may vary by state. Check with your State Insurance Commissioner's Office to see if your state is affected.

CONSOLIDATED OMNIBUS BUDGET RECONCILIATION ACT

If you are no longer able to work, you may be eligible for health care coverage under COBRA (Consolidated Omnibus Budget Reconciliation Act) for up to 18 months. Your employer should be able to provide you with information on COBRA insurance.

RISK POOLS

A number of states sell comprehensive health insurance to state residents with serious medical conditions who can't find a company to insure them. These state programs, sometimes called guaranteed-access programs, or, more commonly, state risk pools, serve people who have pre-existing health conditions who are often denied or have difficulty finding affordable coverage in the private market. They provide a safety net for the "medically uninsurable" population. To find out if your state has a risk pool, contact the state department of insurance by calling directory assistance in your state capitol.

HEALTH MAINTENANCE ORGANIZATIONS

Health maintenance organizations (HMOs) or health care service plans in your community can provide quite comprehensive coverage. Many offer one period of open enrollment each year, where applicants are accepted regardless of health histories.

HELP FROM INDEPENDENT BROKERS

An independent broker may be able to help you locate a reasonable benefit package. Group insurance is usually preferable to individual insurance.

HELP FROM PROFESSIONAL ORGANIZATIONS

You may be able to apply for group insurance through fraternal or professional organizations (such as those for retired persons, teachers, social workers, realtors, etc.). If you are the parent of a school-age child, investigate school insurance. Look for a "guaranteed issue" plan, which means that you cannot be denied.

EMPLOYMENT BENEFITS

If you don't currently have health insurance though your job or your spouse/partner's job, it may be worthwhile to for you or your spouse/partner to consider changing jobs to get better benefits. Larger employers such as Fortune 500 companies or federal, state, or local governments tend to have the best benefits. However, do your research before making a job change: some employers may make employees and their dependents wait before joining a plan, and there may be a period in which pre-existing conditions are not covered.

Disability Insurance

A disability insurance policy pays you a regular income when an illness like cancer or an accident prevents you from doing your job. You may have disability benefits from your employer and/or the government. If not, you may be eligible for SSDI or SSI benefits.

Social Security Disability Insurance

You may qualify for Social Security Disability Insurance (SSDI) if you meet the Social Security Administration's (SSA) definition of disability and have worked long enough in the past to have paid into the social security system. The SSA defines a disability as a physical or mental condition that is expected to last continuously for a year or to cause death. This condition must prevent you from doing any kind of financially meaningful work. To apply for SSDI, contact the SSA at 800-772-1213 to schedule either a phone or face-to-face interview at your local SSA office.

If you are found to be disabled, you will start receiving your check 6 months after the onset of your disability. You may be paid retroactively for up to 12 months. The amount you receive will depend on your previous earnings. You will be eligible for Medicare after you have received disability payments for 24 months. Many people are denied disability on their first application. It is recommended that you appeal this decision if you are denied.

Social Security Income

If you are over 65, disabled, and/or blind, you may qualify for social security income (SSI). This differs from SSDI in that in addition to meeting the Social Security Administration's definition for disability, you must have a limited income and have little in savings or assets (less than $2000 if single, $3000 if married) regardless of how long you have paid into the Social Security system. To see if you are eligible for SSI, contact the SSA at 800-772-1213. You will need to provide financial documentation in addition to the information listed under SSDI, such as payroll slips, insurance policies, mortgage or rent payments, car registration, and burial policies.

If you are found to be eligible, you will receive payment the first of the month after the month in which you applied and were found medically and financially eligible. Because SSI is based on financial need, in most states you can also qualify for food stamps and medical assistance, which includes health and pharmacy coverage. The amount you will receive varies from state to state. If you qualify for SSI, you will also receive Medicaid.

Life Insurance

What will happen to your spouse or partner, children, or other dependents if cancer ends your life prematurely? Are they counting on your paycheck to cover day-to-day needs or future expenses? If so, life insurance can provide your loved ones with income to replace yours until they can live comfortably without it. It can also provide an emergency fund for medical, legal, and funeral costs and can help cover longer-term expenses, such as financing a child's college education or paying off a mortgage or business debts.

Living Benefits From Life Insurance Policies

Life-threatening illnesses and conditions, such as cancer, require extensive medical care and often lead to a need for immediate financial resources. In many states, the value of an individual's life insurance policy can be realized through the acceleration of the policy's death benefit—known as living benefits. These benefits can be accessed several ways, including a viatical (sale of the life insurance policy) and loans from the original insurance company or a third party against the face value of the life insurance policy.

A viatical is the sale of a life insurance policy for cash, which is in turn used to pay for food, shelter, or doctor visits, used to ease the stress of money worries, or used to meet other pressing needs. The process of selling a life insurance policy requires the person insured for a life-threatening illness to sell his or her life insurance policy to the third party. As with any sale, both sides must agree on what is being sold and for how much. A viatical insurance company is a company that buys policies from people with terminal illnesses. After the viatical company buys a policy, the company becomes the new owner and sole beneficiary of the policy. It pays the premiums on the policy as long as the person is alive. When the person dies, all the remaining money from the policy goes to the viatical company.

A viatical transition usually takes place when someone has a limited life expectancy—from less than six months to several years (the life expectancy must be certified by a doctor). A person with cancer who pursues a viatical transaction is probably unable to work, and their household income is likely to be low. To reduce money worries, the patient sells his or her life insurance policy for a lump-sum cash payment—often between 60 and 80 percent of the face value of the policy. The payment is usually tax-free and goes only to the holder of the policy, who can use the money in any way he or she sees fit. The drawbacks of a viatical are that your heirs receive no insurance money, you may not make the best trade available, and the sale is usually not reversible. Before making a decision about life insurance, think over your options carefully. Talk about this matter with a partner, trusted

Before Signing a Contract for a Viatical or Living Benefits

- Get a clear picture of what's involved. Read about viaticals.
- Get professional advice regarding types of living benefits available and their positives and negatives.
- Decide whether a viatical is really the best course of action for you.
- Attempt to verify life expectancy.
- Find out if Medicaid or other benefits will be affected.
- Shop around. Get several bids. Bids can vary from 35 to 80 percent of the policy.
- Find out if the company is a broker. Some companies use their own money to buy policies, but others are brokers. A broker gets a commission from the company and may not act in the best interest of the insured.
- Negotiate to get the best deal you can.

friend, financial advisor, and/or a professional and be sure you exercise caution when proceeding (see above).

Making a Financial Plan

A sound financial plan requires hoping for the best but planning for the worst. Create a financial plan that addresses the highest possible costs that you might encounter. This will give you peace of mind because you'll know you're prepared for whatever might happen.

Developing a financial plan will require that you estimate your sources of income and benefits, estimate your expenses, manage your investments, and plan your estate. Tracking financial issues can be a challenge for anyone. A financial planner can help too.

Cancer treatments may leave you little energy to think about money matters. Don't be too hard on yourself. If it's more difficult to address some topics than others, take on the easier ones first.

Estimate Your Income, Benefits, and Expenses

Determine the sources and amounts of income and benefits you have at your disposal (liquid assets). Make sure to include all regular income, as well as assets that could be sold for cash. Next, estimate your expenses in as much detail as you can. Some of these costs may be hard to estimate. You might want to discuss these issues with your doctor so you can plan accurately. Consider also consulting other people who have been treated for colorectal cancer who have been in a similar situation for information that might be helpful. Use the worksheet in Figure 17.3 on page 302 to help.

Manage Your Savings and Investments

During cancer treatment, it's important to have money available to pay for medical bills. You may worry that you'll be financially unable to meet your treatment costs.

If you have money invested in certificates of deposit, treasury bonds, mutual bonds, or common stock, you may be able to convert some of these to cash. Some investments are easier to cash in than others. Remember that the profit from the sale of stocks and some bonds will be part of your taxable income.

Dealing with cancer often means changing your priorities, including your approach to investing. Before you had cancer, you may have thought about getting a high return on your investments. However, increased return means increased risk. This is not the best time for risk. It's also not the time to think about long-term growth. Right now, your focus should be on your short-term needs and those of your family. Avoid having your money in riskier (or growth-oriented) investments. Instead, choose short-term and limited-term investments that can provide income, such as money market accounts at a bank or a money market mutual fund. Consult a financial advisor about how to best invest your income and maintain your savings.

"It hit us financially, pretty strong. We got by, we just made some adjustments and fortunately, my wife, you know, works, and makes as good as I do, and so together we do fine. With me out of work, it was pretty tough. We were trying to get by on one income and the disability. Some people don't have disability, and they're trying to get by on almost nothing, or one income instead of two. When you have bills that are planning for two incomes, it's pretty tough to get by on just one."

—KEN

Figure 17.3 Income/Benefits and Expenses Worksheet

Estimate Your Income and Benefits	
Your salary	
Your partner's salary or contributions to household	
Other regular income	
List the sources of income you would have if you had to stop working because of your treatment (if any):	
List the market value of each asset that you would consider selling or liquidating:	
Life insurance policies	
Home equity	
Stocks and bonds	
Other	
TOTAL (+) :	

Estimate Your Expenses	
Insurance deductible	
Co-payments	
Keeping in mind your doctor's highest estimates of hospital stays, number of treatment sessions, duration of treatment, and your likely health status, estimate the following costs:	
Highest possible out-of-pocket medical expenses	
Travel costs, flights, lodging, cabs or rental cars, food, and parking related to your medical care	
Greatest possible number of hospital stays	
Prescription drug costs	
Experimental treatments not covered by your insurance	
Complementary treatments not covered by your insurance	
Home healthcare costs	
Services such as babysitting, cooking, or cleaning	
Estimate based on amount of time you expect not to receive a full salary (employed but on medical leave/FMLA, unemployed, or receiving short- or long-term disability insurance)	
Lost wages	
TOTAL (-) :	

Plan Your Estate

Everything you own is part of your estate. This includes your house, car, and jewelry. It also usually includes your life insurance policies, retirement funds, and savings.

Estate planning is essential for everyone, not just those who have cancer. But it's difficult for some people to face. Estate planning can give you peace of mind because it allows you to be in control of your money at all stages of your life. Take care of this part of your financial planning as soon as you feel ready.

If possible, discuss your estate planning needs with an estate attorney. He or she can draw up the necessary documents. Depending on your finances, you may need to set up trusts. Trusts may help protect your assets from taxes and probate costs.

If your finances are simple, the documents could be drafted at a legal clinic or nonprofit group. Call the American Cancer Society (800-ACS-2345/800-227-2345) for names of organizations that can help you.

At minimum, everyone—not just someone with cancer—needs the following estate planning documents. After your documents are in place, it's a good idea to review them from time to time. Check to make sure the information is current and still reflects your wishes.

A Will

Your will directs how and to whom your assets will be distributed. Your will also names a guardian for any minor children and their assets.

Durable Power of Attorney for Finances

A durable power of attorney (DPOA) for finances allows you to name the person who will handle your finances if you are unable to handle them for yourself.

> *"I've taken care of every detail that I need to care of as far as, 'What happens if…?' …I've made sure everything is in order as far as life insurance and wills and all of that."*
>
> —JULIE

Durable Power of Attorney for Health Care

A durable power of attorney for health care or a medical DPOA allows you to name a person who will make decisions about your health care if you are unable to make them yourself. This person is called your health care proxy or agent.

Living Will

The living will allows you to specify the types of medical treatment you would want or not want if you are unable to communicate these choices.

Sources of Financial Help

Serious illnesses such as cancer often lead to a need for immediate financial resources. During treatment, many people find themselves struggling with financial problems.

Without insurance, costs can mount quickly. Even if you have insurance and your plan picks up most of your costs, out-of-pocket expenses can be a burden. If you've found gaps in your coverage, don't hesitate to discuss your needs with your doctor or hospital social worker. You may be pleasantly surprised by the number of organizations that exist to help you and other cancer patients.

If your financial situation is becoming a problem and mounting expenses are putting a strain on your wallet, the following resources may be helpful to you.

Paying Your Bills

Mounting medical and personal bills may add to your stress. Figure out how much you owe and are able to pay. Prioritize the debts that you owe. Work directly with your creditors and try to make payment arrangements when possible with the individual utility agencies, medical providers and mortgage companies. These creditors will often agree to accept smaller payments or a nominal monthly amount.

If credit card debt is an issue, ask your credit card company if you are eligible for a lower interest rate, or transfer you balance to another credit card with a lower interest rate. You may benefit from meeting with a credit counselor. Consumer Credit Counseling Service is a national nonprofit service that offers free and confidential debt counseling. They can help you consolidate your payments and develop a budget and repayment schedule. Contact them at 800-251-2227 or http://www.cccsintl.org.

The Federal Citizen Information Center offers information about managing debt. You can call them toll free at 800-FED-INFO/800-333-4636 or visit their web site at http://www.pueblo.gsa.gov.

Figure 17.4 on page 302 is designed to help you weigh your options.

Prescription Drug Assistance Programs

If you are unable to afford to fill your prescriptions, alert your doctor or a medical social worker. They can connect you with prescription drug assistance programs in your state. In addition, the pharmaceutical companies who manufacture your prescriptions might have their own assistance programs. A list of drug manufacturers that offer such help can be obtained by calling 800-762-4636 or visiting http://www.helpingpatients.org.

Finally, your doctor may be able to provide you with samples of some medications.

Table 17.1 Sources of Cash/Financial Assistance and Related Issues

Sources of Cash	Issues
Assets (sale of stock, real estate, etc)	• May create income tax obligation • May affect qualifying for government benefits
Home equity loan (may be lump sum or line of credit)	• Places home at risk • Must have equity in home • Must make regular payments • Must pass credit check
Family/personal loan	• Requires repayment • May strain family relationships • May require collateral
Policy loan (from life insurance company)	• Death benefit is reduced by the amount of the loan and accrued interest • Must have "cash value" type of policy • Must generally continue premium payments
Accelerated death benefits (life insurance)	• Must keep policy in force • Must be terminally ill (contact insurance company) • May create income tax obligation • May affect qualifying for government benefits
Viatical loan (borrow from investor using life insurance as collateral) OR Viatical settlement (sell life insurance policy to investor)	• May create income tax obligation • Must own policy • Must meet definition of terminally or chronically ill • May affect qualifying for government benefits

Home Equity Loans and Conversions

Home equity is the difference between the home's fair market value and the unpaid balance of the mortgage. Equity increases as the mortgage is paid down and as the property appreciates. A home equity loan allows you to borrow against the value you've built up in your home.

You may be able to convert part of your home's equity into cash if you are at least 62 years old and own your home (or nearly own it). The most common type of equity conversion is called a reverse mortgage. This is a loan against your home that doesn't have to be repaid for as long as you live there. The loan is repaid in the future—usually when the last surviving borrower sells, dies, or moves out of the home. It can provide cash to pay medical bills and other expenses, but it is still considered a loan and includes expenses such as interest charges and service fees. A reverse mortgage can also disqualify you from some government programs. Private, public, and federally insured lenders offer many types of reverse mortgage programs. Contact a financial advisor to find out if a reverse mortgage would help you.

You can get more information about home equity conversion from nonprofit consumer groups, such as the AARP (formerly known as the American Association of Retired Persons).

Retirement

Some people use money from their retirement plan before they retire as a source of cash. You may qualify for hardship provisions in your plan. Contact your financial advisor and/or your human resources office for more information.

Family Loans

Family members can also help pay some of your cancer-related expenses or bills. If you ask for a loan from a relative, outline a repayment period and an interest rate. (Keep in mind that there are federal tax consequences if the person making the loan charges you an interest rate below the minimum federal rate.) It's also important to put the agreement in writing. The tax laws in this area are complicated, so it's a good idea to consult an accountant about family loans.

If you don't think you will be able to repay the loan, ask for a gift instead. Anyone, including a relative, can give a tax-free gift of up to $11,000 per year (as of 2004). Married couples can make a joint tax-free gift of up to $22,000 per year (as of 2004). The allowable amount of tax-free gifting is increasing, so check with an expert for the latest numbers.

In addition, anyone can pay the medical bills of someone else without being subject to the gift limit, if the payment is made directly to the medical facility.

Other Organizations

The American Cancer Society (ACS) has numerous programs that support people with cancer (call 800-ACS-2345/800-227-2345 or visit http://www.cancer.org). Civic and religious organizations may offer financial help or services for people with cancer and their family members. Groups such as the United Way are listed in the yellow pages under "Social Service Organizations." Churches and synagogues may also be able to help with transportation, baby-sitting, and home care services, which may help you financially. The Federal Citizen Information Center offers information about health and money, and it provides many other types of consumer help. You can call them toll free at 800-FED-INFO/800-333-4636 or visit their web site at http://www.pueblo.gsa.gov.

The National Endowment for Financial Education has collaborated with the ACS in developing financial management program for people with cancer. For more information about the program called Taking Charge of Money Matters, call the ACS.

Welfare Office

Contact your county board of assistance, Aid to Families with Dependent Children (AFDC), and the Food Stamps Program for information.

Bankruptcy

If you try but can't make ends meet, you may have to file bankruptcy. Bankruptcy is a complicated area of law, so consult a bankruptcy attorney if you're considering filing for bankruptcy. Legal aid clinics and other nonprofit agencies can also provide advice in this area.

> *"You really need to do your homework in terms of dealing with the medical community, and dealing with the legal community, and dealing with insurance companies to ensure that you get the very best quality care that you can. And there's just you know, learning as much as you can about your situation and what your options are, and not being afraid to ask questions or to demand certain things."*
>
> —SUSAN

Protecting the Bottom Line

Don't make the assumption that because you have cancer you can't stay on top of your work, insurance, or financial situation. As you've read in this chapter, that is not the case. Knowing your rights, your options, and the benefits to which you are entitled—and where to go if you have questions or need assistance—can help make the experience of your cancer treatment easier for you and your loved ones.

CHAPTER EIGHTEEN

FOLLOW UP

David A. Rothenberger, MD

Following up with your doctors after treatment for colorectal cancer serves many purposes. It provides an opportunity for you and your family to pause and look back after the whirlwind of testing, surgery, and chemotherapy or radiation treatments you may have undergone. However, it is also a time to look ahead: to fully understand your prognosis, to plan realistically for the future, and to prevent and/or detect recurrences or new colorectal cancers.

It's also a terrific time to set post-treatment life goals and make changes or improvements to your lifestyle for better overall health (we'll talk more about these in chapter 19). First, you need to work with your health care team to develop short-term and long-term follow-up care plans. It is important that you understand what's involved in follow up, and that you are involved in creating a long-term follow-up plan that fits your particular situation.

> *"Cancer is a lifelong commitment, with the necessary follow-up testing and doctor exams."*
> —DOMINIC

What Is Follow Up?

Follow-up care after treatment of colorectal cancer involves three phases, from short-term to long-term (see Figure 18.1). The first phase is devoted to assuring full recovery from the treatment of your cancer. The second phase involves counseling to discuss your prognosis and to determine whether hereditary factors may have been involved in your case. The third phase involves developing and implementing a long-term cancer follow-up plan. Usually such a long-term plan has two components, one devoted to prevention of a second colorectal cancer in the remaining large intestine and the other devoted to detection of recurrent cancer.

"Make sure you've done your homework, that you know about your disease, that you know about the complications and implications of it, and that you maintain surveillance. You have to be your own best health advocate. You can't depend upon some doctor or some technician somewhere remembering, 'Oh, it's time for your scan, it's time for your blood work, it's time for your colonoscopy.' Make sure you have all your ducks in a row, that you know what tests need to be done at what points in time, and that you know what the expected test results are. And demand to know those test results, good, bad, or indifferent. You have to be the one that's most concerned about your health and your survival. You can't depend on somebody else to do it."

—LOU

As you approach your follow-up care, keep in mind that your follow-up plan is only that: a plan. It is based on what doctors predict will happen in the course of the coming months and years. It can and should change if new circumstances arise. *If you develop new symptoms, such as abdominal or pelvic pain, or if you notice blood in your stool or a new lump in your surgical incision or groin, you should call your doctor immediately.* Do not wait for your next office visit or scheduled follow-up test.

And one final caution: this chapter deals with follow up and monitoring of your health *as it relates to colorectal cancer.* Be sure to get regular check-ups from your primary care physician in addition to your follow-up visits with your cancer care team. Studies show that cancer survivors' other medical problems are often overlooked because of the attention that is paid to the cancer treatment and its effects. You may be at risk for heart disease, diabetes, or other chronic illnesses (*including other types of cancer*) because of your age, genetic profile, or lifestyle choices. Talk to your family doctor about screening for other diseases and consider developing an overall wellness plan. Remember, surviving colorectal cancer is only part of your total health picture.

310

Figure 18.1 The Phases of Follow Up After Colorectal Cancer Treatment

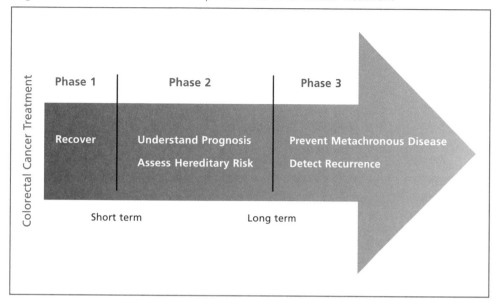

Who's in Charge of Follow Up?

Once your doctors have completed the initial course of cancer treatment, you may be left wondering who'll be in charge of your follow-up care in the near future and in the long term. Some sort of follow up with your doctors is usually recommended, but the extent, type, frequency and goals of follow-up care vary widely.

Most often, a person's recovery from colorectal cancer is straightforward and complications can be managed successfully. Occasionally, worrisome symptoms may arise, and when this happens it may not be clear to you which of your doctors you should call for this type of short-term follow up. For instance, if you develop painful swelling in the calf muscle while at home recovering from surgery and chemoradiation, should you call your surgeon, the medical oncologist, your radiation therapy doctor, or your family doctor? There is no single, correct answer. Before being discharged from the hospital, ask your doctor or nurse for the number you can call 24 hours per day to answer urgent questions.

As for long-term follow-up care, you may assume your doctors will do what they think is best; too often, however, long-term follow-up care is not well planned or well coordinated. If your doctor does not take the responsibility for

Questions to Ask Your Medical Team about Follow-Up Care

- Who is in charge of my follow up after I am discharged from the hospital?
- Whom should I call if I develop a complication from surgery? From radiation? From chemotherapy? What if I can't be certain whom to call?
- Who is going to review the final pathology report with me?
- Who is going to discuss my prognosis?
- Who is in charge of long-term cancer follow up?
- I have relatives who have had cancer. Is it possible that heredity may have caused my cancer? Would that change my risks or change my follow-up care plan?
- What tests are you planning to get? At what intervals? For how many years?
- What if I develop a new symptom or find a lump? Whom do I call?

developing a long-term follow-up plan, check to see if your medical institution has a patient care coordinator nurse available to help. Coordinating care among health care providers can be a challenge, and that responsibility may fall on your shoulders, so be prepared. See above for a list of questions you can ask to help get you started.

Why Do Follow Up?

Follow-up care is offered to patients after treatment for colorectal cancer for two reasons. The first is to monitor the status of the cancer. Regular follow-up visits are aimed at preventing or at least detecting recurrence earlier (when cancer is most responsive to effective treatment) rather than later. The second reason doctors do follow up is to provide information and counseling to you about your prognosis and the role of genetics might have played in your colorectal cancer.

Most doctors and most patients prefer to have a long-term follow-up plan to provide assurance that someone is keeping track of their cancer status, keeping them abreast of new prevention strategies, and keeping them informed about treatment options if the cancer recurs.

A comprehensive follow-up program is focused on five specific goals.

Goal 1: Recover (Short-Term Follow Up)

The goal of short-term follow-up care is to ensure your smooth recovery from colorectal cancer treatment (surgery, chemotherapy, and/or radiation). Depending on the details of your treatment, it may take from six weeks to six months (or more) to fully recover. During that time, you will probably have several outpatient visits so that your doctor can monitor your progress, deal with any side effects of the treatments or complications of surgery, and answer any questions you might have about "getting back to normal" (for example, your level of physical activity, bladder and sexual function, and diet).

Goal 2: Understand Your Prognosis

One of the major purposes of follow up is to provide realistic counseling about your prognosis—the chance of your recovery—after treatment for colorectal cancer (see chapter 6 for a fuller discussion of prognosis). You and your doctor probably discussed your prognosis before your treatment started; now your doctor can use the information gathered during your treatment to refine his or her predictions about your likely health outcome. This information gathered during treatments is used to determine what is called the final pathologic stage (see chapter 5). The final pathologic stage is used to calculate your personal risk of recurrence and your chance of long-term survival.

Who Gives Me the Prognosis?

Although some doctors arrange for a special conference to discuss your prognosis, many assume another member of the health care team will talk to you. There is no formal reporting process. Typically, your surgeon will discuss the final pathologic staging information with you before your discharge from the hospital. You may be told that you will need an appointment with a medical oncologist to discuss the implications of the final reports to decide if other treatment is needed.

To avoid confusion, you may want to ask for a specific time to discuss this information with your doctors. You may want other family members or close friends present to support you and help record what the doctors tell you.

Final Stage and Prognosis

By now you know that a cancer's grade is a measure of how abnormal and aggressive the cancer cells appear to be. If the final stage confirms the stage at diagnosis, your prognosis is the same as it was before treatment, and there usually is no reason to change the treatment or follow-up care plan.

If the final stage is worse than was predicted by pretreatment clinical staging (such as going from a stage II to a stage III cancer), your prognosis is less good. If the final stage is better than predicted by pretreatment staging (such as going from a stage II to a stage I cancer), your prognosis is better.

Final Stage and Treatment

Changes to the stage of your cancer are important to understand because they can affect your treatment or follow-up care plan. For instance, if the clinical stage had been stage II (T2N0M0) at diagnosis, but the final pathology stage after surgery was stage III (T2N1M0), postoperative chemotherapy might now be recommended because the cancer was found to have already spread into the adjacent lymph glands, and chemotherapy might help prevent additional spread and prolong your life.

In some situations, even though your prognosis is worse than it initially appeared, your doctors may not change your therapy. For instance, the change of a stage I (T1N0M0) cancer to a stage I (T2N0M0) cancer may not warrant the addition of chemotherapy to your treatment, but your prognosis with a T2N0M0 cancer is worse than with a T1N0M0 cancer.

What If Curative Treatment Was Not Possible?

Although every patient hopes for the best, it may be that the cancer was so advanced that curative treatment could not be done. Even in these cases, it is still useful to discuss prognosis with the health care team.

Even in cases of advanced cancer, it may be possible to control your disease and maintain a reasonable quality of life for a significant period of time with other treatments. New therapies, including many that are available through clinical trials, now offer the hope of longer survival and good quality of life for those with advanced colorectal cancer (see chapter 13). In some cases, the cancer is so advanced that no curative treatment options remain. In these situations, follow up will focus on palliative care. The goal of palliative care is to ensure the best possible quality of life for people with cancer and their families throughout the course of disease, with a particular emphasis on pain relief and comfort care in the final stages of life. Hospice programs most often provide this type of care.

Goal 3: Assess the Possible Hereditary Influences in Your Cancer

Heredity (the transmission of characteristics from parents to children through genes) is thought to be a major factor in 10 to 25 percent of colorectal cancers.

If you developed colorectal cancer when you were under age 50 years or if you have several first-degree relatives (parents or brothers and sisters) who developed cancer of the colon and rectum or associated cancers, such as ovarian, endometrial (uterine), ureteral or bladder cancers, or if you have many other relatives with cancers, especially at young ages, heredity may have been an important factor in development of your colorectal cancer. This knowledge is important for two reasons—your health and your family's health.

For Your Health

If genetics played a role in your colorectal cancer, you may want to actively seek out testing (also called screening) to detect related cancers early, when they are most likely to be cured. You may even want to consider "prophylactic" surgery to remove the potential site of the next cancer before it develops if you fall into the very high risk category.

For Your Family's Health

Your family's health and well being is another important reason to learn about the role of heredity in your colorectal cancer. If you are concerned that genetics may have been a factor in your cancer, you should gather all available reliable information about cancer and its presence in your family. For each family member, record the type of cancer they had and their age at diagnosis. Once you have put together this medical "family tree," discuss this information with your doctor.

You may want to seek the help of a genetic counselor and/or a doctor with special expertise in hereditary colorectal cancer syndromes who can advise you and your family about your risks, explain genetic tests that may be appropriate in your case, and direct future follow-up care to prevent your development of other cancers.

Having this information could spare your loved ones some of the difficulties you have faced.

Goal 4: Preventing New Colorectal Cancers

One primary goal of your long-term follow-up is to prevent you from developing a new colorectal cancer. Unless your surgeon removed all of your colon and rectum, you are at an increased risk of developing a second cancer in the remaining colorectal tissue sometime in the future, usually years after the initial cancer treatment. This is called developing a metachronous colorectal cancer and is different from a synchronous colorectal cancer, which is a colorectal cancer found at the same time you were found to have the first such cancer but in a different place. It is also different than developing a recurrence or metastasis of the first colorectal cancer, which we'll examine more closely when we discuss goal 5.

Metachronous cancers are new cancers that usually begin as benign polyps that develop slowly in the lining (mucosa) of the remaining large intestine. At the benign polyp stage, almost all can be removed by colonoscopy and polypectomy discussed in chapter 4. Removing such polyps when they are benign prevents the development of metachronous colorectal cancer. Thus, your doctors will probably recommend that you undergo periodic colonoscopy examinations to identify and remove any new polyps before they become cancerous.

Goal 5: Follow Up to Detect Recurrences and Metastasis

The second main goal of your long-term cancer follow-up plan is to identify local recurrences or metastases when it is still possible for you to undergo curative retreatment or at least treatment that can effectively control the disease and help you maintain a reasonable quality of life.

What Is Recurrence?

Recurrence is often defined as a cancer that has come back after treatment. This implies that the cancer was completely wiped out by the treatment and then somehow "magically" returned. What we now know is that recurrent cancer usually develops from incomplete removal of the primary cancer or from cells that spread from the original (primary) cancer to another place in the body. Those cells may grow and become obvious within a few months or years of the original treatment, or, for reasons that are not completely understood, they may remain quiet and undetected for longer periods of time, at which point they grow large enough that they cause symptoms and show up on testing procedures. Therefore, recurrences do not really represent a "magical" return of the cancer but rather a continued growth of cancer that was not completely removed or a reactivation of

316

cancer cells that had previously not bothered the patient and had not been detected by any test.

Recurrences are classified as local if they develop in the tissues at the site where the primary cancer was originally found, regional if they develop in the nearby lymph nodes, and distant or metastatic if they develop at sites far away from the original tumor.

Cure Versus Remission

The term "cure" is often used when a patient has had cancer, receives treatment, and all signs of the cancer disappear. But it is hard for anyone—even the very best doctors—to say with confidence that a person with cancer is ever completely cured.

As you know from the description of recurrence (above), cancer can appear to be gone completely while cancer cells live quietly in hiding.

Therefore, most doctors prefer to use the word "remission" instead of "cure," because "remission" may more accurately portray the real situation: that cancer may recur, even if all tests are clear.

> *"I'm really happy that I'm approaching my 36th birthday in a couple of days now, and I used to always dread my birthdays. I'm happy to be alive and I really appreciate my friends in a way that I didn't before."*
>
> —ADELE

Fear of Recurrence

Recurrence is not inevitable; many patients will never develop recurrence and will live a normal life span. Nonetheless, many patients who are facing the future after surviving treatment of a colorectal cancer are fearful that the cancer will recur. Sometimes this fear becomes overwhelming and can be so strong that counseling is needed to help you regain perspective and move forward with your life.

The best way to manage the fear of recurrence seems to be to talk openly with your doctors and loved ones about your fears. Sometimes, you will find those fears are not based in reality, and you simply need to review your prognosis and understand again why your doctors are optimistic about your long-term survival. At other times, your fears may be based on solid information that confirms your prognosis is guarded and that recurrence is highly likely. While

> *"There's always a feeling of waiting for that other shoe to drop."*
>
> —JACY

you can take some comfort in understanding that such patients do sometimes "beat the odds" and live full and normal lives, it is probably more useful to learn to face such a difficult situation by taking each day at a time.

Dealing With Fear of Recurrence

- Determine whether your fear of recurrence is realistic by reviewing your prognosis with your doctors.
- Review the facts about your case and the likelihood that the cancer will recur.
- Talk with your doctors and your loved ones about your fears.
- Talk with other patients in support groups about your fears.
- Read about colorectal cancer and new treatments that offer hope to patients with recurrence.
- Make proactive changes to improve your health: quit smoking, improve your diet, increase your activity level, and maintain a reasonable weight. (Be sure to discuss such plans with your doctor.) These steps may not prevent recurrence, but they will certainly boost your overall health and sense of well being.
- Consider professional counseling if your fears are interfering with your lifestyle.

Until the recurrence develops, you may feel totally well and can do many of the things you always wanted to but never found the time to do. Experts are available to help you prioritize the time remaining and make the most of your life.

One thing that helps many patients is to understand as much as you can about your disease (see above).

Developing a Personalized Long-Term Cancer Follow-Up Plan

While you are recovering from treatment of your colorectal cancer, you will have had the time to review your cancer status with your doctors. Through such counseling, you will know whether heredity played a role in your cancer, and you should also have a good understanding of your prognosis.

The last phase in follow-up is to work with your health care team to design and put into practice a long-term plan that reflects your needs and your health status.

Recall that this last phase of follow-up involves two goals: goal 4 is to prevent new colorectal cancers, and goal 5 is to detect recurrences as early as possible to ensure the best possible odds of survival.

Your follow-up plan will depend on several factors: what doctors know about colorectal cancer in general, what your doctor knows about your specific health situation, and your philosophy or preferred approach to follow-up care.

General Knowledge About Colorectal Cancer

Doctors have a lot of information about recurrent and metachronous colorectal cancers based on the many cancer patients who have come before you. This general information about how colorectal cancer typically behaves helps doctors shape reasonable long-term follow-up plans for their current patients.

For example, patients treated for colorectal cancer are at an increased risk for developing metachronous colorectal tumors. Thus, your doctor will probably recommend periodic follow-up colonoscopies to detect colon polyps before they develop into metachronous cancer.

Local recurrence after colon cancer resection with adequate margins is uncommon, so this type of screening is not part of most follow up after surgery. However, the rates for local recurrences after rectal cancer resection are higher for a number of reasons, so follow up after resection of a rectal cancer will often include screening for local recurrence on the mucosa (inner lining of the intestine) and in the pelvis outside the bowel wall.

> *"After surgery I had a follow-up every three months, then every six months, and now I go yearly to visit my surgeon. I also go to my gastroenterologist every other year for a colonoscopy. I have been cancer free for five years now."*
>
> —EILEEN

Most local recurrences and metastases develop within the first two to three years after a resection surgery to treat colorectal cancer. As a result, doctors usually recommend that people who have had colorectal cancer resection be screened most intensely in the first three years, with additional tests thereafter. Since patients who have undergone radiation to the pelvis to treat rectal cancer may develop recurrences later than other colorectal cancer patients, the intensive testing period may extend to 6 or more years.

The liver and the lungs are the places where colorectal cancer most often spreads. Therefore, your doctor may screen these sites for metastasis as part of your follow-up care.

Your Unique Situation

No single follow-up plan works for everyone previously treated for colorectal cancer. Your doctors will work with you to design a long-term follow-up plan specifically tailored to your situation. They will pair their general knowledge about recurrent colorectal cancer with an assessment of your overall health status and your willingness to undergo testing and retreatment if recurrence is detected.

For example, if your team of doctors is confident that you were successfully treated for a very early stage colorectal cancer, your follow up will be less intensive than if you underwent curative-intent treatment of a stage III cancer of the rectum that statistically is associated with a higher degree of recurrence. Likewise, if you are relatively young and in otherwise good condition, follow up may be more thorough since retreatment of a recurrence would probably be tolerated and effective. On the other hand, if you are elderly and have numerous other health problems that would make retreatment very risky, follow up is likely to be less extensive.

Your Philosophy of Follow Up

Your approach to health care will also affect your follow-up plan.

People have different philosophies about health care. Some people prefer a "more-is-better" approach to follow up. They want numerous laboratory tests, X-rays, and other studies to be done at short intervals to assure them that their cancer is in remission. They are temporarily reassured by frequent testing and believe this improves their quality of life. Others prefer a "less-is-better" approach to follow up. They believe that the initial treatment for colorectal cancer was their best chance to achieve cure or long-term survival. Frequent testing may cause them anxiety and may negatively affect their quality of life.

Most people fall somewhere between these two extremes. Work with your doctors to design an individualized follow-up plan to detect recurrences that fits your philosophy and makes sense for your specific situation.

Coordinating Your Long-Term Cancer Follow-Up Plan

Follow-up often involves a variety of different types of doctors and—as you will see in a moment—a variety of different tests over the course of several years or more. Some of your follow-up care will probably be done by your local doctors, while part of your follow up will be done by doctors at larger medical centers.

Because so many different doctors may be involved, it is important that your team of physicians communicate with each other. It is also important that they communicate with you. You should have a clear understanding of the long-term plan, and you should also know who should be doing what test and at what interval.

Common Follow-Up Tests

Now that you are educated about the phases of follow-up care after colorectal cancer treatment, what specific tests and procedures can you expect as part of this plan? Follow up most often includes routine office visits, routine blood tests, blood tests to detect specific tumor markers, imaging studies of the lungs and liver, special tests to look for local recurrences, and endoscopic tests.

Office Visits

A long-term plan to detect recurrent cancer usually includes periodic office visits to your doctor. These visits allow your doctor to do a clinical examination and provide you with an opportunity to ask questions. Symptoms such as abdominal pain can be the first signs of recurrence, so pay attention to your body and report any changes to your doctor.

Routine Blood Tests

Although blood tests for hemoglobin and liver function used to be a routine part of follow up for colorectal cancer, they haven't proven very useful, so your doctor may only order these tests if there is a specific reason to do so (such as if the doctor suspects that you might be anemic).

> *"I'm here, I'm alive, my family is here, and my job is here, and it seems to me the best way that I can proceed to go forward is to try not to worry about it every day. I do admit that right before my doctors' checkups I get that anxiety feeling, and I wonder, 'What's my CEA going to look like? Is the doctor going to see something?' But, then, when that's over, I put it out of my mind for the next few months until it's time to go back for another checkup."*
> —PATTI

Blood Tests for Tumor Markers

Tumor markers are substances that can be detected in the blood that may be linked to specific cancers. An example is the prostate-specific antigen or PSA test that doctors use to monitor patients with prostate cancer. For colorectal cancer, the tumor marker that has been most useful is called the carcinoembryonic antigen (CEA).

An elevated CEA level (higher than 5 ng/ml) is often the first indication that someone has recurrent disease. The CEA test is better at detecting liver metastases than lung metastases or local recurrences.

Lung Imaging Studies

Because the lungs are often involved in colorectal cancer metastases, doctors will generally include an imaging study of the lungs—either a chest X-ray or computerized tomography (CT) scan—as part of follow up. This assumes that the patient is in good enough health to tolerate treatment for metastasis if it is detected.

Liver Imaging Studies

Although CT imaging of the liver can detect liver metastases in many patients, such detection does not seem to improve survival rates. For now, the most cost-effective way to screen patients for a liver metastasis is to measure the CEA level. If the patient's CEA level is indeed elevated, then liver imaging tests may follow.

Whether other imaging studies of the liver (such as ultrasound, magnetic resonance imaging, or positron emission tomography) will have a role to play in routine follow-up needs further study.

Imaging Studies for Local Recurrence

Some people who have been treated for colorectal cancer are more prone to recurrence than others. Certain tumor characteristics and certain findings on pathology and postoperative reports are linked to an increased the risk of local recurrence. In such cases, the risk of local recurrence is high enough that it makes sense to routinely test the patient for early signs of local recurrence. (Again, the doctor will do this only if he or she thinks that the patient is a good candidate for retreatment if a local recurrence is found.)

Follow-up tests to screen for local recurrence usually include imaging studies, such as an endorectal ultrasonography or magnetic resonance imaging study and a CT scan of the pelvis, to detect a local pelvic recurrence. Estimates vary, but many experts recommend testing every three to four months for the first three years and then every six months for the next three years.

Endoscopic Tests for Local Recurrence

The chances of a local recurrence after colon resection are fairly low, so the doctor will probably only order endoscopic tests to selectively evaluate worrisome symptoms such as intestinal bleeding or a lump detected during abdominal examination.

However, the chances of a local recurrence after resection of a rectal cancer are higher, so your doctor may perform a digital rectal exam (DRE) and do a proctoscopy or flexible sigmoidoscopy to help identify local recurrence.

What Happens if Recurrence, Metastasis, or a Second Cancer Is Detected?

Finding out that your cancer has returned or spread, or that a second cancer has developed, can be extremely upsetting. You may feel betrayed by your body and even your doctors: didn't you feel better? Didn't they say you were doing fine? It is normal to feel grief, anger, disappointment, sadness, and fear. The thought of going through treatment again can add to these feelings.

Coping

Although it will not be easy, you can face the challenges ahead. You've probably already resolved some of the practical issues of delaying with colorectal cancer, and you know what to expect from your health care team and from treatment. Reconnect with your support team and let your loved ones know you'll be counting on them to help you get through this again. Use the strategies you used to help you cope with your initial diagnosis. (See chapter 7 for more information on coping with a diagnosis.)

Depending on how much time has passed since your initial diagnosis, you may also want to re-educate yourself about available treatment options, including clinical studies (see chapter 13). Exciting advances in cancer treatment are happening all the time.

More Testing

If any of the follow-up tests mentioned in the previous section suggest recurrence, your doctors will begin the cancer detection process anew. They will attempt to confirm the recurrence by doing a biopsy of the tissue. They will also order other diagnostic tests to rule out additional sites of recurrence and to determine the extent (stage) of the recurrent disease.

> *"There is no easy way to hear the news that you have cancer or that it has recurred (I have heard that four or five times now). Just when I start to believe that the new treatment (surgery, chemo or radiation) is working, a new symptom pops up like a bad penny and the tests start all over again only to show that the cancer cells are growing again in either the same spot or a new location. I can honestly say that no matter how many times you hear it, you will always have some sort of grief reaction, even if it is for a short period."*
> —KRIS

Treatment or Care Plan

With this new information, your health care team will modify your follow-up plan to manage the recurrent cancer. This might include chemotherapy and radiation (if not previously given) and/or additional surgery if the patient is strong enough to tolerate these treatments. If the recurrence is too advanced for treatment with curative intent, the focus will switch to palliative care, with its emphasis on managing pain and preserving quality of life.

CHAPTER NINETEEN

LIVING WELL AFTER CANCER

Amy Kelly

Finding out you had colorectal cancer was undoubtedly upsetting. But you may discover some surprising and positive aspects of this otherwise difficult and painful experience. Perhaps you have emerged from the experience with a new-found sense of wisdom and strength, a renewed commitment to life goals, a deeper sense of meaning and purpose, and possibly the resolve to reach out to others. This chapter is all about making the most of life after colorectal cancer.

Survivorship

You may hear the terms survivor, five-year survival rate, and remission in reference to you or your cancer, and you may wonder what they mean.

Survivor is not a medical term; it's a word adopted by cancer advocates. It can have several different meanings. Some people use the word to refer to anyone who has been diagnosed with cancer. For example, someone living with cancer may be considered a "survivor." Some people use the term

> *"When I was younger, 'cancer' was a word that was whispered. Now, I tell everyone I have cancer. I AM A SURVIVOR."*
> —LAURA

when referring to someone who has completed cancer treatment, and still others call a person a survivor if he or she has lived several years past a cancer diagnosis.

> *"Find some way to associate yourself with cancer survivors. You need to see people who have been there. You need to meet people who have lived three years, six years, ten years, twelve years. To be a survivor, you need to believe that you can survive."*
> —COLLEEN

The American Cancer Society believes that each individual has the right to define his or her own experience with cancer and considers a survivor to be anyone who defines himself or herself this way, from the time of diagnosis through the balance of his or her life.

For doctors and scientists, the five-year survival rate refers to the percentage of people who are alive five years after a cancer diagnosis. Five-year and 10-year rates are used as a standard way of discussing the chances that a person might live a certain length of time after being diagnosed with cancer. Medical professionals use survival rates to help them understand how cancer affects the life expectancy of people who have been diagnosed with tumors of a similar type and stage (see chapter 6 for more information).

Remission is the complete disappearance of the signs and symptoms of cancer, which usually occurs in response to a specific form of cancer treatment. It's the period during which a disease is under control and there is no evidence that the cancer exists. However, a remission does not always mean that there has been a cure or a permanent disappearance of cancer.

It's impossible to pinpoint a moment when one has "survived" cancer. Therefore, most people who have had cancer are monitored indefinitely to ensure that if the disease returns, it is found and treated as soon as possible. This uncertainty is one reason some people with cancer are uncomfortable with the term "survivor" and don't use it. Others with cancer consider being a survivor a state of mind rather than a scientific measure of their life with the disease and embrace the word.

Setting Post-Treatment Life Goals

People who have faced cancer share a unique appreciation of time and the desire to make every day count. Before you find yourself immersed in daily commitments and routines, or with new resolutions in danger of fading into the background, set down on paper the goals most important to your happiness and satisfaction.

Some people may want to help others who are going through the challenges of colorectal cancer treatment by taking part in a support group or by raising awareness about colorectal cancer screening by talking to relatives and friends. Others find volunteering with nonprofit organizations like the American Cancer

Society or political action groups who lobby on behalf of increased funding for colorectal cancer research a rewarding experience.

Many see the period after treatment as a time to recapture the satisfying lives they had before cancer's interruption. Others have discovered new goals and dreams through their cancer journey. You may want to take this opportunity to take stock of your personal life, revisit your individual goals and desires, and resolve to take steps to achieve them, whatever they may be.

Lifestyle Changes and Improvements

As research advances, more people with colorectal cancer are living long, healthy lives, which means they need to adjust to life beyond cancer. The period after treatment may be viewed as a time for new beginnings or a chance to make lifestyle improvements. One of the best ways to do this is to commit to living a balanced lifestyle that includes eating a healthy diet, maintaining an appropriate weight, staying physically active, restricting alcohol intake, and avoiding tobacco products.

> *"I found that my cancer is not only a cross, and this might sound odd, but it's also a gift. Once you've been diagnosed with a serious illness, you realize all the beautiful things that are around you. Your priorities shift very quickly."*
> —MAURA

Diet

Treatment for any type of cancer can affect your digestive system and result in unintended weight loss. Having colorectal cancer makes this even more challenging, because this type of cancer is located in your gastrointestinal tract. The cancer itself and the treatment are likely to have an impact on your digestive system. For this reason, you need to pay close attention to what you eat to be sure your body is well nourished. This may seem like a daunting task, especially if you are experiencing a change in your bowel habits from surgery, chemotherapy or radiation therapy; a lack of appetite; and/or a change in your taste for certain foods you once enjoyed.

> *"You realize how fragile life is: no matter how wonderful things might be on Monday, you could find out on Tuesday some horrible news that changes everything. Given that, are there things you want to do differently?"*
> —SUSAN

But eating well during and after cancer treatment can help you better tolerate the effects of treatment and recover more quickly. Here are some tips for healthy eating after cancer:

- Check with your doctor for any food or diet restrictions.
- Ask your dietitian to help you create a nutritious, balanced eating plan.
- Choose a variety of foods from all the food groups.
- Try to eat at least five to seven servings a day of fruits and vegetables, including citrus fruits and dark green and deep yellow vegetables.
- Eat plenty of high-fiber foods, such as whole-grain breads and cereals.
- Buy a new fruit, vegetable, low-fat food, or whole-grain product each time you shop for groceries.
- Reduce your intake of red meat and processed meat.
- Choose low-fat milk and dairy products.
- Avoid salt-cured, smoked, and pickled foods.
- Decrease the amount of fat in your meals by baking or broiling foods, and limit your consumption of trans-fatty acids.

Studies have shown that nutrition and physical activity can have an impact on cancer prevention, but their affect on preventing recurrence is unclear. We do know, though, that a diet rich in vegetables, whole grains, legumes, and fruits will help to build a stronger body, make recovery quicker, and lead to an overall health benefit.

An ideal nutrition and wellness plan will rebuild the strength in your muscles and help correct problems with organ function and the effects of your treatment such as anemia. A dietitian and members of your healthcare team can help you to design a plan that meets your needs. Most hospitals have dietitians on staff; if not, ask other members of your health care team, including your oncologist or nurse, about your nutritional needs and goals.

Obesity

Changes in dietary patterns and exercise habits related to cancer treatment may cause unexpected weight gain as well. In addition, some people are overweight before their cancer diagnosis. It is important to talk to your doctor about your target body mass index (BMI), which takes both weight and height into account (see page 23 for a chart to help you calculate your BMI). Your doctor will have suggestions on how to achieve this target body mass index after treatment and the pace at which this should be achieved.

Physical Activity

After cancer treatment, it is important to regain or improve your pretreatment fitness level and increase your strength. Most of us are aware that exercise improves our quality of life. For people who have had cancer, it can have a positive influence on lung capacity, heart rate, and lean body mass. For the general population, the American Cancer Society recommends at least 30 minutes of moderate physical activity at least five days per week. Before starting any exercise plan—especially after cancer treatment—it is important that you talk to your health care team.

Exercise can have other positive effects. Exercise helps your body to produce new red blood cells and may also help strengthen the immune system. It helps you regain strength and flexibility, maintain your ideal weight, and can even help control stress and moderate depression. Exercise programs should include aerobic exercise (increases the heart rate and the amount of oxygen your body uses), strength training using weights, and flexibility exercises. Even a small amount of these activities, when performed regularly, can provide noticeable benefits to your body and its healing after cancer treatment.

You don't need to join a gym to incorporate exercise into your daily routine. Here are some examples of how you can become more aerobically active in your every day life:

- Skip the elevator and use the stairs.
- If possible, walk or bike to wherever you need to go.
- On your lunch break, walk to local park and have a picnic lunch.
- Take a ten-minute break at work to stretch at your desk.
- Go dancing with your loved one or a friend.
- Take an active vacation such as a canoe or hiking trip.
- Wear a pedometer every day. Try to work up to 10,000 steps per day.
- Join a community sports league like softball, basketball, or tennis.
- If you have a treadmill or exercise bike at home, use it while you watch your favorite TV show.

Treatment may make you fatigued, and sometimes you will be unable to be physically active for a long period of time after treatment. Do not push yourself. You will build your endurance back slowly over time. Please consult your doctor before beginning any exercise routine or increasing your physical activity. Becoming physically fit is a long-term goal and should be done gradually.

Alcohol

Heavy alcohol use may contribute to colorectal cancer risk (and certainly causes harmful effects on overall health). Drinking alcohol only in moderation (maximum of two drinks per day for men and one drink per day for women) is a smart way to decrease these consequences and may reduce your risk of heart disease and stroke. You should discuss this with your doctor to determine what is appropriate for you.

Tobacco

Recent studies indicate that smokers are 30 to 40 percent more likely than non-smokers to die from colorectal cancer. Almost everyone knows that smoking causes cancers in sites in the body that come in direct contact with the smoke, such as the mouth and lungs. What you may not know is that some cancer-causing chemical agents are swallowed and can lead to digestive system cancers, such as colorectal cancer. Some of these substances are also absorbed into the bloodstream and can increase the risk of developing other cancers.

If you are a smoker, talk to your health care team about getting help to quit. There are many smoking cessation (quitting) programs available that your health care team will be able to discuss with you. For example, the American Cancer Society's Quitline nearly doubles a smoker's chances of quitting successfully compared with the use of self-help materials alone. Call 800-ACS-2345/800-227-2345 to receive phone counseling and support.

The sooner you quit, the greater the health benefits. Almost immediately, a person's blood circulation begins to improve, dangerous carbon monoxide levels begin to drop, and pulse rate and blood pressure begin to normalize.

Sexuality and Relationships

Through all that a colorectal cancer diagnosis has brought to your life, sex may very well be the last thing on you or your partner's mind. Changes to your body shape and your self-image as a result of your colorectal cancer diagnosis and treatment may affect your desire and/or your ability to have rewarding sexual relations. This is a very normal reaction to what you've been through. When you feel you're ready to take this step, talk to your doctor—he or she can provide support and helpful suggestions for regaining intimacy with your partner.

Couples

Cancer happens to a couple, not just the survivor. Each of you will react and cope with it in different ways. For many couples, talking about sex after a cancer diagnosis is not easy. If you do not talk about it though, you both will be guessing as to what the other is thinking and feeling.

Some couples can do this without professional help. However, you may find it helpful to talk to a therapist. A cancer diagnosis can force you to make adjustments in many aspects of your life—including your intimate relationships. A therapist can help you focus on what is important to you and your partner. You may be feeling that your partner is not sexually attracted to you because of your ostomy or scars from surgery. Meanwhile, your partner may just be waiting for you to initiate the activity for fear of pushing you into doing something you are just too exhausted or not ready to do.

Colorectal cancer sometimes involves an ostomy. This can be a constant reminder to your partner and yourself that you had cancer, which can counteract any desires for sexual activity. Some may find their ostomy bag makes them feel unattractive, and their partners may be afraid of dislodging the bag or hurting their loved one. Both of these can easily be misinterpreted as rejection. Even the thought of rejection can cause someone to avoid sexual intimacy. See chapter 16 for specific information and tips for regaining intimacy and having sex after an ostomy.

Even for those who don't have an ostomy, cancer and its treatment can have a major impact on sexual activity. In men, there may be nerve damage that can affect the ability to have an erection. For some, this may heal over time, and for others there could be permanent damage. This doesn't have to mean the end of your sex life. Nerve damage can be treated through penile injections and implants and constriction devices. Your doctor can refer you to an urologist to discuss your options.

Some women find intercourse painful after surgery for colorectal cancer. Adhesions, or scar tissue, can develop after surgery. Movement during intercourse can pull on the scar tissue and cause pain. Kegel exercises, which involve flexing or squeezing then relaxing the muscles used to control the flow of urine, may offer some relief. Another option is the use of vaginal dilators. Both of these methods should be discussed with your doctor. Women who are treated for cancer may enter menopause prematurely because of chemotherapy. The most common problems affecting woman's sexuality in menopause are vaginal dryness and infections of the vagina and urinary tract. Both are related to the loss of estrogen and can cause pain during sex. Your doctor can help you to find solutions to these issues.

Cancer and cancer treatment can also affect your libido and level of desire. There may be many times when you simply don't feel like having intercourse but want some physical closeness with your partner. Many couples find intimacy through kissing, hugging, and lying in each other's arms. You may also consider sensual massage, fondling, oral sex, and mutual stimulation. Intimacy is more than sex. It is spending time with the one you love, whether that's taking a walk or going on a date. This can be a special time to rekindle the feelings you had when you first started your courtship. There are no rules. Take it at your own pace. As long as you communicate with each other, these steps will lead to a satisfying intimate relationship for you and your partner that may even exceed what it was before cancer.

Single and Dating

Cancer happens to single men and women, too. Cancer may bring additional concerns about dating. Dating is challenging enough without having to discuss a cancer diagnosis. It is up to you to reveal information about your cancer, and you can take it at your own pace. As in any other personal issue, you may want to wait until you have developed some trust in this new person and there is a possibility of a deeper relationship. If you anticipate a sexual encounter may take place, it's probably a good idea to introduce the subject before sexual contact occurs.

Don't let your cancer diagnosis define you. It isn't who you are. If someone rejects you after you reveal your experiences with colorectal cancer to him or her, the problem is theirs, not yours. Would you really want to be with someone who responds that way anyway?

For many, having cancer may create anxiety, depression, and feelings of helplessness. Thoughts of recurrence may overshadow everyday activities, including sexuality. Sexual desires may take time to resurface and become important. Be patient and give yourself time to work through feelings of anxiety and discomfort. Professional help is an option, and there are many resources to turn to.

Your doctor may not bring up the subject with you, but you should feel comfortable starting the conversation with him or her. They can help you understand what is normal and what is not after treatment. If you are uncomfortable talking with your doctor about these issues, another member of the health care team, such as a social worker or nurse, may be easier for you to talk to.

> "I reviewed my life quite thoroughly shortly after my diagnosis. Like most people, I have had my ups and downs, and my troubles and my trauma, and very bad financial times and emotional times through my life. But there have been so many wonderful things. In my review of my life, I have come to the conclusion that I have been given a much better life than I ever possibly imagined when I was young. I have been blessed with a wonderful family, a lovely caring wife and, much to my surprise, after my diagnosis, I had friends and relatives and caring people coming out of the woodwork, giving me love and emotional support. This has continued right up until this particular time. My feeling is that, if I have to depart this earth, I will go with a smile on my face because I have been truly blessed."
>
> —RICHARD

Finding Meaning

Cancer came into your life without warning. It has probably affected every part of your daily life. The end of cancer treatment can be both exciting and challenging. Now that treatment is over, though, it is time to move on to a time where cancer treatment isn't a part of your daily vocabulary. However, you will never forget cancer's impact or the way it has changed your life.

There is no normal way to deal with a life after cancer. Everyone's definition of normal is different. And what was normal before cancer has changed significantly. Normal may now include making changes in your diet, your activities, and your relationships with friends and loved ones. Each person reacts differently to his or her experience with cancer. It is most important to find what works for you, makes you feel fulfilled, and brings you joy.

Faith and Spirituality

A cancer diagnosis can affect your faith and spirituality. It may test your faith, or it may be what gets you through. The way cancer affects faith or religion is different for everyone. It is common to question one's faith after cancer. Some turn away from their religion because they feel it has deserted them. Some rely on their faith more than ever and draw strength from their religious beliefs. Spirituality helps some get them through the day.

There are many ways to find meaning through faith:

> *"My faith in God and the support of my husband, family and church friends helped me to make it through the tough times."*
> —DIANNE

- Meditate or pray to help ease stress.
- Seek out spiritual or religious materials that can help you feel more connected to a higher power.
- Talk to your religious leader about your concerns and fears.
- Participate in religious activities to meet new people.
- Talk to other members of your house of worship who have had similar experiences.

Getting Involved

As you may know by now, colorectal cancer is highly preventable and quality of life after a colorectal cancer diagnosis can remain high. By sharing your experience with others, you can help spread these messages, which may even save the lives of loved ones, friends, or strangers. You may have avoided screening because of fear or embarrassment; you may have dismissed rectal bleeding as hemorrhoids; your doctor may never have discussed the need for screening; or you may not have known you had a family history of polyps or colorectal cancer. Whatever the reason, you can get involved to make sure someone else doesn't have to hear the words *you have colorectal cancer.*

Family First

Start with your own family. You are probably familiar with a family tree but may never have thought of using a family tree as a tool to help future generations assess their risk and maintain their health. Begin with your own health history and go on from there. Every holiday and family reunion is an opportunity to fill in your family tree with more information. Make copies and enlist the help of other family members. Pass on the information to all of your living relatives and encourage them to do the same. Your experience with colorectal cancer may very well save the lives of your children's children and so on.

> *"Since 1997, I have been the direct cause of about 27 colonoscopies, including my brother, my sister, and all four sons. And three in my family, and four others outside of my family, had precancerous polyps removed."*
> —PETE

Speak Out in Your Community

You have relationships and encounters with many people every day—in your workplace, your neighborhood, your gym, and your house of worship. Most of these people probably do not know the risk factors of colorectal cancer. Take these daily interactions as opportunities to educate them about the importance of knowing their risk factors and being screened for colorectal cancer.

> *"Each of us has a unique circle of influence. You can talk with the folks in your church groups and your civic groups and your business where you work, so that the subject becomes talked about. By talking about it and getting people to understand about it—that colorectal cancer is preventable, that they can do something to prevent it—this will go a long ways to eradicating the disease."*
> —ERNESTINE

Become a Mentor

Don't you wish you knew then what you know now? Consider becoming a mentor to people just beginning the journey you have just been through. Many community hospitals and national colorectal cancer organizations, such as the Colon Cancer Alliance and the United Ostomy Association (UOA), have mentor programs. Find out more about the Colon Cancer Alliance Buddy Program at http://www.ccalliance.org/patient/buddy/buddy.html and the UOA visitor program at http://www.uoa.org/chapters_visiting.htm. Your experience can help those newly diagnosed with colorectal cancer.

Become an Advocate

An advocate is someone who uses their voice as a tool to speak out on a subject that matters to them. The colorectal cancer community needs advocates. You can get involved in many ways if you are interested. Here are some areas of advocacy you might consider:

- Encourage Congress to allocate more dollars to cancer research.
- Get the media to raise awareness or cover issues relating to colorectal cancer such as screening.
- Lobby drug companies to apply more research to the development of new treatment options.

Do you feel strongly about something that you experienced through your journey with colorectal cancer? If so, make it known. You can make a difference.

Moving On

Not everyone feels compelled to use their experience with colorectal cancer as a reason to remain involved with colorectal cancer causes. Some people want to move past cancer. You have every right to make this disease a closed chapter in the book of your life. You have been through so much because of this disease; you are not required to become a community activist or even talk about your experience publicly. Your only obligation is to yourself and to do what makes you happy and fulfilled.

> *"There hasn't been enough education, enough talk to the public about colon cancer. I know, to me, any kind of cancer is cancer. I've never looked at one being worse than the other. When I hear about all these, the fundraising projects that breast cancer gets, and all the TV advertising I see for breast cancer, I get kind of jealous, I guess. I just feel like, why not talk a little bit about my kind of cancer? There are an awful lot of people out there with colon cancer. You just don't hear enough about it."*
>
> —PAT

Facing the Future

Today, colorectal cancer no longer has to be a death sentence. Cure rates continue to improve as new medicines and treatments are discovered. Doctors cannot predict how long a person will live. They can only make an educated guess based on what they have seen in other people in comparable situations. Even for a poor prognosis, new research advances and discoveries can offer hope.

After treatment ends, you still will need to address issues relating to your cancer. These include lifelong monitoring (see chapter 18 on recurrence and follow up) and the emotional and physical impact cancer has left on you and your loved ones. Without a doubt, cancer does leave a mark on everyone affected by it. You may not realize the full force of its impact all at once. Things may appear months or even years after treatment is over.

> "In a lot of ways I feel like I'm lucky to have had cancer. Not so much the disease, but the experience that went along with it. Because when someone says 'cancer,' I don't think of the disease anymore. I think of a time in my life that had tremendous, tremendous growth."
> —LIZETTE

Use the ways discussed in this chapter and throughout this book to help move past a life consumed with cancer and to find your own way to bring normalcy back to your life. You may be able to work through the emotional aspects of this on your own or you may need professional counseling to help you. Don't be afraid to ask for help.

As you face the future, make every moment count. That is all each of us can do.

CHAPTER TWENTY

WHEN YOUR LOVED ONE HAS COLORECTAL CANCER

Michelle Rhiner RN, MSN, NP, CHPN
Neal Slatkin, MD, DABPM

A diagnosis of colorectal cancer affects not only the person with the diagnosis but also family members, loved ones, friends, neighbors, and coworkers—everyone involved in the person with cancer's extended support system. Although family members and caregivers may not experience the physical effects of treatment, the emotional challenge of watching a loved one struggle is very real. Loved ones often want to help, but may not know what to expect, what to say, what to do, or how to cope with the emotional and practical challenges that a diagnosis of colorectal cancer may raise.

What You Can Expect

It is well-established in the medical literature that people who have a family caregiver and a good support network generally cope better and have better overall outcomes than those who do not, so your role is an important one.

Throughout the cancer experience, from diagnosis through the various treatments offered, you and your loved one will face numerous physical, emotional, and spiritual challenges. The support you can offer the person with colorectal cancer will be essential, and there are many things you can do—large and small—to help.

As you support the person with cancer through his or her diagnosis, treatment, and recovery, you will be confronted with an array of emotions that can, at times, seem overwhelming. You'll need to deal with your own changing emotions and responses while you help the person with cancer cope with the shifting circumstances and challenges of his or her illness.

> "At the time of my first cancer experience I was fortunate to be surrounded by a very loving and supportive family. My wife and two young sons helped me to ride through the emotional roller coaster and return to a full and active life. Support also came flooding in from extended family and friends, as well as from the medical professionals who saw me through this ordeal. The family physician that worked with me to produce an accurate and early diagnosis became a lifelong friend."
> —DICK

This chapter offers an overview of some of the more common concerns of the patient and family caregiver. We'll discuss the many ways you can support and care for your loved one, keys to good communication, the importance of taking care of yourself, the role of the family caregiver in a patient's treatment, transitioning to recovery, and last but not least, life after cancer.

This guide will help you and the one you love face colorectal cancer *together*.

Supporting the Person With Cancer

When a person faces a serious illness like colorectal cancer, knowing that people around them care is extremely important. People can offer many different kinds of support, and patients are very fortunate if they have a network of friends and loved ones who can provide this full spectrum of support.

> "It's not just the cancer patient that has to deal with the cancer; it's the family and the friends also. It's not just one person that's affected, it's your whole world and relationships that are affected."
> —JACY

Consider the many ways in which you and others can help. For example, the person with cancer might need emotional support, which may come in the form of a friend offering a shoulder to cry on or a respected family member offering assurance that good decisions are being made about treatment options.

The person with cancer may also require physical support, such as help with tasks of everyday living: help bathing or dressing while the patient is recovering from surgery, or cleaning the house and doing laundry when he or she feels too fatigued.

Practical help can come in the form of volunteering to run errands (such as taking a child to and from soccer practice) or performing helpful tasks like walking the dog or grocery shopping and cooking meals.

Colleagues and coworkers can offer professional support, taking on a few extra work-related tasks when the person with cancer needs to take time off from work to receive treatment or focus on recovery.

Social support is a big help too: spending time with your friend or loved one chatting, playing cards or watching movies, or visiting them during hospital stays. Even a card or a short note can boost their spirits.

> *"I think sometimes it may be tougher for the caregiver, or the wife or relative, than it is for the patient."*
>
> —PETE

Spiritual support might be a shared understanding about values and belief systems. If it is compatible with his or her belief system, you may want to pray with or on behalf of the person with cancer.

In addition to offering physical, emotional, practical, and/or spiritual support there are other ways you can help the person with colorectal cancer, as loved one, family caregiver, or trusted friend.

Understanding the Needs of Your Loved One

The most important way you can support someone you care about when they have cancer is to listen to their needs and respond accordingly. For example, you may have a burning desire to discuss all possible treatment scenarios (even worst-case ones) the minute the patient is diagnosed, but he or she may need time to absorb the information before talking about it. Follow the lead of the person with cancer and be sensitive to their unique needs and personal preferences. Respect their wishes.

Educate Yourself

You can also support the person with colorectal cancer by learning more about the disease. Educate yourself about the type of colorectal cancer your loved one has been diagnosed with, how the treatment they have decided upon will work, and the possible effects and outcomes of this disease. Familiarizing yourself with this information will ensure that your loved one has an informed and understanding "sounding board"

> *"I learned so much about the cancer patient's definition of 'quality of life.' As a nurse, I had often entered into discussions with other professionals about 'quality of life.' What a narrow perspective I had until I took this cancer journey with my daughter. The fight, whatever it entailed, was worth every effort to her. The experience was often brutal and other times it was glorious. We experienced a closeness afforded only to people who fight a battle together. We celebrated, mourned, rejoiced, and learned to wring every ounce out of life we could in a very short period of time."*
>
> —SUE

when he or she is ready to discuss the illness. Your interest in their condition confirms to them how much you care.

Sources of Information

Books such as this one can be helpful in obtaining a general overview of the diagnosis of cancer, the various treatment options, and emotional and practical issues. There are also a variety of print and electronic materials that can help. See chapter 9 for more information.

Participating in Your Loved One's Health Care

Another way you can support the person with cancer is to play an active role in his or her health care. Loved ones and family caregivers can go to medical appointments with the patient to offer support, advocate for the patient, and provide a second set of ears.

> "My wife is a tremendous asset to me. She is a fantastic caregiver, she is very knowledgeable, and she works diligently to make sure that all my appointments are made, my blood tests are done on time and they get to the right people. And, she makes sure that I have the right kind of food and she pushes me to exercise. So, she is an excellent caregiver. I'm so happy and proud that I have her to share this difficulty with me."
>
> —RICHARD

Family caregivers can also provide valuable information to the health care team about the patient's condition, including reporting levels of discomfort, appetite, and sleep habits.

As a loved one or caregiver, you may meet several people from different disciplines that will be involved in the patient's care. You can count on these people to help identify your needs and lend assistance to the person with cancer and to you, the family caregiver. Members of this team might include doctors, nurses, clinical social workers, chaplains, psychologists, and rehabilitation professionals.

Communication

The strain of dealing with cancer can make communication between friends and family members difficult. Even couples who have been able to "talk about anything" may find it difficult to talk about cancer, yet positive communication is an essential part of facing the challenges cancer can pose and supporting the person with cancer.

Talking About Cancer With Your Loved One

There can be many barriers to open and honest communication when a person you love is diagnosed with cancer. The family caregiver and the person with cancer each have his/her own concerns.

You may be reluctant to bring up the subject, because you don't know what to say, or because you think you might upset or depress the person with cancer. You might be afraid to face the many fears that have crossed your mind, such as whether the person with cancer will ever fully recover, or if you will be able to assume primary responsibility for family or financial matters. You may simply feel overwhelmed by all that needs to be done.

The person with cancer may also be reluctant to communicate openly. He or she may be overwhelmed by the importance of choosing the best treatment option for his or her circumstances, or may fear the complications or side effects of treatment. Other worries might include lost time from work, loss of control, and being "diminished" in one's stature or role. Grave thoughts about cancer recurrence and fears about death may seem too frightening to share.

Many caregivers and patients alike are hesitant to discuss their real concerns for fear that these, may in turn, frighten their loved one, causing them needless distress. Each may then withdraw from open and honest discussion, trying instead to "protect" the other from any new or additional worry. Yet inadequate communication may only compound these burdens. Failure to clearly communicate one's fears, needs, and frustrations—however well-intentioned these efforts are—may lead to feelings of isolation and increased psychological pain. By not expressing your feelings or by discouraging open communication with your loved one, opportunities may be lost to identify and resolve problems or to solicit additional information that might reduce some worry.

> *"I don't know that I could have gotten through the fears and the treatment without my husband. And, if anything, it strengthened our relationship. He's just wonderful, and I just couldn't have done it without him. We often talk about the cancer. It's not an 'I,' it's a 'we.' It's definitely strengthened our family."*
>
> —JANET

Here are some ways you can encourage positive communication:

- Start slowly. Discussions about important issues are always difficult. Don't feel like you have to rush. And don't let silences scare you away from talking. It can be hard to find the right words to describe feelings. Begin by opening up the lines of communication, asking "How do you feel about...?" Starting off this way shows that it's okay for your loved one who has cancer to open up to you emotionally.

341

- Listen without judging. Avoid saying, "You shouldn't…" or "Don't say that." Allow your loved one to express himself/herself and don't trivialize what he or she is feeling. If you're uncertain about the meaning of what's said to you, ask for clarification. Repeat what you hear back to your loved one in your own words, so that he or she knows you understand what has been said.
- Be honest. Discuss real and projected events and share emotional reactions to those events. Don't pretend that you don't feel upset or fearful if you do.
- Express your feelings. "I'm afraid of losing you" is a way to express your concern that your loved one may die. Let the person with cancer know how much you care.
- Resist the urge to assure your loved one with statements like, "You'll be fine," "Everything's going to be okay," or "Don't worry." These statements may be untrue, and the person with cancer is likely to know it. Saying such things may indicate that you don't want to think about the unpleasantness of cancer, and that he or she can't truly confide in you.
- Understand that men and women often communicate in different ways, and make allowances for those differences. It may be helpful to openly discuss differences in your communication styles.
- Remember that you don't have to agree with your loved one. Two people aren't always in the same emotional state or at the same level of acceptance at the same time. There's no simple answer to many problems, especially if they are long-standing.
- Consider seeking help from an uninvolved party such as a clergy member, therapist, or someone else you're comfortable with, and allow that person to guide conversations that are difficult for you.

Talking About Cancer With Health Care Professionals

Having cancer exposes patients and caregivers to an unfamiliar vocabulary, and communicating with doctors, nurses, and specialists can be challenging. See chapter 8 for tips for improving communication with the members of your loved one's health care team.

Taking Care of Yourself

Caregiving—especially for extended periods of time—can be an exhausting task. It can be an even greater strain if you are also trying to balance caregiving with other important responsibilities, such as work and parenting. Some factors that may affect the intensity of the experience include the patient's stage of illness and prognosis, the amount of physical and emotional care the he or she requires, the duration of his or her illness, the site or sites of cancer involvement, the side effects of treatment, the patient's own coping mechanisms and levels of stress, and the quality of the caregiver's and patient's relationship before the cancer diagnosis.

Sometimes, family caregivers get so absorbed in the act of caring for the person with cancer that they forget to look after their own well being.

Potential Reactions

Caregiving and offering support to someone with cancer who is close to you can elicit a wide variety of reactions, both emotional and physical.

It is not uncommon to have feelings of anger, depression, guilt, anxiety, hopelessness, and fear while caring for someone with cancer. The experience of these emotions can seem like a rollercoaster ride. See chapter 7 for specific tips on coping with these emotions.

Both the patient and their caregiver may experience powerful emotional reactions to cancer, and one person's emotional state certainly affects the other. For example, patients' feelings of guilt, worries that they are being overly burdensome, or resentment over the loss of role, function, and decision-making autonomy may cause them to lash out, leaving caregivers to feel that their best efforts and sacrifices are being misunderstood, resented, or unappreciated.

> *"It was extremely difficult. There were days when I was lonely. There were days when I was angry, and some days I was angry at her. I was angry at her for getting sick. I was angry at her for not feeling well enough that day to talk with me or interact with me."*
> —SUSAN

Some caregivers may even develop physical symptoms in unconscious sympathy with their loved one or as a reaction to their own stress and anxiety over the illness, its treatment, and uncertain outcomes.

Tips for Taking Care of Yourself

Remember: you cannot be a good caregiver or a source of strength to the person with cancer if you yourself are falling apart. Here are some tips for taking care of yourself:

- Take care of your physical health. Eat well, exercise regularly, and get adequate rest. These factors contribute to a positive attitude, restore your energy, and provide the stamina you will need to support the person with cancer through whatever challenges they may face.

- Take care of your emotional health. The experience of cancer may bring to the surface long-neglected or repressed emotions. Over the long term, if these feelings are left unaddressed, they can become a major strain on the relationship. When strong emotions are denied, they have a way of appearing in distorted forms or being explosively expressed at surprising times. Attempts to deny, filter, or dismiss these emotions can lead to overall sadness, depression, and isolation. Talk with your loved one about your emotions in a candid manner, involving third parties such as a social worker, psychiatrist or psychologist, or member of the clergy when appropriate.

> "I think sometimes for people who get wrapped up in care-giving, it's also hard to ask other people for something they need. And that's the other thing I learned: first you have to take care of yourself, and secondly, you shouldn't be afraid to ask other people for help."
> —SUSAN

- Seek outside help if you need it. Sometimes people who do the supporting need support themselves. If you find that you are having trouble balancing responsibilities or coping with the situation, turn to your other family members and members of your extended support network (friends, neighbors, or members of your house of worship, for example). Don't be afraid or embarrassed to ask for help. Professional counseling can also help, as can attending a support group for caregivers or family members of people with cancer.

Support Groups

Support groups can either be of a general type focusing on the problems of patients with a wide variety of cancers, or they can be specifically focused on a particular type of cancer, such as colorectal cancer. Support groups vary considerably in their composition and leadership, and they may be open-ended with members joining at any time or may have a specific beginning and end with a defined group of patients and/or caregivers. Some groups are limited to patients or to caregivers alone, while others are open to both. In general, groups that are led by an experienced health care professional tend to be the most beneficial.

> "It's good to talk with other people who are going through the same thing that you're going through."
> —JUDY

Support groups can give loved ones and caregivers a forum for expressing their feelings, and can affirm to those who feel isolated that they are not alone. Support groups can also be a place to get practical information on coping with personal and family conflicts from those who have shared a similar experience and may understand first hand what you are going through. However, support groups should not be relied upon as one's exclusive source of information on cancer or how best to deal with cancer. Individual experiences and disease vary widely, even for specific tumor types.

Online Support

Some Internet web sites on cancer also offer message boards and real-time "web chats" that encourage cancer patients and caregivers to electronically interact and exchange information with others experiencing cancer. It is important to be discriminating about any advice given by other patients or caregivers. Check all information you come across in these forums with your health care provider.

Providing Physical Care and Support

Depending on the patient's medical condition and needs, the family caregiver may play many roles. You may be required to assist with practical tasks, such as assisting with ostomy care, ordering prescriptions and supplies, providing transportation to doctor's appointments, and assuming responsibility for household tasks formerly done by the patient (childcare, managing the finances, keeping the household running, etc.). You may also provide emotional support, playing the role of cheerleader.

One of your most important functions will be to provide physical comfort and medical care under the direction of the patient's health care team. This might involve dispensing medications, monitoring symptoms, and knowing when to call the doctor.

Delivering Medication

All medications can have potentially troublesome or unpleasant side effects. Managing these symptoms is essential if the patient is going to stick to the prescribed treatment plan, be it chemotherapy or pain management.

When treatment regimens call for many medications with complicated dosing schedules, it is easy for both caregivers and patients to become confused. It often falls upon the caregiver to organize the medicines and to create a schedule for their use. For times when the primary caregiver may not be available, it is important that a written list of all medications is available to the patient as well as to other caregivers. This list should include the names, the dose, and the administration schedule for each medicine.

Pain

A full explanation of pain and other symptoms and side effects associated with cancer and its treatment can be found in chapter 15. However, there are a few important points a caregiver needs to know to ensure the patient receives adequate pain relief.

Pain is a common symptom of cancer, and one often dreaded by patients and caregivers. Yet most pain can be treated. Unrelieved pain is often associated with decreased activity, withdrawal from social relationships, insomnia, anxiety, and depression. Pain may arise from the cancer itself; from cancer treatments, such as radiation therapy or surgery; or even, in the case of opiate pain medications, from unrecognized constipation. It is important for the caregiver to be aware of the various potential causes of pain, so that it is not automatically assumed that pain represents worsening cancer.

Since only the person who is experiencing the pain can describe its intensity and characteristics, it is important to help the person with cancer to accurately report their pain severity.

Caregivers can also assist in pain management by allaying the patient's reluctance to use certain types of medications.

Emotional Pain/ Distress

It is common for patients to use the word "pain" almost as a shorthand notation to communicate the total suffering of their illness. Every pain experienced by humans has both physical and emotional components. For example, patients who are highly anxious and distressed are likely to experience higher levels of pain than patients who are not so distressed.

Having cancer is a stressful experience. Being upset and worried are part of the process. However, sometimes distress can become so excessive that it interferes with the patient's treatment or his or her ability to cope. Since people with cancer can be reluctant to discuss this type of distress with their health care providers, caregivers can be a big help in recognizing when other factors of distress may be contributing to the pain experience and by bringing these considerations to the attention of the health care team.

Transitioning to Recovery

You have been through the "hard part"—the numerous diagnostic tests and treatments associated with colorectal cancer. You are survivors! Now it is time to try to regain a sense of normalcy. Both you and the patient should realize however, that things might not go back to the way they were before the cancer. There may be reminders, such as scars or symptoms of pain or fatigue that may be present to some extent for many months or years to come. There may be additional challenges, such as resuming sexual activity after an ostomy (see chapter 16). All of these changes may be distressing to both patient and caregiver, and the challenge will be to define a new "normal" for both of you.

Part of this new normal may be establishing new habits (like making a commitment to a healthful lifestyle) or new rituals or traditions (such as attending services at your house of worship or spending more time with family). Many people also find it helpful to mark special events—like birthdays, anniversaries, and other milestones—as a way of celebrating life.

The process of adjusting to life after cancer is part of survivorship. Sometimes, survivorship can as stressful as the acute treatment period. Many patients and caregivers experience a form of "post-traumatic stress" once the flurry of the initial cancer treatment has passed.

Even when a good adjustment is being made, you and your loved one may share fears of cancer recurrence, even in the face of apparently successful treatment and multiple reassurances. Each series of follow-up scans and the appearance of new symptoms, no matter how ordinary or benign, may trigger recurrent symptoms of anxiety. See chapter 18 for more information.

If you find it difficult to move beyond your experience with cancer, seek out a support group where you can feel free to share your experience with others who have gone through it as well. If your fears or anxieties persist, seek the help of a mental health professional.

Life After Cancer

You have helped someone you care about get through cancer treatment. Take time to realize what a valuable contribution you have made.

For some caregivers, their contribution never seems to be great enough, and they are filled with remorse at not having done more. Life after cancer means putting such matters aside for both patient and caregiver. It also means putting aside any sense of disappointment with friends or relatives whose contribution may not have filled your expectations. It is important to remember that cancer remains a frightening disease to many, and even talking about the subject of cancer makes many people uncomfortable.

Some family members and friends feel that facing cancer with their loved one has deeply enriched their lives by giving them the opportunity to show love and appreciation to someone who has done so much for them in the past. Providing care and support to someone with cancer can also bring with it a feeling of satisfaction and confidence by highlighting inner strengths that you didn't realize you had.

After such an experience you may feel closer to your family members and develop a better understanding of how important your family is to your overall well being. Assuming such an important role in your family during a crisis may have also allowed you to open doors to new friends and relationships as you talked to people who faced similar problems, or you may have grown closer to distant relatives as you shared updates and tasks.

As your partner or loved one makes changes to his or her lifestyle—such as changes in diet and exercise—you may want to join in, not only to continue your support but to look toward your own future health and reduce your cancer risk.

As your loved one begins to look to the future and the rest of his or her life, you will probably begin to focus on yours as well. You can start setting new goals such as taking a postponed vacation or refocusing some of your energy at work.

You and your loved one can make new plans for yourselves and your family and look forward to creating new memories and dreams for the future.

> *"On the surface it seems a bit illogical. Yet I've heard hundreds of cancer patients frame their experience with cancer as a positive force in their lives. Since I've arrived at that same conclusion, I can now understand it fully. A cancer diagnosis requires us to take that step back and examine our very mortality as it hangs in the balance. Many patients who eventually recover actually come close to death during treatment, and no one comes away from that unchanged. I have sensed new perspectives on what is really important in life, a revised value system and even a new approach to living life day to day."*
>
> —DICK

RESOURCES

ABOUT THE RESOURCES

Listings in this section represent organizations that operate on a national level and provide some type of service or resource to consumers related to cancer, cancer research, colorectal cancer specifically, or public health. This list is designed to offer a starting point for seeking information, support, and needed resources. Most of the organizations listed here can be contacted via phone, fax, e-mail, or web site. Many of the web sites provide much of the same information that is available by postal mail. Some organizations are solely web-based and will require Internet access. Keep in mind that new web sites appear daily while old ones expand, move, or disappear entirely. Some of the web sites or content outlined below may change. Often, a simple Internet search will point to the new web site for a given organization. The American Cancer Society web site provides links to outside sources of cancer information as well (http://www.cancer.org; click on Cancer Resource Center).

There is a vast amount of information on the Internet. This information can be very valuable to the public in making health decisions. However, since any group or individual can publish on the Internet, it is important to consider the credentials and reputation of the organization providing information. Internet information should not be a substitute for medical advice.

The American Cancer Society does not necessarily endorse the agencies, organizations, corporations, and publications represented in this resource guide. This guide is provided for assistance in obtaining information only.

American Cancer Society Resources

AMERICAN CANCER SOCIETY
Toll-Free: 800-ACS-2345
Web site: http://www.cancer.org

The American Cancer Society is the nationwide community-based volunteer health organization dedicated to eliminating cancer as a major health problem by preventing cancer, saving lives and diminishing suffering from cancer, through research, education, advocacy, and service. For more information about colorectal cancer,

educational materials (*Spanish materials are available*), patient programs, and services within your community, call 800-ACS-2345/ 800-227-2345 or visit http://www.cancer.org to locate your division office for your state or region. The publications listed in the front of this book are available for sale through the Society's toll-free number and web site and include information about caregiving, couples facing cancer, pain control, and making informed decisions about treatment and end of life care.

General Cancer Resources

AMERICAN SOCIETY OF CLINICAL ONCOLOGY (ASCO)
People Living with Cancer
1900 Duke Street, Suite 200
Alexandria, VA 22314
Toll-Free: 888-651-3038
Phone: 703-797-1914
Fax: 703-299-1044
E-mail: contactus@plwc.org, help@plwc.org, or privacy@plwc.org
Web site: http://www.plwc.org

The ASCO is an international medical society representing about 10,000 cancer specialists involved in clinical research and patient care. People Living With Cancer, the patient information website of ASCO, provides oncologist-approved information on more than 50 types of cancer and their treatments, clinical trials, coping, and side effects. Additional resources include a *Find an Oncologist* database, live chats, message boards, a drug database, and links to patient support organizations. The site is designed to help people with cancer make informed health care decisions.

ASSOCIATION OF CANCER ONLINE RESOURCES (ACOR)
173 Duane Street, Suite 3A
New York NY 10013-3334
Phone: 212-226-5525
Web site: http://www.acor.org

The goal of this online community is to provide information and support to people with cancer and those who care for them through the creation and maintenance of cancer-related Internet mailing lists and credible web-based resources.

ASSOCIATION OF COMMUNITY CANCER CENTERS (ACCC)
11600 Nebel Street, Suite 201
Rockville, MD 20852-2557
Phone: 301-984-9496
Fax: 301-770-1949
Web site: http://www.accc-cancer.org

This national organization includes more than 600 medical centers, hospitals, and cancer programs. This web site contains a searchable database of cancer centers listed by state as well as information about oncology drugs (registration is required), and specific cancers.

CANCER RESEARCH INSTITUTE (CRI)
681 Fifth Avenue
New York, NY 10022
Toll-Free: 800-99-CANCER (800-992-2623)
Phone: 212-688-7515
Fax: 212-832-9376
Web site: http://www.cancerresearch.org

An institute funding cancer research and providing public information on cancer immunology and cancer treatment, the CRI helps patients locate immunotherapy clinical trials and offers a cancer reference guide and other informational booklets.

HEREDITARY CANCER INSTITUTE
Creighton University
2500 California Plaza
Omaha, NE 68178
Phone: 402-280-2942
Web site: http://medicine.creighton.edu/hci/

The Hereditary Cancer Institute provides information about hereditary cancer risk factors and offers genetic counseling. It is devoted to cancer prevention resulting from identification of hereditary cancer syndromes, including the study of Lynch syndrome, also known as hereditary nonpolyposis colorectal cancer (HNPCC) syndromes.

NATIONAL CANCER INSTITUTE (NCI)
NCI Public Inquiries Office
Building 31, Room 10A03
31 Center Drive, MSC 2580
Bethesda, MD 20892-2580
Toll-Free: 800-4-CANCER (800-422-6237)
Web site: http://www.cancer.gov

This government agency provides cancer information through several services (see list below). The Physicians' Data Query (PDQ) database contains a directory of 10,000 doctors whose practices center on cancer treatment. *Spanish-speaking staff and Spanish materials are available.*

CANCERLIT (Bibliographic Database)
Web site: http://www.cancer.gov/ cancerinfo/literature

This searchable site is maintained by the NCI and contains cancer articles published in medical and scientific journals, books, government reports, and articles that were presented at national meetings. A link to the Physicians' Data Query (PDQ) search engine is provided, which allows you to search for clinical trials by state, city, and type of cancer.

CancerTrials
Web site:
  http://www.cancer.gov/clinicaltrials

Maintained by the NCI, this site offers information about ongoing cancer clinical trials and explanations of what a trial is and what is involved. A link to the PDQ search engine allows you to search for clinical trials by state, city, and type of cancer.

CancerFax
Fax: 301-402-5874
CancerFax includes information about cancer treatment, screening, prevention, and supportive care. To obtain a contents list, dial the fax number from a fax machine handset and follow the recorded instructions.

Cancer Topics
Web site:
  http://cancer.gov/cancerinformation
Web site (Spanish version):
  http://www.cancer.gov/espanol
Web site (online ordering):
  https://cissecure.nci.nih.gov/ncipubs/

This comprehensive web site contains information on diagnosis, treatment, support, resources, literature, clinical trials, prevention and risk factors, and testing. The PDQ section provides a treatment option overview for patients and addresses treatment options for colon or rectal cancer by stages (800-4-CANCER/800-422-6237 or http://www.cancer.gov/cancertopics/pdq/ treatment/colon/patient/ or http://www.cancer.gov/cancertopics/pdq/ treatment/rectal/patient/). Up to 20 publications can be ordered online. The publications list is searchable. *Some publications are available in Spanish.*

Cancer Information Service (CIS)
Toll-Free: 800-4-CANCER
  (800-422-6237)
Web site: http://cis.nci.nih.gov

The CIS provides information to consumers and health care professionals. The web site contains a wealth of information including pamphlets and brochures on cancer diagnosis, treatment, research, and prevention. *Spanish-speaking staff members are available.*

Center to Reduce Cancer Health Disparities
6116 Executive Boulevard
Suite 602 MSC 8341
Rockville, MD 20852
Phone: 301-496-8589
Fax: 301-435-9225
E-mail: crchd@mail.nih.nci.gov
Web site: http://crchd.nci.nih.gov/

The Center to Reduce Cancer Health Disparities is the keystone of NCI's efforts to reduce the unequal burden of cancer in our society. As the organizational locus for these efforts, the center directs the implementation of and supports initiatives that advance understanding of the causes of health disparities and develops and integrates effective interventions to reduce or eliminate these disparities. The web site includes patient, family, and caregiver information, news and updates, and other information.

NATIONAL CENTER FOR COMPLEMENTARY AND ALTERNATIVE MEDICINE (NCCAM)
Toll-Free: 888-644-6226
Web site: http://altmed.od.nih.gov

The NCCAM, part of the National Institutes of Health (NIH), facilitates research and evaluation of unconventional medical practices and distributes this information to the public. Their web site provides information on some complementary and alternative methods promoted as treatments for different diseases.

NATIONAL COMPREHENSIVE CANCER NETWORK (NCCN)
50 Huntingdon Pike, Suite 200
Rockledge, PA 19046
Toll-Free: 800-909-NCCN (800-909-6226)
Phone: 215-728-4788
Fax: 215-728-3877
Web site: http://www.nccn.org

The NCCN is a nonprofit organization that is an alliance of 19 cancer centers. The American Cancer Society has partnered with NCCN to translate the NCCN Clinical Practice Guidelines into a patient-friendly resource with easy-to-understand information for patients and family members (see chapter 9). Call the American Cancer Society for the latest guidelines or view them online at either http://www.cancer.org or http://www.nccn.org.

NATIONAL LIBRARY OF MEDICINE (INCLUDES MEDLINE)
Web site: http://www.nlm.nih.gov

This National Institutes of Health web site provides a search engine for health, medical, and scientific literature and research as well as links to other government resources. Medline (http://medlineplus.gov/) is a searchable site with health information from the National Library of Medicine about conditions including cancer. It includes lists of hospitals and physicians, a medical encyclopedia and a medical dictionary, information on prescription and nonprescription drugs, health information from the media, and links to thousands of clinical trials. *Spanish materials are available*.

PubMed
Web site:
http://www.ncbi.nlm.nih.gov/PubMed

As part of the National Library of Medicine (NLM), this web site provides access to literature references in Medline and other databases, with links to online journals. The site is searchable by key word.

ONCOLINK
OncoLink Editorial Board
University of Pennsylvania Cancer Center
3400 Spruce Street-2 Donner
Philadelphia, PA 19104-4283
Web site: http://www.oncolink.com

This web site provides information on cancer including educational materials about colorectal cancer, support groups, financial questions, and other resources for people with cancer.

Colorectal Cancer Resources

COLON CANCER ALLIANCE
175 Ninth Avenue
New York, NY 10011
Toll-free: 877-422-2030 (Helpline)
Fax: 425-940-6147
Web site: http://www.ccalliance.org/

The Colon Cancer Alliance (CCA), a national patient advocacy organization and the official patient support partner of the National Colorectal Cancer Research Alliance (NCCRA), is dedicated to ending the suffering caused by colorectal cancer. The Colon Cancer Alliance brings the voices of survivors to battle colorectal cancer through patient support, education, research, and advocacy. CCA provides information about colorectal cancer; patient support services, including a helpline, survivor stories, buddy program and online chats; a resource center; local chapters called *Voices*; annual CRC conferences; and opportunities for grassroots advocacy work.

COLORECTAL CANCER COALITION (CCC)
4301 Connecticut Avenue NW, Suite 404
Washington, DC 20008
Phone: 202-244-2906
E-mail: info@c-three.org
Web site: http://www.c-three.org

The Colorectal Cancer Coalition is a non-profit advocacy organization dedicated to reducing suffering and death caused by colorectal cancer. The coalition's goals are to advocate for research for better screening, better diagnosis, and better treatments; back policy reform through grassroots movements; and raise awareness so people know that colorectal cancer is "preventable, treatable, and beatable."

COLORECTAL CANCER NETWORK
PO Box 182
Kensington, MD 20895-0182
Phone: 301-879-1500

Fax: 301-879-1901
Web site: http://www.colorectal-cancer.net/

The Colorectal Cancer Network has three main functions: to provide a support network, to lead aggressive awareness, screening, and early detection programs, and to promote legislative action. Support groups, listservs, chat rooms, matching list that connects newly diagnosed patients with long-term survivors, colorectal cancer and other relevant links, literature, awareness pins and t-shirts are available online.

HEREDITARY COLON CANCER
M. D. Anderson Cancer Center
Box 243
1515 Holcombe Boulevard
Houston, TX 77030
Web site:
  http://www3.mdanderson.org/depts/hcc/

This site provides information on genetic testing, genetic counseling, support resources, screening, and prevention for individuals and families with hereditary conditions associated with an increased risk of colon cancer.

NATIONAL COLORECTAL CANCER RESEARCH ALLIANCE (NCCRA)
Phone: 800-872-3000
Web site: http://www.nccra.org

The National Colorectal Cancer Research Alliance (NCCRA), a program of the Entertainment Industry Foundation, communicates the seriousness of colorectal cancer and encourages preventive testing. The NCCRA supports public education and medical research to develop better tests, treatments, and cures for colorectal cancer. NCCRA was founded by NBC *Today* show co-anchor Katie Couric, cancer activist Lilly Tartikoff, and the Entertainment Industry Foundation (EIF).

NATIONAL COLORECTAL CANCER ROUNDTABLE (NCCRT)

Phone: 404-329-5705
Fax: 404-248-1780
E-mail: ksharpe@cancer.org
Web site: http://www.nccrt.org/

The National Colorectal Cancer Roundtable (NCCRT) is a national coalition of public, private, and voluntary organizations whose mission is to advance colorectal cancer control efforts by improving communication, coordination, and collaboration among health agencies, medical-professional organizations, and the public. The ultimate goal of the roundtable is to increase the use of proven colorectal cancer screening tests among the entire population for whom screening is appropriate.

Professional Organizations, Licensing, and Certifying Boards

AMERICAN BOARD OF MEDICAL SPECIALTIES

1007 Church Street, Suite 404
Evanston, IL 60201-5913
Phone: 866-ASK-ABMS (for verification of a doctor's credentials)
Phone: 847-491-9091
Fax: 847-328-3596
Web site: http://www.abms.org

The American Board of Medical Specialties maintains a list of all board-certified doctors, including surgeons and oncologists. These doctors have demonstrated that they have the knowledge and training necessary to practice their medical specialty. To find a board-certified specialist near you or to check the certification of a doctor, contact the ABMS or check your local library for a copy of *The Official American Board of Medical Specialties Directory of Board Certified Medical Specialists.*

American Board of Colon and Rectal Surgery (ABCRS)

20600 Eureka Road, Suite 600
Taylor, MI 48180
Phone: 734-282-9400
Fax: 734-282-9402
E-mail: admin@abcrs.org
Web site: http://www.abcrs.org/

The American Board of Colon and Rectal Surgery is a member board of the American Board of Medical Specialties. The ABCRS develops and maintains high standards for certification in the specialty of colon and rectal surgery. For a fee, and with a signed permission release form from the physician, the board will verify a physician's certification.

AMERICAN COLLEGE OF SURGEONS

633 North St. Claire Street
Chicago, IL 60611-3211
Toll-free: 800-621-4111
Phone: 312-202-5000
Fax: 312-202-5001
E-mail: postmaster@facs.org
Web site: http://www.facs.org/

The American College of Surgeons has a member database that can be searched by name, location, and medical specialty. It can be found online at http://web.facs.org/acs-dir/default_public.cfm.

AMERICAN GASTROENTEROLOGICAL ASSOCIATION
National Office
4930 Del Ray Avenue
Bethesda, MD 20814
Phone: 301-654-2055
Fax: 301-654-5920
E-mail: info@gastro.org or
   webmaster@gastro.org
Web site: http://www.gastro.org/

The American Gastroenterological Association (AGA) is a professional organization for physicians and scientists who research, diagnose and treat disorders of the gastrointestinal tract and liver. Founded in 1897, the AGA is dedicated to the mission of advancing the science and practice of gastroenterology.

AMERICAN MEDICAL ASSOCIATION
515 North State Street
Chicago, IL 60610
Toll-free: 800-621-8335
Web site: http://www.ama-assn.org/

The American Medical Association maintains a database called Physician Select that lists every licensed doctor in the United States. It includes information on each doctor's training, specialty, gender, and office location. For some doctors, it also lists office hours, health plan participation, and hospital affiliations. To search Physician Select, visit http://dbapps.ama-assn.org/aps/amahg.htm.

AMERICAN PSYCHOLOGICAL ASSOCIATION (APA)
750 First Street, NE
Washington, DC 20002-4242
Toll-Free: 800-374-2721
Phone: 202-336-5500
Web site: http://www.apa.org

This organization has a Division on Health Psychology that addresses a range of health issues including cancer. The APA provides a hotline that patients can use to obtain literature and discuss psychological conditions and referrals to state psychological associations to locate a psychologist in a specific area. The APA web site provides a help center with information about psychological issues. *Spanish-speaking staff members are available.*

AMERICAN SOCIETY OF CLINICAL ONCOLOGY (ASCO)
1900 Duke Street, Suite 200
Alexandria, VA 22314
Toll-Free: 888-651-3038
Phone: 703-797-1914
Fax: 703-299-1044
Web site: http://www.asco.org/

The American Society of Clinical Oncologists has a member database that includes the names and affiliations of over 15,000 oncologists worldwide. To search the database online, visit http://www.asco.org/ac/1,1003,_12-002215,00.asp.

AMERICAN SOCIETY OF COLON AND RECTAL SURGEONS
85 West Algonquin Road, Suite 550
Arlington Heights, IL 60005
Phone: 847-290-9184
Fax: 847-290-9203
E-mail: ascrs@fascrs.org
Web site: http://www.fascrs.org/

The American Society of Colon and Rectal Surgeons (ASCRS) is a national association of colon and rectal surgeons and other surgeons dedicated to advancing and promoting the science and practice of the treatment of patients with diseases and disorders affecting the colon, rectum, and anus.

AMERICAN SOCIETY OF GASTROINTESTINAL ENDOSCOPY (ASGE)
1520 Kensington Road, Suite 202
Oak Brook, IL 60523
Toll-free 866-305-ASGE
Phone: 630-573-0600
Fax: 630.573.0691
E-mail: info@asge.org
Web site: http://www.askasge.org

ASGE is a professional organization dedicated to endoscopy and the prevention of colorectal cancer through proper screening. It promotes excellence in gastrointestinal endoscopy. The web site includes information for patients on endoscopic procedures in English and Spanish.

JOINT COMMISSION ON ACCREDITATION OF HEALTHCARE ORGANIZATIONS (JCAHO)
One Renaissance Boulevard
Oakbrook Terrace, IL 60181
Toll-Free (for filing complaints about a
   health care organization): 800-994-6610
Phone: 630-792-5000
Fax: 630-792-5005
Web site: http://www.jcaho.org

This is an independent nonprofit organization that evaluates and accredits more than 19,500 health care organizations in the United States, including hospitals, health care networks, and health care organizations that provide home care, long-term care, behavioral health care, and laboratory and ambulatory care services. JCAHO provides information to the public about accreditation status and selecting quality care. Performance reports of accredited organizations and guidelines for choosing a health care facility are available to the public and can be obtained by calling JCAHO or visiting their web site.

NATIONAL ASSOCIATION OF SOCIAL WORKERS
750 First Street NE, Suite 700
Washington, DC 20002-4241
Toll-Free: 800-638-8799
Phone: 202-408-8600
Fax: 202-336-8340
Web site: http://www.naswdc.org

This organization is concerned with advocacy, work practice standards and ethics, and professional standards for agencies employing social workers. The web site provides a national register of clinical social workers for local referrals. *Spanish-speaking staff members are available.*

ONCOLOGY NURSING SOCIETY (ONS)
501 Holiday Drive
Pittsburgh, PA 15220-2749
Phone: 412-921-7373
Fax: 412-921-6565
Web site: http://www.ons.org

This organization is a national membership organization of registered nurses involved in oncology care whose mission is to promote professional standards for oncology nursing, research, and education. Nonmembers can access the ONS web site to find information about cancer treatment, survivorship, and end-of life issues.

Patient and Family Services

AARP (FORMERLY THE AMERICAN ASSOCIATION OF RETIRED PERSONS)
Dept. # 258390
P.O. Box 40011
Roanoke, VA 24022
Toll-Free: 800-456-2277
Web site: http://www.aarp.org
Web site (for Pharmacy Service):
  http://www.aarppharmacy.com

The AARP is a nonprofit membership organization with a commitment to older adults. It provides a variety of services to its members including information on managed care, Medicare, Medicaid, long-term care, and other issues of interest. Membership is open to anyone 50 years of age or older. The web site includes information on a member pharmacy service that offers discounts on drugs used for cancer treatment and pain relief.

AIRLIFELINE
50 Fullerton Court, Suite 200
Sacramento, CA 95825
Toll-Free: 877-AIR-LIFE
Phone: 916-641-7800
Fax: 916-641-0600
Web site: http://www.airlifeline.org

A nonprofit charitable organization, AirLifeLine provides free flights to patients who can't afford the cost of commercial airfare when traveling to a medical facility.

AMERICAN CANCER SOCIETY HOPE LODGES
Toll-free: 800-ACS-2345

The Hope Lodge is a temporary residential facility providing sleeping rooms and related facilities for people with cancer who are undergoing outpatient treatment and their family members. Approval from a physician or referring agency is necessary.

AMERICANS WITH DISABILITIES ACT (ADA)
United States Department of Justice
950 Pennsylvania Avenue, NW
Civil Rights Division
Disability Rights Section-NYAV
Washington, D.C. 20530
Phone: 800-514-0301
Fax: 202-307-1198
Web site: http://www.ada.gov

Specialists at the ADA information line answer questions about titles II and III of the ADA. The ADA web site includes a text version of the ADA and available publications. Many publications can be ordered through the automated fax system; call the information line for directions. *Spanish-speaking staff and Spanish materials are available.*

CANCER CARE, INC.
275 Seventh Avenue
New York, NY 10001
Toll-Free (Counseling): 800-813-HOPE
(800-813-4637)
Phone: 212-712-8080
Fax: 212-712-8495
Web site: http://www.cancercare.org
Web site (Spanish version): http://www.
  cancercare.org/EnEspanol/EnEspanolmain.cfm

A nonprofit social service agency, Cancer Care, Inc. provides counseling and guidance to help people with cancer, their families, and friends cope with the impact of cancer. The web site includes detailed information on specific cancers and cancer treatment, cancer pain, clinical trials, a searchable database of regional and national resources, and links to other sites. The organization also provides videos, free support groups (online, telephone, and face-to-face), workshops, seminars and clinics, a newsletter, and other publications to interested consumers. *Spanish-speaking staff members are available.*

CANCER HOPE NETWORK

Two North Road
Chester, NJ 07930
Toll-free: 877-HOPENET
E-mail: info@cancerhopenetwork.org
Web site: http://www.cancerhopenetwork.org/

Cancer Hope Network is a not-for-profit
organization that provides free and confidential one-on-one support to people with
cancer and their families. They match
patients with cancer and/or family members
with trained volunteers who have themselves
undergone and recovered from a similar
cancer experience.

HEALTH INSURANCE ASSOCIATION
OF AMERICA

555 13th Street, NW, Suite 600 East
Washington, DC 20004
Toll-Free: 800-879-4422
Phone: 202-824-1600
Fax: 202-824-1722
Web site: http://www.hiaa.org

This association represents most United
States health insurance companies. The web
site contains insurance guides and general
insurance information, and an annual directory and survey of hospitals, along with
other information.

HOSPICE LINK

Hospice Education Institute, Suite 2
190 Westbrook Road
Essex, CT 06426
Toll-free: 800-331-1620
Phone: 860-767-1620 (in Alaska and
  Connecticut)

Hospice Link is a nonprofit service that
provides information on hospice care and
refers patients with cancer and their families
to local hospice programs.

I CAN COPE

American Cancer Society
Toll-Free: 800-ACS-2345
Web site: http://www.cancer.org

This educational program is provided in a
supportive environment for adults with cancer and their loved ones. The program offers
several courses designed to help participants
cope with their cancer experience by
increasing their knowledge, positive attitude,
and skills. The program is conducted by
trained health care professionals in communities throughout the United States, often
with hospital co-sponsorship, as well as in
other countries. It offers straightforward
cancer information and answers to questions
about human anatomy, cancer development,
diagnosis, treatment, side effects, new
research, communication, emotions, sexuality,
self-esteem, and community resources.
The program also provides information,
encouragement, and practical hints through
presentations and class discussions. All classes
are free.

LOOK GOOD... FEEL BETTER (LGFB)

American Cancer Society
Toll-Free: 800-395-LOOK
Web site: http://www.cancer.org

The Look Good...Feel Better program is a
community-based, free, national service that
teaches female patients with cancer beauty
techniques to help restore their appearance
and self-image during chemotherapy and
radiation treatments. For men, LGFB
provides a brochure for men undergoing
chemotherapy or radiation treatment. The
brochure also features a tear-out sheet
containing steps to help men with skin care
and other information.

MAKE TODAY COUNT

Mid-American Cancer Center
1235 East Cherokee,
Springfield, MO 65804-2263
Toll-Free: 800-432-2273
Phone: 417-885-2273
Fax: 417-888-8761

This is a support organization for people
affected by cancer or other life-threatening
illness.

358

MEDICARE HOTLINE
Department of Health and Human Services
Toll-Free: 800-MEDICARE (800-633-4227)
Web site: http://www.medicare.gov

The official U.S. Government site for Medicare provides information on eligibility, enrollment, premiums, coverage, payment and billing, insurance, prescription drugs, and frequently asked questions. Call the toll-free number to receive information about local services. Visit http://www.medicare.gov/Health/ColonCancer.asp for the most up-to-date information on Medicare coverage for colorectal cancer screening.

NATIONAL FAMILY CAREGIVERS ASSOCIATION (NFCA)
10400 Connecticut Avenue, Suite 500
Kensington, MD 20895-3944
Toll-Free: 800-896-3650
Phone: 301-942-6430
Fax: 301-942-2302
Web site: http://www.nfcacares.org

This organization is a national, nonprofit, membership association whose mission is to promote caregiving through education and advocacy. NFCA publishes *Take Care!* a newsletter (free for family caregivers) that includes can-do advice, helpful resources, and stories about family caregivers. The NFCA provides referrals to national resources for caregivers and offers a bereavement kit for caregivers. The NFCA web site provides a report on the status of family caregivers and ten tips for family caregivers.

NATIONAL HOSPICE AND PALLIATIVE CARE ORGANIZATION (NHCPO)
1700 Diagonal Road, Suite 625
Alexandria, VA 22314
Toll-Free: 800-658-8898
Phone: 703-837-1500
Fax: 703-837-1233
E-mail: nhpco_info@nhpco.org
Web site: http://www.nhpco.org/

The National Hospice and Palliative Care Organization is the largest nonprofit membership organization representing hospice and palliative care programs and professionals in the United States. The NHPCO is committed to improving end-of-life care and expanding access to hospice care with the goal of enhancing quality of life for people who are dying and their loved ones.

NATIONAL SELF-HELP CLEARINGHOUSE
Graduate School and University Center of the City University of New York
365 Fifth Avenue, Suite 3300
New York, NY 10016
Phone: 212-817-1822
Fax: 212-817-2990
Web site: http://www.selfhelpweb.org

This nonprofit organization provides access to regional self-help services.

PARTNERSHIP FOR CARING: AMERICA'S VOICES FOR THE DYING
1620 Eye Street NW, Suite 202
Washington, DC 20006
Toll-Free: 800-989-9455 (Hotline)
Phone: 202-296-8071
Fax: 202-296-8352
E-mail: pfc@partnershipforcaring.org
Web site: http://www.partnershipforcaring.org

Partnership for Caring: America's Voices for the Dying is a national, nonprofit organization that partners individuals and organizations with the goal of improving how society cares for dying people and their loved ones. Services include: counseling via their 24-hour hotline; publications and videos; information about speaking with family and friends about end-of-life issues; advance directives (living wills and/or medical powers of attorney forms) tailored to each state's legal requirements; and information about state laws on issues such as refusing medical treatment, withdrawing life supports, honoring advance directives, and managing pain.

PARTNERSHIP FOR PRESCRIPTION ASSISTANCE
Toll-free: 888-4PPA-NOW (888-477-2669)
Web site: http://www.pparx.org

Through the Partnership for Prescription Assistance, pharmaceutical companies, health care providers, patient advocacy organizations, and community groups combine their efforts to increase enrollment in patient assistance programs. These programs provide free or discounted medicines to those who do not have prescription coverage. The Partnership for Prescription Assistance program provides access to more than 275 public and private patient assistance programs, including more than 150 programs offered by pharmaceutical companies. Call or go to the web site to determine which patient assistance programs you qualify for, and you can download applications online. The American Cancer Society is a national partner in this program. *Information is available in Spanish.*

PHARMACEUTICAL RESEARCH AND MANUFACTURERS ASSOCIATION OF AMERICA (PHRMA)
1100 15th Street, NW, Suite 900
Washington, DC 20005
Phone: 202-835-3400
Fax: 202-835-3414
Web site: http://www.phrma.org

PHRMA provides information about member pharmaceutical companies and drugs that are currently available, in use in clinical trials, or under development. The web site includes a directory of patient assistance programs for prescription drugs and a database of new medications for cancer and other diseases.

SOCIAL SECURITY ADMINISTRATION
Department of Health and Human Services
Toll-Free: 800-772-1213
Web site: http://www.ssa.gov

Call the toll-free number to receive information about local services or visit the web site to learn more about benefits, disability, and other frequently asked-about topics.

TRICARE (FORMERLY CHAMPUS)
Web site: http://www.tricare.osd.mil

TRICARE is part of the military health care system. The web site offers a link to TRICARE regional offices and a list of phone numbers.

WELLNESS COMMUNITY
919 18th Street NW, Suite 54
Washington, DC 20006
Toll-Free: 888-793-WELL
Phone: 202-659-9709
Fax: 202-659-9301
E-mail: help@thewellnesscommunity.org
Web site:
  http://www.thewellnesscommunity.org

The Wellness Community is a nonprofit organization whose mission is to help people with cancer and their families enhance their health and well being by providing a professional program of emotional support, education, and hope. Support groups are facilitated by licensed psychotherapists. Bereavement support groups are also available. Referrals are provided to their 25 facilities across the nation. The web site has information about relaxation, talking with children when a parent has cancer, a study sponsored by the Wellness Community investigating the benefits of a professionally facilitated, online support group for women with breast cancer.

WESTIN HOTEL GUESTROOM FOR CANCER PATIENTS
Toll-Free: 800-ACS-2345
Web site: http://www.cancer.org

In cooperation with the American Cancer Society, participating Westin hotels will provide overnight accommodations when cancer patients must travel considerable distances from their homes to receive treatment. Some rooms are free; however, some only offer reduced rates. Contact the Society for more information.

Ostomy Care and Supplies

UNITED OSTOMY ASSOCIATION, INC.
Web site: http://www.uoa.org

UOA web site provides information for people with intestinal or urinary diversions. The web site also includes ostomy tips, FAQs, and information on local chapters with support groups.

WOUND, OSTOMY, AND CONTINENCE NURSES SOCIETY (WOCN)
WOCN Society National Office
4700 West Lake Ave
Glenview, IL 60025
Toll-free: 888-224-WOCN
Fax: 866-615-8560
Web site: http://www.wocn.org/

In addition to serving people with ostomies with care and rehabilitation, ostomy nurses coordinate patient care, teach nursing personnel in hospitals and clinics, and work closely with the nursing and medical professions to improve the quality of ostomy rehabilitation programs. The WOCN national office can provide information and refer you to an ostomy nurse in your area.

INTERNATIONAL OSTOMY ASSOCIATION (IOA)
International Ostomy Association Office
102 Allingham Gardens
Toronto, ON M3H 1Y2
Canada
Phone: 416-633-6783
Fax: 416-633-6712
Web site: http://www.ostomyinternational.org/

The International Ostomy Association provides information regarding ostomy associations worldwide.

Survivorship

CANCER SURVIVORS NETWORK
American Cancer Society
1599 Clifton Road, NE
Atlanta, GA 30329-4251
Toll-Free: 800-ACS-2345
Web site: http://www.acscsn.org

This network provides an online community that welcomes cancer survivors, friends, and families to share and communicate with others with similar interests and experiences. The program offers a vibrant community of real people supporting one another and sharing personal experiences with cancer. The web site enables registered members to have live, private chats, to create personal web pages to share experiences, thoughts, and wisdom, to help people create personal support communities of people who share common concerns and interests, and offers information about resources.

CANCERVIVE
1875 Century Park East, Suite 700
Los Angeles, CA 90067
Phone: 310-203-9232
Web site: http://www.cancervive.org/
   index2.html

Cancervive provides emotional support, education, and advocacy to assist survivors facing life after cancer.

NATIONAL COALITION FOR CANCER SURVIVORSHIP (NCCS)
1010 Wayne Avenue, Suite 770
Silver Spring, MD 20910
Toll free: 877-NCCS-YES (877-622-7937)
Phone: 301-650-9127
Fax: 301-565-9670
E-mail: info@canceradvocacy.org
Web site: http://www.canceradvocacy.org

The NCCS is a survivor-led advocacy organization working in the area of cancer survivorship and support. NCCS seeks to empower survivors by educating all those affected by cancer and speaking out on issues related to quality cancer care. The web site offers links to online cancer resources, support groups, survivorship programs, a newsletter, and an audio program that teaches skills to help people with cancer meet the challenges of illness.

Cancer in Diverse Populations

CENTER TO REDUCE CANCER HEALTH DISPARITIES (CRCHD)
National Cancer Institute
6116 Executive Boulevard
Suite 602 MSC 8341
Rockville, MD 20852
Phone: 301-496-8589
Fax: 301-435-9225
E-mail: crchd@mail.nih.nci.gov
Web site: http://crchd.nci.nih.gov

The CRCHD was created in 2001 to carry out NCI's Strategic Plan for Reducing Cancer Health Disparities. NCI's goal is to nearly triple the funding for cancer health disparities in four years. Research will investigate social, cultural, environmental, biological, and behavioral determinants of cancer disparities across the cancer control continuum from prevention to end-of-life care.

GAY AND LESBIAN MEDICAL ASSOCIATION (GLMA)
459 Fulton Street, Suite 107
San Francisco, CA 94102
Phone: 415-255-4547
Fax: 415-255-4784
E-mail: info@glma.org
Web site: http://www.glma.org

The Gay and Lesbian Medical Association is a national organization of doctors, dentists, therapists, and chiropractors who understand and are sensitive to the needs of gay, lesbian, bisexual, transgendered, or intersex people. GLMA is committed to ensuring equality in health care for patients and health care professionals. GLMA achieves its goals by using medical expertise in professional education, public policy work, patient education and referrals, and the promotion of research. To locate a GLMA member, visit: http://services.glma.org/referrals/

INTERCULTURAL CANCER COUNCIL (ICC)
6655 Travis, Suite 322
Houston, TX 77030-1312
Phone: 713-798-4617
Fax: 713-798-6222
E-mail: info@iccnetwork.org
Web site: http://iccnetwork.org/

The Intercultural Cancer Council is a non-profit organization that promotes policies, programs, partnerships, and research to eliminate the unequal burden of cancer among racial and ethnic minorities and medically underserved populations in the United States and its associated territories. The web site provides cancer fact sheets on different medically underserved populations (such as African Americans, Asian Americans, and Hispanics/Latinos), as well as cancer news updates.

SPECIAL POPULATIONS NETWORKS FOR CANCER AWARENESS, RESEARCH, AND TRAINING

National Cancer Institute
6116 Executive Boulevard
Suite 602 MSC 8341
Rockville, MD 20852
Phone: 301-496-8589
Fax: 301-435-9225
Web site: http://crchd.nci.nih.gov/spn

The purpose of the special populations networks is to build relationships between large research institutions and community based programs and to find ways of addressing important questions about the burden of cancer in minority communities. The major goal is to build infrastructure to promote cancer awareness within minority and medically underserved communities and to launch from these communities more research and cancer control activities aimed at specific population subgroups. Currently the special populations' network consists of 18 projects in 15 states.

RACIAL AND ETHNIC APPROACHES TO COMMUNITY HEALTH (REACH)

Centers for Disease Control and Prevention
1600 Clifton Road
Atlanta, GA 30333
Toll-Free: 800-311-3435
Phone: 404-639-3311
Public Inquiries: 404-639-3534
Web site: http://www.cdc.gov/reach2010

The REACH program funds community coalitions to develop and implement activities to reduce the level of disparities in one or more of six priority areas, which include breast and cervical cancer screening. The program emphasizes the importance of working more closely with communities to identify culturally sensitive implementation strategies.

Other Organizations Providing Health Information and Support

AGENCY FOR HEALTHCARE RESEARCH AND QUALITY (AHRQ)

Publications Clearinghouse
P.O. Box 8547
Silver Springs, MD 20907-8547
Toll-Free: 800-358-9295
Web site: http://www.ahrq.gov

The AHRQ, an office within the US Department of Health and Human Services' Public Health Service, is responsible for supporting research designed to improve the quality of health care, reduce its cost, and broaden access to essential services. One of AHRQ's highest priorities is providing consumers with science-based, easily understandable information that will help them make informed decisions about their own personal health care, including selection of the highest quality health plans and most appropriate health care services.

THE AMERICAN GERIATRICS SOCIETY FOUNDATION FOR HEALTH IN AGING (FHA)
Toll-Free: 800-563-4916
Web site: http://www.healthinaging.org/
public_education/

The FHA's patient education resources were developed in collaboration with the American Geriatrics Society (AGS) and are based on the new major AGS clinical practice guideline for health care providers entitled *The Management of Persistent Pain in Older Persons*. The FHA web site provides practical and easy-to-use tools to help older adults and their caregivers better manage persistent pain in consultation with their physicians and other health care providers, including: a pain diary and a medication and supplement diary, guides to pain medications, how to assess pain in those with dementia, and information about eldercare at home. Materials may be downloaded and printed from the web site. Call to obtain hard copies or to place bulk orders.

MEMORIAL SLOAN-KETTERING CANCER CENTER (MSKCC)
AboutHerbs
Web site: http://www.mskcc.org/mskcc/html/
11570.cfm

Memorial Sloan-Kettering Cancer Center's *AboutHerbs* web site provides information for consumers about herbs, botanicals, and alternative or unproven cancer therapies, including details about adverse effects, interactions, and potential benefits or problems.

QUACKWATCH
Web site: http://www.quackwatch.com

This web site provides a guide to fraudulent claims about alternative medicines and questionable health products. The site is searchable by keyword.

UNIVERSITY OF TEXAS M. D. ANDERSON CANCER CENTER COMPLEMENTARY/INTEGRATIVE MEDICINE (CIMER)
Web site: http://www.mdanderson.org/
departments/CIMER/

M. D. Anderson Cancer Center's Complementary/Integrative Medicine Education Resources (CIMER) web site is offered to help patients and physicians decide how best to integrate complementary therapies into their care under the direction of informed physicians to enhance patient wellness and quality of life and avoid harm. Although the site is not staffed to respond to patient inquires, it contains useful information on a variety of complementary therapies, answers to frequently asked questions, and videos, presentations, recommended reading, and related links.

WORLD HEALTH ORGANIZATION (WHO)
WHO Publications Center USA
49 Sheridan Avenue
Albany, NY 12210
Phone: 202-974-3000
Fax: 202-974-3663
Web site: http://www.who.org

The WHO is an agency of the United Nations that promotes technical cooperation for health among nations, carries out programs to control and eradicate disease, and strives to improve the quality of human life. The WHO web site includes data on cancer, a list of publications, and links to related web sites. *Spanish materials are available.*

References

Introduction

American Cancer Society. Cancer facts and figures 2005. Available at http://www.cancer.org/downloads/STT/CAFF2005PWSecured4.pdf. Accessed February 4, 2005.

Seffrin JR. "Colon Cancer Campaign" e-mail message from CEO of American Cancer Society to staff, February 7, 2005.

Chapter 1

American Cancer Society. *Cancer Control State of the Science Guide*. Atlanta, GA: American Cancer Society; 2002.

American Cancer Society. Cancer facts and figures 2004. Available at http://www.cancer.org/downloads/STT/CAFF_finalPWSecured.pdf. Accessed August 20, 2004.

American Cancer Society. Cancer facts and figures 2005. Available at http://www.cancer.org/downloads/STT/CAFF2005PWSecured4.pdf. Accessed February 4, 2005.

American Cancer Society. Cancer facts and figures for African-Americans 2005-2006. Available at http://www.cancer.org/downloads/STT/CAFF2005AAv4PWSecured.pdf. Accessed February 7, 2005.

American Cancer Society. *Cancer: What Causes It, What Doesn't*. Atlanta, GA. American Cancer Society; 2003.

American Cancer Society. *Colon Testing Can Save Your Life!* Atlanta, GA. American Cancer Society; 2001.

American Cancer Society. Detailed guide: colon and rectum cancer. What is colorectal cancer? Available at http://www.cancer.org/docroot/CRI/content/CRI_2_4_1x_What_Is_Colon_and_Rectum_Cancer.asp?sitearea=CRI. Accessed July 2, 2004.

CancerNetwork.com. What is colorectal cancer? http://cancernetwork.com/myths/colon/Col02.htm. Accessed August 16, 2004.

Couric K. Colon cancer in women: the need for awareness. *Obstet Gynecol*. 2004;104(5 Pt 1): 910-912.

Fletcher RH. Patient information: screening for colon cancer. In: Rose BD, Rush JM. *UpToDate*. Available at http://patients.uptodate.com/topic.asp?file=cancer/6968. Accessed June 17, 2004.

Itzkowitz SH. Colonic polyps and polyposis syndromes. In: Feldman M, Friedman LS, Sleisenger MH. *Gastrointestinal and Liver Disease*. 7th ed. New York: Elsevier Science; 2002.

Janne PA, Mayer RJ. Chemoprevention of colorectal cancer. *N Engl J Med*. 2000;342:1960-1968.

Jemal A, Murray T, Ward E, et al. Cancer statistics, 2005. *CA Cancer J Clin*. 2005;55:10-30.

Levin B. *Colorectal Cancer: A Thorough and Compassionate Resource for Patients and Their Families*. Atlanta, GA: American Cancer Society; 1999.

CancerNetwork.com. Myths and facts about colorectal cancer. Available at http://cancernetwork.com/myths/colon/Col02.htm. Accessed August 20, 2004.

People Living with Cancer: An ASCO web site. Cancer type: colorectal. Available at http://www.peoplelivingwithcancer.org/plwc/MainConstructor/1,1744,_04-003-00_12-001043-00_17-001029-00_18-0025980-00_19-000-00_20-001-00_21-008,00.asp?ArticleId=25980&ArticleBodyId=0&ShowHead=&PageNo=1&cancer_type_id=3&state=. Accessed August 20, 2004.

Seifeldin R, Hantsch JJ. The economic burden associated with colon cancer in the United States. *Clin Ther*. 1999;21:1370-1379.

Jemal A, Tiwari RC, Murray T, et al. Cancer statistics, 2004. *CA Cancer J Clin*. 2004;54:8-29.

Wu JS, Fazio VW. Colon cancer. *Dis Colon Rectum*. 2000;43:1473-1486.

CHAPTER 2

Adami H, Trichopoulos D. Obesity and mortality from cancer. *N Engl J Med*. 348:1623-1624.

American Cancer Society and National Comprehensive Cancer Network. Colon and rectal cancer: treatment guidelines for patients, version III/September 2003. Atlanta, GA: American Cancer Society; 2003. Available at http://www.cancer.org/downloads/CRI/F9409.00.pdf. Accessed September 2, 2004.

American Cancer Society and National Comprehensive Cancer Network. Colon and rectal cancer: treatment guidelines for patients, version IV/February 2005. Atlanta, GA: American Cancer Society; 2005. Available at http://www.nccn.org/patients/patient_gls/_english/_colon/contents.asp. Accessed May 3, 2005.

American Cancer Society. Cancer facts and figures 2002. Available at: http://www.cancer.org/downloads/STT/CancerFacts&Figures2002TM.pdf. Accessed September 2, 2004.

American Cancer Society. Cancer facts and figures 2004. Available at: http://www.cancer.org/downloads/STT/CAFF_finalPWSecured.pdf. Accessed September 2, 2004.

American Cancer Society. Cancer facts and figures 2005. Available at: http://www.cancer.org/downloads/STT/CAFF2005PWSecured4.pdf. Accessed February 10, 2005.

American Cancer Society. Colorectal cancer facts and figures—Special edition 2005. Available at: http://www.cancer.org/docroot/STT/content/STT_1x_Colorectal_Cancer_Facts_and_Figures_-_Special_Edition_2005.asp. Accessed March 15, 2005

American Cancer Society. Cancer prevention and early detection facts and figures 2004. Available at: http://www.cancer.org/downloads/STT/CPED2004PWSecured.pdf. Accessed September 2, 2004.

American Cancer Society. *Cancer: What Causes It, What Doesn't*. Atlanta, GA: American Cancer Society; 2003.

American Cancer Society. Detailed guide: colon and rectum cancer. Available at: http://www.cancer.org/docroot/CRI/CRI_2_3x.asp?dt=10. Accessed July 2, 2004.

American Cancer Society. Detailed guide: colon and rectum cancer. Available at: http://documents.cancer.org/107.00/107.00.pdf. Accessed September 9, 2004.

American Cancer Society. Estrogen replacement may lower colorectal cancer risk. Available at http://www.cancer.org/docroot/NWS/content/NWS_1_1x_Estrogen_Replacement_May_Lower_Colorectal_Cancer_Risk.asp. Accessed October 22, 2004.

American Cancer Society. Obesity linked to cancer, other chronic disease risk: overeating and inactivity lead to obesity and chronic diseases. Available at http://www.cancer.org/docroot/NWS/content/update/NWS_1_1xU_Obesity_Linked_to_Cancer__Other_Chronic_Disease_Risk.asp. Accessed October 22, 2004.

American Cancer Society. The complete guide: nutrition and physical activity. Available at: http://www.cancer.org/docroot/PED/content/PED_3_2X_Diet_and_Activity_Factors_That_Affect_Risks.asp. Accessed August 31, 2004.

Bingham S, Riboli E. Diet and cancer—the European Prospective Investigation into Cancer and Nutrition. *Nat Rev Cancer*. 2004; 4:206-215.

Bruce WR, Giacca A, Medline A. Possible mechanisms relating diet to colorectal cancer risk. *IARC Sci Publ*. 2002;156:277-281.

Calle EE, Kaaks R. Overweight, obesity and cancer: epidemiological evidence and proposed mechanisms. *Nat Rev Cancer*. 2004;4:579-591.

Calle EE, Rodriguez C, Walker-Thurmond K, Thun MJ. Overweight, obesity, and mortality from cancer in a prospectively studied cohort of US adults. *N Engl J Med*. 2003;348:1625-1638.

CancerNetwork.com. Myths and facts about colorectal cancer: what causes colorectal cancer? Available at: http://cancernetwork.com/myths/colon/Col03.htm. Accessed August 16, 2004.

Chao A, Thun MJ, Connell CJ, et al. Meat consumption and risk of colorectal cancer. *JAMA*. 2005;293:172-182.

Chlebowski RT, Wactawski-Wende J, Ritenbaugh C, et al. for the Women's Health Initiative Investigators. Estrogen plus progestin and colorectal cancer in postmenopausal women. *N Engl J Med*. 350:991-1004. Available at http://content.nejm.org/cgi/content/short/350/10/991. Accessed October 22, 2004.

Colditz G, Cannuscio C, Frazier A. Physical activity and reduced risk of colon cancer: implications for prevention. *Cancer Causes Control*. 1997;8:649-667.

Feskanich D, Ma J, Fuchs CS, et al. Plasma vitamin D metabolites and risk of colorectal cancer in women. *Cancer Epidemiol Biomarkers Prev*. 2004;13:1502-1508.

Giardiello FM, Brensinger JD, and Petersen GM. AGA technical review on hereditary colorectal cancer and genetic testing. *Gastroenterology*. 2001;121:198-213.

Giovannucci E, Ascherio A, Rimm EB, et al. Physical activity, obesity, and risk for colon cancer and adenoma in men. *Ann Intern Med*. 1995;122:327-334.

Giovannucci E, Colditz GA, Stampfer MJ, et al. A prospective study of cigarette smoking and risk of colorectal adenoma and colorectal cancer in US women. *J Natl Cancer Inst*. 1994;86:192-199.

Giovannucci E, Rimm EB, Stampfer MJ, et al. 1994. A prospective study of cigarette smoking and risk of colorectal adenoma and colorectal cancer in US men. *J Natl Cancer Inst*. 1994;86:183-191.

Hawk ET, Umar A and Viner JL. Colorectal cancer chemoprevention—an overview of the science. *Gastroenterology*. 2004;126:1423-1447.

Johns LE, Houlston RS. A systematic review and meta-analysis of familial colorectal cancer risk. *Am J Gastroenterol*. 2001;96:2992-3003.

Kim DH, Smith-Warner SA, Hunter DJ. Pooled analysis of prospective cohort studies on folate and colorectal cancer. Pooling Project of Diet and Cancer Investigators (abstract). *Am J Epidemiol*. 2001;153(suppl):S118.

Lamprecht SA, Lipkin M. Chemoprevention of colon cancer by calcium, vitamin D and folate: molecular mechanisms. *Nat Rev Cancer*. 2003;3;601-614.

Martinez ME, Giovannucci E, Spiegelman D, Hunter DJ, Willett WC, Colditz GA. Leisure-time physical activity, body size, and colon cancer in women. Nurses' Health Study Research Group. *J Natl Cancer Inst*. 1997;89:948-955.

Mason JB. Nutritional chemoprevention of colon cancer. *Semin Gastrointest Dis*. 2002;13:143-153.

McKay B. Obesity is linked to cancer risk: extra weight sharply increases likelihood of disease in breast, colon and organs. *Wall Street Journal*. August 24, 2004:D1.

National Cancer Institute. Cholesterol-lowering statins may protect against colorectal cancer. Available at: http://www.nci.nih.gov/cancertopics/prevention-genetics-causes/statins-and-colorectal-cancer0604. Accessed August 23, 2004.

National Cancer Institute. Colorectal cancer (PDQ): prevention. Available at: http://www.nci.nih.gov/cancertopics/pdq/prevention/colorectal/patient. Accessed February 2, 2004.

Platz EA, Willett WC, Colditz GA, Rimm EB, Spiegelman D, Giovannucci E. Proportion of colon cancer risk that might be preventable in a cohort of middle-aged US men. *Cancer Causes Control*. 2000;11:579-558.

Singh GK, Miller BA, Hankey BF, Feuer EJ, Pickle LW. Changing area socioeconomic patterns in U.S. cancer mortality, 1950-1998: Part I—All cancers among men. *J Natl Cancer Inst*. 2002;94:904-915.

Slattery ML. Diet, lifestyle, and colon cancer. *Semin Gastrointest Dis*. 2000;11:142-146.

Solomon CH, Pho LN, Burt RW. Current status of genetic testing for colorectal cancer susceptibility. *Oncology* (Huntingt). 2002;16:161-171; discussion 176, 179-180.

CHAPTER 3

American Cancer Society. ACS News Center. Potential for reducing colon cancer risk not being realized. October 24, 2001. Available at: http://www.cancer.org/docroot/NWS/content/NWS_2_1x_Potential_for_Reducing_Colon_Cancer_Risk_Not_Being_Realized.asp. Accessed August 31, 2003.

American Cancer Society. Detailed guide: colon and rectum cancer. Can colorectal polyps and cancer be found early? Available at: http://www.cancer.org/docroot/CRI/content/CRI_2_4_3X_Can_colon_and_rectum_cancer_be_found_early.asp. Accessed September 7, 2003.

American Cancer Society. Frequent questions about colonoscopy and sigmoidoscopy. Available at: http://www.cancer.org/docroot/CRI/content/CRI_2_6x_Frequent_Questions_About_Colonoscopy_and_Sigmoidoscopy.asp. Accessed August 16, 2003.

American Cancer Society. Tools and strategies to increase colorectal cancer screening rates: a practical guide for health insurance plans. Available at http://www.cancer.org/docroot/PRO/content/PRO_1_1_Tools_and_Strategies_to_Increase_Colorectal_Cancer_Screening_Rates.asp. Accessed April 21, 2005.

Bond J. Screening for colorectal cancer: is there progress for early detection? *Pract Gastroenterol.* 2004;28:48-60.

Centers for Disease Control and Prevention. Colorectal cancer: the importance of prevention and early detection. Available at: http://www.cdc.gov/cancer/colorctl/colorect.htm. Accessed September 7, 2003.

Centers for Disease Control and Prevention. Colorectal cancer questions and answers. Available at http://www.cdc.gov/cancer/screenforlife/qanda.htm. Accessed August 16, 2003.

Coyle C. Virtual colonoscopy & DNA stool testing: the future of colon cancer screening? Available at: http://www.oncolink.com/types/article.cfm?c=5&s=11&ss=83&id=7020. Accessed September 9, 2003.

Levin B, Brooks D, Smith R, Stone A. Emerging technologies in screening for colorectal cancer: CT colonography, immunochemical fecal occult blood tests, and stool screening using molecular markers. *CA Cancer J Clin.* 2003;53:44-55.

Levin B, Smith RA, Feldman GE, Colditz GA, et al, for National Colorectal Cancer Roundtable. Promoting early detection tests for colorectal carcinoma and adenomatous polyps: a framework for action: the strategic plan of the National Colorectal Cancer Roundtable [published erratum appears in: *Cancer.* 2002;95:2580] *Cancer.* 2002;95:1618-1628.

OncoLink. Colon cancer: the basics. Available at: http://www.oncolink.com/types/article.cfm?c=5&s=11&ss=81&id=7336. Accessed August 16, 2003.

Pignone M, Rich M, Teutsch S, Berg A, Lohr K. Screening for colorectal cancer in adults at average risk: a summary of evidence for the U.S. preventive services task force. *Ann Intern Med.* 2002;137:132-141.

Rex D. Current colorectal cancer screening strategies: overview and obstacles to implementation. *Rev Gastroenterol Disord.* 2004; 2(suppl 1):S2-S11.

Rex D, Johnson D, Lieberman D, Burt R, Sonnenberg A. Colorectal Cancer Prevention 2000: screening recommendations of the American College of Gastroenterology. *Am J Gastroenterol.* 2000;95:868-877.

Winawer S, Fletcher R, Rex D, et al, for the Gastrointestinal Consortium Panel. Colorectal cancer screening and surveillance: clinical guidelines and rationale—update based on new evidence. *Gastroenterol.* 2003;124:544-560.

CHAPTER 4

Ahsan H, Neugut AI, Garbowski GC, et al. Family history of colorectal adenomatous polyps and increased risk for colorectal cancer. *Ann Intern Med.* 1998;128:900-905.

American Cancer Society and National Comprehensive Cancer Network. Colon and rectal cancer: treatment guidelines for patients, version III/September 2003. Available at http://www.cancer.org/downloads/CRI/F940 9.00.pdf. Accessed September 2, 2004.

American Cancer Society and National Comprehensive Cancer Network. Colon and rectal cancer: treatment guidelines for patients, version IV/February 2005. Available at http://www.nccn.org/patients/patient_gls/_english/_colon/contents.asp. Accessed May 3, 2005.

American Cancer Society. Detailed guide: colon and rectum cancer what is colorectal cancer? Available at http://www.cancer.org/docroot/CRI/content/CRI_2_4_1x_What_Is_Colon_and_Rectum_Cancer.asp?sitearea=CRI. Accessed July 2, 2004.

Burt RW. Screening of patients with a positive family history of colorectal cancer. *Gastrointest Endosc Clin N Am.* 1997;7:65-79.

Eyre H, Lange DP, Morris LB, eds. *Informed decisions: the complete book of cancer diagnosis, treatment, and recovery.* 2nd ed. Atlanta, GA: American Cancer Society; 2002.

Fuchs CS, Giovannucci EL, Colditz GA, Hunter DJ, Speizer FE, Willett WC. A prospective study of family history and the risk of colorectal cancer. *N Engl J Med.* 1994;331:1669-1674.

Murphy GP, Lawrence W Jr, Lenhard RE Jr, eds. *American Cancer Society Textbook of Clinical Oncology.* 2nd ed. Atlanta, GA: American Cancer Society; 1994.

Slattery ML, Kerber RA. Family history of cancer and colon cancer risk: the Utah Population Database. *J Natl Cancer Inst.* 1994;86:1618-1626.

Slattery ML, Levin TR, Ma K, Goldgar D, Holubkov R, Edwards S. Family history and colorectal cancer: predictors of risk. *Cancer Causes Control.* 2003;14:879-887.

Willett CG. *American Cancer Society Atlas of Clinical Oncology. Cancer of the Lower Gastrointestinal Tract.* Hamilton, ON, Canada: BC Decker; 2001.

CHAPTER 5

American Cancer Society. Detailed guide: colon and rectum cancer. Available at: http://documents.cancer.org/107.00/107.00.pdf. Accessed September 9, 2004.

American Cancer Society and National Comprehensive Cancer Network. Colon and rectal cancer: treatment guidelines for patients, version III/September 2003. Available at http://www.cancer.org/downloads/CRI/F9409.00.pdf. Accessed September 2, 2004.

American Cancer Society and National Comprehensive Cancer Network. Colon and rectal cancer: treatment guidelines for patients, version IV/February 2005. Available at http://www.nccn.org/patients/patient_gls/_english/_colon/contents.asp. Accessed May 3, 2005.

Corman ML, ed. Colon and rectal surgery. 4th ed. Philadelphia: Lippincott Williams & Wilkins; 1998.

Church JM, Gibbs P, Chao MW, Tjandra JJ. Optimizing the outcome for patients with rectal cancer. *Dis Colon Rectum.* 2003;46:389-402.

Gordon PH, Nivatvongs S, eds. *Principles and Practice of Surgery for the Colon, Rectum, and Anus.* 2nd ed. St. Louis: Quality Medical Publishing; 1999.

Greene FL, Page DL, Fleming ID, et al. *American Joint Committee on Cancer (AJCC) Cancer Staging Manual.* 6th ed. New York: Springer-Verlag; 2002.

Levin B. *Colorectal Cancer: A Thorough and Compassionate Resource for Patients and Their Families.* Atlanta, GA: American Cancer Society; 1999.

Rothenberger DA. Colorectal cancer. Preface. *Surg Oncol Clin N Am.* 2000;9:xvii-ix.

CHAPTER 6

American Cancer Society. Cancer facts and figures 2004. Available at: http://www.cancer.org/downloads/STT/CAFF_finalPWSecured.pdf. Accessed September 2, 2004.

American Cancer Society. Cancer facts and figures 2005. Available at http://www.cancer.org/downloads/STT/CAFF2005PWSecured4.pdf. Accessed February 4, 2005.

American Cancer Society. Colorectal cancer facts and figures—Special edition 2005. Available at: http://www.cancer.org/docroot/STT/content/STT_1x_Colorectal_Cancer_Facts_and_Figures_-_Special_Edition_2005.asp. Accessed March 15, 2005.

American Cancer Society. Detailed guide: colon and rectum cancer. Available at: http://documents.cancer.org/107.00/107.00.pdf. Accessed September 9, 2004.

American Cancer Society. Detailed guide: colon and rectum cancer (revised). Available at: http://www.cancer.org/docroot/CRI/CRI_2_3x.asp?rnav=cridg&dt=10. Accessed February 27, 2005.

American Cancer Society and National Comprehensive Cancer Network. Colon and rectal cancer: treatment guidelines for patients, version III/September 2003. Atlanta, GA: American Cancer Society; 2003. Available at http://www.cancer.org/downloads/CRI/F9409.00.pdf. Accessed September 2, 2004.

American Cancer Society and National Comprehensive Cancer Network. Colon and rectal cancer: treatment guidelines for patients, version IV/February 2005. Atlanta, GA: American Cancer Society; 2005. Available at http://www.nccn.org/patients/patient_gls/_english/_colon/contents.asp. Accessed May 3, 2005.

DeVita VT, Hellman S, Rosenberg SA, eds. Cancer: Principles and Practices of Oncology, 6th ed. Philadelphia: Lippincott Williams & Wilkins; 2001:1230-1238.

Greene FL, Page DL, Fleming ID, et al. American Joint Committee on Cancer (AJCC) Cancer Staging Manual. 6th ed. New York: Springer-Verlag; 2002.

Kato I, Severson RK, Schwartz AG. Conditional median survival of patients with advanced carcinoma: surveillance, epidemiology, and end results data. Cancer. 2001;92:2211-2219.

O'Connell JB, Maggard MA, Ko CY. Colon cancer survival rates with the new American Joint Committee on Cancer Sixth Edition staging. J Natl Cancer Inst. 2004;96:1420-1425.

Smith RE, Colangelo LH, Wieand S, Begovic M, Wolmark N. Randomized trial of adjuvant therapy in colon carcinoma: 10-year results of NSABP protocol C-01. J Natl Cancer Inst. 2004;96:1128-1132.

CHAPTER 7

American Cancer Society. After diagnosis: a guide for patients and families. Pamphlet 9440. Atlanta, GA: American Cancer Society.

American Cancer Society. Caring for the patient with cancer at home: a guide for patients and families. Pamphlet 4656. Atlanta, GA: American Cancer Society.

American Cancer Society. Coping with cancer in everyday life. Available at http://www.cancer.org/docroot/MBC/MBC_4x_Coping Cancer.asp?sitearea=MBC. Accessed December 22, 2004.

American Cancer Society. It helps to have friends: when mom or dad has cancer. Pamphlet 4654. Atlanta, GA: American Cancer Society.

American Cancer Society. Listen with your heart: talking with the person who has cancer. Pamphlet 4557. Atlanta, GA: American Cancer Society.

Centers for Disease Control and Prevention. Cancer survivorship—United States, 1971-2001. MMWR Morb Mortal Wkly Rep. 2004; 53:526-529.

Holland JC, Lewis S. The Human Side of Cancer: Living With Hope, Coping With Uncertainty. New York: HarperCollins; 2000.

National Cancer Institute. Taking Time: Support for People with Cancer and the People Who Care About Them. NIH Publication No. 04-2059. Washington, DC: US Department of Health and Human Services; 2003.

CHAPTER 8

Agency for Healthcare Quality and Research. Your guide to choosing quality health care: summary. Available at http://www.ahrq.gov/consumer/qntool.htm. Accessed December 22, 2004.

American Cancer Society. Communication with medical professionals. Available at: http://www.cancer.org/docroot/ETO/eto_7_1.asp. Accessed December 22, 2004.

Beaver K, Bogg J, Luker KA. Decision-making role preferences and information needs: a comparison of colorectal and breast cancer. *Health Expect.* 1999;2:266-276.

Dimick JB, Cowan JA, Upchurch GR, Colletti LM. Hospital volume and surgical outcomes for elderly patients with colorectal cancer in the United States. *J Surg Res.* 2003;114:50-56.

Dorrance HR, Docherty GM, O'Dwyer PJ. Effect of surgeon specialty interest on patient outcome after potentially curative colorectal cancer surgery. *Dis Colon Rectum.* 2000;43: 492-498.

Hodgson DC, Fuchs CS, Ayanian JZ. Impact of patient and provider characteristics on the treatment and outcomes of colorectal cancer. *J Natl Cancer Inst.* 2000;93:501-515.

Hodgson DC, Zhang W, Zaslavsky AM, Fuchs CS, Wright WE, Ayanian JZ. Relation of hospital volume to colostomy rates and survival for patients with rectal cancer. *J Natl Cancer Inst.* 2003;95:708-716.

McArdle CS, Hole DJ. Influence of volume and specialization on survival following surgery for colorectal cancer. *Br J Surg.* 2004;91:610-617.

Rabeneck L, Davila JA, Thompson M, El-Serag HB. Surgical volume and long-term survival following surgery for colorectal cancer in the Veterans Affairs Health-Care System. *Am J Gastroenterol.* 2004;99:668-675.

Salkeld G, Solomon M, Short L, Butow PN. A matter of trust—patients' views on decision-making in colorectal cancer. *Health Expect.* 2004;7:104-114.

Schrag D, Cramer LD, Bach, PB. Influence of hospital procedure volume on outcomes following surgery for colon cancer. *JAMA.* 2000;284:3028-3035.

Schrag D, Panageas KS, Riedel E, et al. Hospital and surgeon procedure volume as predictors of outcome following rectal cancer resection. *Ann Surg.* 2002;236:583-592.

Sanders T. Do bowel cancer patients participate in treatment decision-making? Findings from a qualitative study. *Eur J Cancer Care.* 2003; 12:166-175.

Smith JAE, King PM, Lane RHS, Thompson MR. Evidence of the effect of 'specialization' on the management, surgical outcome, and survival from colorectal cancer in Wessex. *Br J Surg.* 2003;90:583-592.

CHAPTER 9

American Cancer Society and National Comprehensive Cancer Network. Colon and rectal cancer: treatment guidelines for patients, version III/September 2003. Atlanta, GA: American Cancer Society; 2003. Available at http://www.cancer.org/downloads/CRI/F9409.00.pdf. Accessed September 2, 2004.

American Cancer Society and National Comprehensive Cancer Network. Colon and rectal cancer: treatment guidelines for patients, version IV/February 2005. Atlanta, GA: American Cancer Society; 2005. Available at http://www.nccn.org/patients/patient_gls/_english/_colon/contents.asp. Accessed May 3, 2005.

American Cancer Society. Detailed guide: colon and rectum cancer treatment by stage of colon cancer. Available at: http://www.cancer.org/docroot/CRI/content/CRI_2_4_4X_Treatment_by_Stage_of_Colon_Cancer_10.asp?sitearea=. Accessed April 6, 2005.

Barry MJ. Health decision aids to facilitate shared decision making in office practice. *Ann Intern Med.* 2002;136:127-135.

Coulter, A, Entwistle, V, Gilbert, D. Sharing decisions with patients: is the information good enough? *BMJ.* 1999, January 30;318: 318-322. Available at http://bmj.bmjjournals.com/cgi/content/full/318/7179/318. Accessed April 6, 2004.

Elit L. Receiving curative treatment session-consideration of patient preference in determining cancer treatment. Available at http://www.bccancer.bc.ca/NR/rdonlyres/ecknekjfbqclftarnh55llgebejspz2kpe34brfoewn72jphptnhhq5xib4q3yjfouirckrj5s7ezj/07ReceivingCurative.pdf Accessed April 1, 2004.

Gattellari M, Voigt KJ, Butow PN, Tattersall MH. When the treatment goal is not cure: are cancer patients equipped to make informed decisions? *J Clin Oncol.* 2002;20:503-513. Available at http://www.jco.org/cgi/content/full/20/2/503. Accessed April 6, 2004.

Huang QR. Creating informed consumers and achieving shared decision making. *Aust Fam Physician.* 2003;32:335-341.

Lee SJ, Back AL, Block SD, Stewart SK. Enhancing physician-patient communication. In: *American Society of Hematology Education Program Book;* 2002:464-483. Available at: http://www.asheducationbook.org/cgi/content/full/2002/1/464. Accessed April 6, 2004.

Leighl N, Gattellari M, Butow P, Brown R, Tattersall MH. Discussing adjuvant cancer therapy. *J Clin Oncol.* 2001;19:1768-1778.

Medical News Today. Web sites can give patients info they need for decisions. Available at http://www.medicalnewstoday.com/index.php?newsid=5505. Accessed April 6, 2004.

Mulay M. *Making the Decision: A Cancer Patient's Guide to Clinical Trials.* Sudbury, MA: Jones and Bartlett Publishers; 2001.

Napa Valley Cancer Resource Guide. Elaine Mackie Charitable Trust. Available at http://www.elainemackietrust.org/html/rbook_index.htm. Accessed April 12, 2004.

Renneker M. No stone unturned: seeking optimal cancer care. The Jenifer Altman Memorial Lecture. Bolinas, CA: Commonweal; 1999. Available at http://www.commonweal.org/programs/lectures/altman.html. Accessed April 12, 2004.

Say RE, Thomson R. The importance of patient preferences in treatment decisions—challenges for doctors. *BMJ.* 2003;327:542-545. Available at http://bmj.bmjjournals.com/cgi/content/full/327/7414/542. Accessed April 6, 2004.

CHAPTER 10

American Cancer Society. Detailed guide: colon and rectum cancer. What is colorectal cancer? Available at http://www.cancer.org/docroot/CRI/content/CRI_2_4_1x_What_Is_Colon_and_Rectum_Cancer.asp?sitearea=CRI. Accessed July 2, 2004.

American Cancer Society and National Comprehensive Cancer Network. Colon and rectal cancer: treatment guidelines for patients, version III/September 2003. Atlanta, GA: American Cancer Society; 2003. Available at http://www.cancer.org/downloads/CRI/F9409.00.pdf. Accessed August 23, 2004.

American Cancer Society and National Comprehensive Cancer Network. Colon and rectal cancer: treatment guidelines for patients, version IV/February 2005. Atlanta, GA: American Cancer Society; 2005. Available at http://www.nccn.org/patients/patient_gls/_english/_colon/contents.asp. Accessed May 3, 2005.

Fine AP. Laparoscopic colon surgery. Miami, FL: Society of Laparoendoscopic Surgeons. Available at http://www.sls.org/i4a/pages/index.cfm?pageid=3358. Accessed September 16, 2004.

gihealth.com. What is a colon polyp? Available at http://www.gihealth.com/html/education/colonpolyps.html. Accessed September 15, 2004.

Levin B. *Colorectal Cancer: A Thorough and Compassionate Resource for Patients and Their Families.* Atlanta, GA: American Cancer Society; 1999.

Medina M. Laparoscopic surgery. Miami, FL: Society of Laparoendoscopic Surgeons. Available at http://www.sls.org/i4a/pages/index.cfm?pageid=3294. Accessed September 16, 2004.

Weiser MR. Laparoscopic colorectal surgery for cancer: is it ready for prime time? Available at http://www.cancernews.com/articles/laparoscopiccancersurgery.htm. Accessed September 16, 2004.

Willett CG. *American Cancer Society Atlas of Clinical Oncology. Cancer of the Lower Gastrointestinal Tract.* Hamilton, ON, Canada: BC Decker; 2001.

CHAPTER 11

American Cancer Society. Detailed guide: colon and rectum cancer. What is colorectal cancer? Available at http://www.cancer.org/docroot/CRI/content/CRI_2_4_1x_What_Is_Colon_and_Rectum_Cancer.asp?sitearea=CRI. Accessed July 2, 2004.

American Cancer Society and National Comprehensive Cancer Network. Colon and rectal cancer: treatment guidelines for patients, version III/September 2003. Atlanta, GA: American Cancer Society; 2003. Available at http://www.cancer.org/downloads/CRI/F9409.00.pdf. Accessed August 23, 2004.

American Cancer Society and National Comprehensive Cancer Network. Colon and rectal cancer: treatment guidelines for patients, version IV/February 2005. Atlanta, GA: American Cancer Society; 2005. Available at http://www.nccn.org/patients/patient_gls/_english/_colon/contents.asp. Accessed May 3, 2005.

Anonymous. Improved survival with preoperative radiotherapy in resectable rectal cancer. Swedish Rectal Cancer Trial [published erratum appears in *N Engl J Med.* 1997;336:1539]. *N Engl J Med.* 1997;336:980-987.

Anonymous. Prolongation of the disease-free interval in surgically treated rectal carcinoma. Gastrointestinal Tumor Study Group. *N Engl J Med.* 1985;312:1465-1472.

Krook JE, Moertel CG, Gunderson LL, et al: Effective surgical adjuvant therapy for high-risk rectal carcinoma. *N Engl J Med.* 1991; 324:709-715.

Levin B. *Colorectal Cancer: A Thorough and Compassionate Resource for Patients and Their Families.* Atlanta, GA: American Cancer Society; 1999.

Sauer R, for the German Rectal Cancer Group. Adjuvant verses neoadjuvant combined modality treatment for locally advanced rectal cancer: first results of the German Rectal Cancer Study (CAO/ARO/AIO-94). *Int J Radiat Oncol Biol Phys.* 2003;57:S124-S125.

CHAPTER 12

Ackerman NB. The blood supply of experimental liver metastases. IV. Changes in vascularity with increasing tumor growth. *Surgery.* 1974; 75:589-596.

American Cancer Society. Cancer drug guide: 5-fluorouracil. Available at http://www.cancer.org/docroot/CDG/content/CDG_5-fluorouracil.html. Accessed September 24, 2004.

American Cancer Society. Cancer drug guide: bevacizumab. Available at http://www.cancer.org/docroot/CDG/content/CDG_bevacizumab.html. Accessed September 24, 2004.

American Cancer Society. Cancer drug guide: capecitabine. Available at http://www.cancer.org/docroot/CDG/content/CDG_capecitabine.html. Accessed September 24, 2004.

American Cancer Society. Cancer drug guide: cetuximab. Available at http://www.cancer.org/docroot/CDG/content/CDG_cetuximab.html. Accessed September 24, 2004.

American Cancer Society. Cancer drug guide: irinotecan. Available at http://www.cancer.org/docroot/CDG/content/CDG_irinotecan.html. Accessed September 24, 2004.

American Cancer Society. Cancer drug guide: leucovorin calcium. Available at http://www.cancer.org/docroot/CDG/content/CDG_leucovorin_calcium.html. Accessed September 24, 2004.

American Cancer Society. Cancer drug guide: oxaliplatin. Available at http://www.cancer.org/docroot/CDG/content/CDG_oxaliplatin.html. Accessed September 24, 2004.

American Cancer Society. What are the different types of chemotherapy drugs? Available at http://www.cancer.org/docroot/ETO/content/ETO_1_4X_What_Are_The_Different_Types_Of_Chemotherapy_Drugs.asp?sitearea=ETO. Accessed September 24, 2004.

Andre T, Boni C, Mounedji-Boudiaf L, et al. Oxaliplatin, fluorouracil, and leucovorin as adjuvant treatment for colon cancer. *N Engl J Med.* 2004;350:2343-2351.

Cassidy J, Scheithauer W, McKendrick M. Capecitabine (X) vs bolus 5-FU/leucovorin (LV) as adjuvant therapy for colon cancer (the X-ACT study): efficacy results of a phase III trial. *J Clin Oncol.* 2004 ASCO Annual Meeting Proceedings (post-meeting edition). 2004;22 Suppl):a3509.

Cassidy J, Tabernero J, Twelves C, et al. XELOX (capecitabine plus oxaliplatin): active first-line therapy for patients with metastatic colorectal cancer. *J Clin Oncol.* 2004;22:2084-2091.

Cunningham D, Pyrhonen S, James RD, et al. Randomised trial of irinotecan plus supportive care versus supportive care alone after fluorouracil failure for patients with metastatic colorectal cancer. *Lancet.* 1998;352:1413-1418.

Douillard JY, Cunningham D, Roth AD, et al. Irinotecan combined with fluorouracil compared with fluorouracil alone as first-line treatment for metastatic colorectal cancer: a multicentre randomised trial. *Lancet.* 2000; 355:1041-1047.

Eng C, Abbruzzese J. The efficacy and expectations of capecitabine monotherapy. *Am J Oncol Rev.* 2003;2(suppl 3):8-14.

Goldberg RM, Sargent DJ, Morton RF, et al. A randomized controlled trial of fluorouracil plus leucovorin, irinotecan, and oxaliplatin combinations in patients with previously untreated metastatic colorectal cancer. *J Clin Oncol.* 2004;22:23-30.

Goldberg RM. Current approaches to first-line treatment of advanced colorectal cancer. *Clin Colorectal Cancer.* 2004;4(Suppl 1):S9-S15.

Hurwitz H, Fehrenbacher L, Novotny W, et al. Bevacizumab plus irinotecan, fluorouracil, and leucovorin for metastatic colorectal cancer. *N Engl J Med.* 2004;350:2335-2342.

Jemal A, Murray T, Samuels A, Ghafoor A, Ward E, Thun MJ. Cancer statistics, 2003. *CA Cancer J Clin.* 2003;53:5-26.

Kemeny MM, Adak S, Gray B, et al. Combined-modality treatment for resectable metastatic colorectal carcinoma to the liver: surgical resection of hepatic metastases in combination with continuous infusion of chemotherapy—an intergroup study. *J Clin Oncol.* 2002;20:1499-1505.

Kemeny N, Huang Y, Cohen AM, et al. Hepatic arterial infusion of chemotherapy after resection of hepatic metastases from colorectal cancer. *N Engl J Med.* 1999;341:2039-2048.

Mattison LK, Ezzeldin H, Carpenter M, Modak A, Johnson MR, Diasio RB. Rapid identification of dihydropyrimidine dehydrogenase deficiency by using a novel 2-13C-uracil breath test. *Clin Cancer Res.* 2004;10:2652-2658.

Mazumdar M, Smith A, Schwartz LH. A statistical simulation study finds discordance between WHO criteria and RECIST guideline. *J Clin Epidemiol.* 2004;57:358-365.

Mitchell EP. Oxaliplatin with 5-FU or as a single agent in advanced/metastatic colorectal cancer. *Oncology (Huntingt).* 2000;14:30-32.

Moertel CG, Fleming TR, Macdonald JS, et al. Intergroup study of fluorouracil plus levamisole as adjuvant therapy for stage II/Dukes' B2 colon cancer. *J Clin Oncol.* 1995;13:2936-2943.

Monetti F, Casanova S, Grasso A, Cafferata MA, Ardizzoni A, Neumaier CE. Inadequacy of the new Response Evaluation Criteria in Solid Tumors (RECIST) in patients with malignant pleural mesothelioma: report of four cases. *Lung Cancer.* 2004;43:71-74.

Piedbois P, Michiels S. Survival benefit of 5-FU/LV over 5-FU bolus in patients with advanced colorectal cancer: an updated meta-analysis on 2,751 patients. *Proc Am Soc Clin Oncol.* 2003;22:294, abstr 1180.

Rougier P, Van Cutsem E, Bajetta E, et al. Randomised trial of irinotecan versus fluorouracil by continuous infusion after fluorouracil failure in patients with metastatic colorectal cancer [published erratum appears in *Lancet.* 1998;352:1634]. *Lancet.* 1998;352: 1407-1412.

Sadahiro S, Suzuki T, Ishikawa K, et al. Recurrence patterns after curative resection of colorectal cancer in patients followed for a minimum of ten years. *Hepatogastroenterology*. 2003;50:1362-1366.

Saltz LB, Cox JV, Blanke C, et al. Irinotecan plus fluorouracil and leucovorin for metastatic colorectal cancer. Irinotecan Study Group. *N Engl J Med*. 2000;343:905-914.

Saltz LB, Niedzwiecki D, Hollis D. Irinotecan plus fluorouracil/leucovorin (IFL) versus fluorouracil/leucovorin alone (FL) in stage III colon cancer (intergroup trial CALGB C89803). *J Clin Oncol*., 2004 ASCO Annual Meeting Proceedings (post-meeting edition). 2004;22(suppl):3500.

Scheithauer W, McKendrick J, Begbie S, et al. Oral capecitabine as an alternative to i.v. 5-fluorouracil-based adjuvant therapy for colon cancer: safety results of a randomized, phase III trial. *Ann Oncol*. 2003;14:1735-1743.

Tournigand C, Andre T, Achille E, et al. FOLFIRI followed by FOLFOX6 or the reverse sequence in advanced colorectal cancer: a randomized GERCOR study. *J Clin Oncol*. 2004;22:229-237.

Van Cutsem E, Findlay M, Osterwalder B, et al. Capecitabine, an oral fluoropyrimidine carbamate with substantial activity in advanced colorectal cancer: results of a randomized phase II study. *J Clin Oncol*. 2000;18:1337-1345.

Van Cutsem E, Twelves C, Cassidy J, et al. Oral capecitabine compared with intravenous fluorouracil plus leucovorin in patients with metastatic colorectal cancer: results of a large phase III study. *J Clin Oncol*. 2001;19:4097-4106.

CHAPTER 13

American Cancer Society. Detailed guide: colon and rectum cancer. What's new in colorectal cancer research and treatment? Available at http://www.cancer.org/docroot/CRI/content/CRI_2_4_6X_Whats_new_in_colon_and_rectum_cancer_research_and_treatment.asp?sitearea=. Accessed November 2, 2004.

American Cancer Society. Clinical trials: what you need to know. Available at http://www.cancer.org/docroot/ETO/content/ETO_6_3_Clinical_Trials__Patient_Participation.asp. Accessed May, 2004.

Bhatnagar A, Carmichael J, Cosgriff T. A randomized, double-blind, placebo controlled phase III study of monoclonal antibody 3H1 plus 5-fluorouracil (5-FU)/leucovorin (LV) in stage IV colorectal carcinoma. *Proc Am Soc Clin Oncol*. 2003;22:260 (abstr 1041).

Cunningham D, et al. Cetuximab (C225) alone or in combination with irinotecan (CPT-11) in patients with epidermal growth factor receptor (EGFR)-positive, irinotecan-refractory metastatic colorectal cancer (MCRC). *N Engl J Med*. In press.

Fields AL, Keller AM, Schwartzberg L. Edrecolomab (17-1A antibody) (EDR) in combination with 5-fluorouracil (FU) based chemotherapy in the adjuvant treatment of stage III colon cancer: Results of a randomised North American phase III study. *Proc Am Soc Clin Oncol*. 2002;21;128a (abstr 508).

Foon KA, John WJ, Chakraborty M, et al. Clinical and immune responses in advanced colorectal cancer patients treated with anti-idiotype monoclonal antibody vaccine that mimics the carcinoembryonic antigen. *Clin Cancer Res*. 1997;3:1267-1276.

Foon KA, John WJ, Chakraborty M, et al. Clinical and immune responses in resected colon cancer patients treated with anti-idiotype monoclonal antibody vaccine that mimics the carcinoembryonic antigen. *J Clin Oncol*. 1999;17;2889-2895.

Foon KA. Vaccine strategies for colorectal cancer. In: Saltz L, editor. *Colorectal Cancer*. Totowa, NJ: Humana Press Inc.; 2002:795-810.

Grem JL, Jordan E, Robson ME, et al. Phase II study of fluorouracil, leucovorin, and interferon alfa-2a in metastatic colorectal carcinoma. *J Clin Oncol*. 1993;11;1737-1745.

Hamid O, Varterasian ML, Wadler S, et al. Phase II trial of intravenous CI-1042 in patients with metastatic colorectal cancer. *J Clin Oncol*. 2003;21:1498-1504.

Hao Desiree, Rowinsky EK, Smetzer LA, et al. A phase I and pharmacokinetic study of intravenous (IV) p53 gene therapy with RPR/INGN-201 in patients (pts) with advanced cancer. *Proc Am Soc Clin Oncol.* 2001;20; (abstr 1045).

Harris JE, Ryan L, Hoover HC Jr, et al. Adjuvant active specific immunotherapy for stage II and III colon cancer with an autologous tumor cell vaccine: Eastern Cooperative Oncology Group Study E5283. *J Clin Oncol.* 2000;18;148-157.

Hoover HC Jr, Brandhorst JS, Peters LC, et al. Adjuvant active specific immunotherapy for human colorectal cancer: 6.5-year median follow-up of a phase III prospectively randomized trial. *J Clin Oncol.* 1993;11:390-399.

Hurwitz H, Fehrenbacher L, Novotny W, et al. Bevacizumab plus irinotecan, fluorouracil, and leucovorin for metastatic colorectal cancer. *N Engl J Med.* 2004;350:2335-2342.

National Cancer Institute. Learning about clinical trials. Available at: http://www.cancer.gov/clinicaltrials/learning. Accessed May, 2004.

Punt CJ, Nagy A, Douillard JY, et al. Edrecolomab alone or in combination with fluorouracil and folinic acid in the adjuvant treatment of stage III colon cancer: a randomised study. *Lancet.* 2002;360:671-677.

Reid TR, Sze D, Galanis E, et al. Intra-arterial administration of a replication-selective adenovirus ONYX-015 in patients with colorectal carcinoma metastatic to the liver: safety, feasibility and biologic activity. *Proc Am Soc Clin Oncol.* 2003;22:198 (abstr 793).

Rosen LC, Li WW. Angiogenesis and colorectal cancer: from the laboratory to the clinic. In: Saltz L, editor. *Colorectal Cancer.* Totowa, NJ: Humana Press Inc.; 2002:739-758.

Rosenberg AH, Loehrer PJ, Needle MN, et al. Erbitux (IMC-C225) plus weekly irinotecan (CPT-11), fluorouracil (5FU) and leucovorin (LV) in colorectal cancer (CRC) that expresses the epidermal growth factor receptor (EGFr). *Proc Am Soc Clin Oncol.* 2002;21: (abstr 536).

Saltz LB, Meropol NJ, Loehrer PJ Sr, et al. Phase II trial of cetuximab in patients with refractory colorectal cancer that expresses the epidermal growth factor receptor. *J Clin Oncol.* 2004;22:1201-1208.

Schoffski P, Lutz MP, Folprecht G, et al. Cetuximab (C225) plus irinotecan (CPT-11) plus infusional 5FU-folinic acid (FA) is safe and active in metastatic colorectal cancer (MCRC), that expresses epidermal growth factor receptor (EGFR). *Proc Am Soc Clin Oncol.* 2002;21:(abstr 633).

Venook AP, Bergsland EK, Ring E, et al. Gene therapy of colorectal liver metastases using a recombinant adenovirus encoding wt p53 (SCH 58500) via hepatic artery infusion: a phase I study. *Proc Am Soc Clin Oncol.* 1998; 17:(abstr 1661).

Wadler S, Lembersky B, Atkins M, et al. Phase II trial of fluorouracil and recombinant interferon alfa-2a in patients with advanced colorectal carcinoma: an Eastern Cooperative Oncology Group study. *J Clin Oncol.* 1991;9: 1806-1810.

Weir HK, Thun MJ, Hankey BF, et al. Annual report to the nation on the status of cancer, 1975-2000, featuring the uses of surveillance data for cancer prevention and control [published erratum appears in: *J Natl Cancer Inst.* 2003;95:1641]. *J Natl Cancer Inst.* 2003;95: 1276-1299.

Wolmark N, Bryant J, Smith R, et al. Adjuvant 5-fluorouracil and leucovorin with or without interferon alfa-2a in colon carcinoma: National Surgical Adjuvant Breast and Bowel Project protocol C-05. *J Natl Cancer Inst.* 1998;90:1810-1816.

CHAPTER 14

Alimi D, Rubino C, Pichard-Leandri E, et al. Complementary and Alternative Medicine Use Among Adults: United States, 2002. CDC Advance Data Report #343. Atlanta, GA: Centers for Disease Control and Prevention; 2004.

Cassileth B. *Complementary Therapies to Ease the Way During Cancer Treatment and Recovery* [pamphlet]. New York: Memorial Sloan-Kettering Cancer Center; 2004.

Cassileth BR, Vickers AJ, Deng G, Vickers AJ, Yeung KS. *PDQ Integrative Oncology: Complementary Therapies in Cancer Care.* Hamilton, ON, Canada: BC Decker, Inc., 2005.

Hill C. Analgesic effect of auricular acupuncture for cancer pain: a randomized, blinded, controlled trial. *J Clin Oncol.* 2003;21:4120-4126.

Memorial Sloan-Kettering Cancer Center. About herbs, botanical and other products. Available at http://www.mskcc.org/mskcc/html/11570.cfm. Accessed December 16, 2004.

Vickers A. Alternative cancer cures: "unproven" or "disproven"? *CA Cancer J Clin.* 2004;54: 110 118.

CHAPTER 15

American Cancer Society. *American Cancer Society's Guide to Pain Control: Understanding and Managing Cancer Pain.* Rev. ed. Atlanta, GA: American Cancer Society; 2004.

American Cancer Society. Cancer drug guide: 5-fluorouracil. Available at http://www.cancer.org/docroot/CDG/content/CDG_5-fluorouracil.html. Accessed September 24, 2004.

American Cancer Society. Cancer drug guide: bevacizumab. Available at http://www.cancer.org/docroot/CDG/content/CDG_bevacizumab.html. Accessed September 24, 2004.

American Cancer Society. Cancer drug guide: capecitabine. Available at http://www.cancer.org/docroot/CDG/content/CDG_capecitabine.html. Accessed September 24, 2004.

American Cancer Society. Cancer drug guide: cetuximab. Available at http://www.cancer.org/docroot/CDG/content/CDG_cetuximab.html. Accessed September 24, 2004.

American Cancer Society. Cancer drug guide: irinotecan. Available at http://www.cancer.org/docroot/CDG/content/CDG_irinotecan.html. Accessed September 24, 2004.

American Cancer Society. Cancer drug guide: leucovorin calcium. Available at http://www.cancer.org/docroot/CDG/content/CDG_leucovorin_calcium.html. Accessed September 24, 2004.

American Cancer Society. Cancer drug guide: oxaliplatin. Available at http://www.cancer.org/docroot/CDG/content/CDG_oxaliplatin.html. Accessed September 24, 2004.

American Cancer Society. *Eating Well, Staying Well During and After Cancer.* Atlanta, GA: American Cancer Society; 2004.

American Cancer Society. Symptoms and side effects. Available at http://www.cancer.org/docroot/MBC/MBC_2_Side_Effects.asp?sitearea=MBC. Accessed October 21, 2004.

American Cancer Society and National Comprehensive Cancer Network. Colon and rectal cancer: treatment guidelines for patients, version III/September 2003. Atlanta, GA: American Cancer Society; 2003. Available at http://www.cancer.org/downloads/CRI/F9409.00.pdf. Accessed August 23, 2004.

American Cancer Society and National Comprehensive Cancer Network. Colon and rectal cancer: treatment guidelines for patients, version IV/February 2005. Atlanta, GA: American Cancer Society; 2005. Available at http://www.nccn.org/patients/patient_gls/_english/_colon/contents.asp. Accessed May 3, 2005.

American Cancer Society/National Comprehensive Cancer Network. Nausea and vomiting: treatment guidelines for patients, version I/January 2001. Available at http://www.cancer.org/downloads/CRI/NCCN_nausea.pdf. Accessed October 26, 2004.

American Cancer Society/National Comprehensive Cancer Network. Cancer-related fatigue and anemia: treatment guidelines for patients, version II/May 2003. Available at http://www.cancer.org/downloads/CRI/944601%20-%20Fatigue%20and%20Anemia%20(En).pdf. Accessed October 26, 2004.

Aventis Pharmaceuticals, Inc. How do I know if I have peripheral neuropathy? A common side effect of anticancer treatments. Patient Information and Weekly Diary, Bridgewater, NJ: Aventis Pharmaceuticals; 2002.

Klemm P, Miller MA, Fernsler J. Demands of illness in people treated for colorectal cancer. *Oncol Nurs Forum*. 2000;27:633-639.

Lewis SM, Heitkamper, MM, Dirksen SR. Medical-surgical nursing. Assessment and management of clinical problems. St Louis: CV Mosby Co.; 2004.

Sargent C, Murphy D. What you need to know about colorectal cancer. *Nursing* 2003;33: 37-41.

Shelton BK. Introduction to colorectal cancer. *Semin Oncol Nursing*. 2002;18(suppl 2);2-12.

CHAPTER 16

American Cancer Society. *Colostomy: A Guide*. Booklet; Code# 4703.00. Available at http://documents.cancer.org/6397.00/6397.00.pdf. Accessed September 24, 2004.

Brewer B. *Diet & Nutrition Guide*. United Ostomy Association.

Mullen BD and McGinn, KA. *The Ostomy Book: Living Comfortably With Colostomies, Ileostomies and Urostomies*. Bull Publishing Company. 1992.

Turnbull GB. *Intimacy, Sexuality and an Ostomy*. United Ostomy Association.

United Ostomy Association, Inc. Colostomy Guide, Rev. ed. Irvine, CA: United Ostomy Association; 2004.

United Ostomy Association, Inc. Colostomy fact sheet. http://www.uoa.org/ostomy_facts_colostomy.htm. Accessed September 17, 2004.

United Ostomy Association, Inc. Ileostomy fact sheet. http://www.uoa.org/ostomy_facts_ileostomy.htm. Accessed September 17, 2004.

United Ostomy Association, Inc. Ostomy FAQs. Available at http://www.uoa.org/ostomy_faqs.htm. Accessed September 17, 2004.

United Ostomy Association, Inc. Sex and the female ostomate fact sheet. Available at http://www.uoa.org/ostomy_facts_woman.htm. Accessed September 17, 2004.

United Ostomy Association, Inc. Sex and the male ostomate fact sheet. Available at http://www.uoa.org/ostomy_facts_man.htm. Accessed September 17, 2004.

United Ostomy Association, Inc. Sex and the single ostomate fact sheet. Available at http://www.uoa.org/ostomy_facts_single.htm. Accessed September 17, 2004.

United Ostomy Association, Inc. What is an ostomy? Available at http://www.uoa.org/ostomy_main.htm. Accessed September 17, 2004.

CHAPTER 17

American Cancer Society. A *Breast Cancer Journey: Your Personal Guidebook*, 2nd ed. Atlanta, GA: American Cancer Society; 2003.

American Cancer Society. *When the Focus Is on Care: Palliative Care and Cancer*. Atlanta, GA: American Cancer Society; 2004.

CHAPTER 18

American Cancer Society. Close follow-up after colon cancer recommended: doctors want to prevent cancer's return. Available at http://www.cancer.org/docroot/NWS/content/NWS_1_1x_Close_Follow-Up_After_Colon_Cancer_Recommended.asp. Accessed January 27, 2005.

American Cancer Society. Detailed guide: colon and rectum cancer. What happens after treatment? Available at http://www.cancer.org/docroot/CRI/content/CRI_2_4_5x_What_happens_after_treatment_10.asp?sitearea=. Accessed January 27, 2005.

Cancer survivors' other medical problems often neglected. *CA Cancer J Clin*. 2005;55:3-4. Available at http://caonline.amcancersoc.org:80/cgi/content/full/55/1/3?etoc. Accessed January 20, 2005.

The Oncology Group. Follow-up care for colorectal cancer patients. Available at http://www.cancernetwork.com/myths/colon/Col06.htm. Accessed August 16, 2004.

CHAPTER 19

American Cancer Society. Alcohol and Cancer PDF. Available at: http://www.cancer.org/downloads/PRO/alcohol.pdf. Accessed May 16, 2004.

American Cancer Society. Nutrition after treatment ends. Available at http://www.cancer.org/docroot/MBC/content/MBC_6_2X_Nutrition_after_treatment_ends.asp?sitearea=MBC. Accessed May 20, 2004.

American Cancer Society. What are the risk factors for colorectal cancer? Available at http://www.cancer.org/docroot/CRI/content/CRI_2_4_2X_What_are_the_risk_factors_for_colon_and_rectum_cancer.asp?sitearea=CRI. Accessed May 1, 2004.

Bloch A, Cassileth B, Homes M, Thomson C, eds. *Eating Well, Staying Well: During and After Cancer.* Atlanta, GA: American Cancer Society; 2004.

Bostwick, DG, Crawford ED Higano, CS, Roach M, eds. *American Cancer Society's Complete Guide to Prostate Cancer.* Atlanta, GA: American Cancer Society; 2005.

Fincannon J, Bruss K. *Couples Confronting Cancer: Keeping Your Relationship Strong.* Atlanta, GA: American Cancer Society; 2003.

Living with Colorectal Cancer. New York: Colon Cancer Alliance; 2000.

National Cancer Institute. Questions and answers about smoking cessation. Available at http://cis.nci.nih.gov/fact/8_13.htm. Accessed May 3, 2004.

CHAPTER 20

American Cancer Society. *A Breast Cancer Journey: Your Personal Guidebook,* 2nd ed. Atlanta, GA: American Cancer Society; 2004.

American Cancer Society and National Comprehensive Cancer Network. Distress: treatment guidelines for patients. Available at http://www.cancer.org/docroot/CRI/content/CRI_2_4_7x_NCCN_Distress_Treatment_Guidelines_for_Patients.asp. Accessed January 19, 2005.

American Pain Foundation. *Pain Notebook, 2004.* Baltimore, MD: American Pain Foundation; 2004. Available at http://www.painfoundation.org/downloads/Notebook.pdf

Davies B. (2001) Supporting families in palliative care. In: Rolling Ferrell B, Coyle N, ed. *Textbook of Palliative Nursing.* New York: Oxford University Press; 2001:363-373.

Fincannon JL, Bruss KV. *Couples Confronting Cancer: Keeping Your Relationship Strong.* Atlanta, GA: American Cancer Society; 2003.

Given BA, Given CW, Kozachik S. (2001). Family support in advanced cancer. *CA Cancer J Clin.* 51:213-231.

Houts PS, Bucher JA. *Caregiving: A Step-by-Step Resource for Caring for the Person with Cancer at Home.* Atlanta, GA: American Cancer Society; 2003.

GLOSSARY

A

Abdominoperineal resection with permanent colostomy: a process in which the surgeon removes a portion or all of the sigmoid colon, the entire rectum, the adjacent mesentery, and the anus. A permanent colostomy is constructed and the patient wears a pouch to collect stool and gas from the colon.

Ablation: techniques that use microwaves, freezing, burning, or other similar methods to destroy a cancer without resecting (removing) it.

Acupressure: a traditional Chinese medical treatment that uses finger pressure applied in a massage-like fashion to treat symptoms.

Acupuncture: a traditional Chinese medical treatment that uses the insertion of tiny needles into the skin to treat symptoms.

Acute effects: temporary side effects that occur while a person with colorectal cancer is receiving therapy.

Adenocarcinomas: cancers of the glandular cells that line the inside layer of the wall of the colon and rectum. Almost all colorectal cancers are adenocarcinomas.

Adenoma: *see adenomatous polyps.*

Adenomatous polyps: these polyps are common and are the most likely of all polyp types to become cancers. Also called adenomas. *See also tubular adenoma and villous adenoma.*

Adhesions: this term implies scar tissue on the outer surface of a segment of the bowel that can cause it to stick to other segments of bowel or other nearby organs. This may occasionally cause mechanical obstruction of the intestines.

Adjuvant chemotherapy: chemotherapy given in addition to surgery to destroy microscopic tumor cell deposits and thereby improve treatment outcomes.

Adjuvant therapy: treatment that is used in addition to the primary therapy to increase its effectiveness (for example, chemotherapy after surgery).

Alkylating agent: a chemical agent that works directly on DNA during all phases of the cell cycle to prevent the cancer cell from reproducing. An example of an alkylating agent used as a chemotherapy for colorectal cancer is oxaliplatin (Elotaxin).

Alternative therapies: ineffective and sometimes harmful interventions falsely touted as "cures" for cancer, alternative therapies typically involve diets, vitamins, and unusual drugs and are often delivered at special clinics that may be located outside the Unites States to avoid usual regulations that govern the safety of drugs and procedures as well as the training of medical staff. It is important to distinguish alternative therapies, which can be harmful, from complementary therapies, which are generally helpful.

Anal verge: the junction between the anal canal and anal skin.

Analgesic: pain medicine.

Anastomosis: the process of surgically connecting the two ends of intestine left after the cancerous tissue is removed. The place where the two parts of the intestinal tract are joined is also called the anastomosis.

Anemia: a deficiency in the size or number of red blood cells. A low red blood cell count means less oxygen is carried to the body's cells, which can make a person feel tired or weak.

Anesthesia: medication that reduces feeling, such as pain, during the operation.

Angiogenesis: the growth of new blood vessels.

Angiography: the process of X-raying blood vessels.

Anorexia: loss of, or poor appetite, often resulting in weight loss.

Anterior resection with anastomosis: a process in which the surgeon does a radical "sphincter-sparing" proctectomy. The sigmoid colon, rectum, and the associated mesentery are resected to a point at least one to three inches below the rectal cancer. After the proctectomy, the surgeon does an anastomosis between the colon and the stump of the rectum.

Antiangiogenesis drugs: medicines that block the growth of new blood vessels in tumors.

Antimetabolite: a drug that is very similar to natural chemicals in a normal biochemical reaction in cells but is different enough to interfere with the normal division and functions of cells. Examples of antimetabolites used to treat colorectal cancer are 5-fluorouracil (5-FU, Adrucil, Fluorouracil) and capecitabine (Xeloda).

Anus: the opening at the end of the digestive tract where stool (feces) is excreted.

Ascending colon: the portion of the colon that extends upward from the cecum on the right side of the body.

Astler-Coller staging system: a modification of the Dukes staging system that uses letters A through D as a code for the extent of the cancer.

B

Barium enema with air contrast: *see double-contrast barium enema.*

Benign: noncancerous.

Biomodulator: a biologic agent that mimics some of the natural signals that the body uses to regulate growth. A biomodulator used in the treatment of colorectal cancer is leucovorin (Folinic acid).

Biopsy: the surgical removal of a small piece of tissue, which is then examined under a microscope to see if cancer cells are present.

BMI: *see body mass index.*

Body mass index (BMI): a ratio of weight to height used to determine if a person is overweight.

Bolus: a single injection of medicine.

Botanicals: include whole or parts of the plant (in contrast, pharmaceutical agents include a single compound that may be either synthetic or plant-derived). Producers of these products are not required to prove safety and effectiveness.

Bowel prep: before endoscopic procedures, the colon must be thoroughly cleansed to allow for thorough inspection. This may involve using large volumes of fluids (PEG prep), small doses of liquid laxatives combined with large volumes of clear liquids, or a laxative in tablet form along with large volumes of clear liquids.

Brachytherapy: a type of internal radiation that uses radioactive seeds or pellets to deliver high doses of radiation directly to a tumor.

C

Carcinoembryonic antigen (CEA): a tumor marker for colorectal cancer. Everyone has some CEA in their blood, but people with colon cancer will often have higher levels. This level is often used as a rough guide to monitor recurrence of cancer and as a marker of response to treatment.

Carcinogens: substances that can lead to an increased risk of cancer development.

CEA: *see carcinoembryonic antigen.*

Cecum: the first part of the large intestine, which receives the small intestinal contents. The cecum is located in the lower right part of the abdomen and has the appendix attached to it.

Chemoprevention: the use of medicines or nutritional supplements to prevent or inhibit tumor growth and/or to prevent the formation of invasive cancer from a precancerous state.

Chemopreventive agents: substances that may protect the body from cancer development.

Chemoradiation: chemotherapy and radiation combined for even greater anticancer effect.

Chemotherapy regimen: the selection of chemotherapy drug(s), method of administration, dose, and schedule for treatment.

Chemotherapy: medicine that kills existing cancer cells.

Clinical nurse specialist (CNS): a nurse who has a master's degree and specializes in such areas as oncology, psychiatry, and critical care nursing.

Clinical stage: an estimate of the cancer's stage that is established before treatment.

Clinical trials: research studies in people to determine whether new drugs or treatments are safe and effective.

Colectomy: removal of a portion of the colon. Can be partial, subtotal, or total. *See resection.*

Colon: the main part of the large intestine, made up of the cecum, the ascending colon (right segment), the transverse colon (middle section), the descending colon (left segment), the sigmoid colon (S-shaped segment just above the rectum).

Colonoscope: a longer version of a sigmoidoscope, the colonoscope is a thin, flexible, lighted tube that is inserted through the rectum into the colon. It can be hooked up to a video camera and display monitor to allow a doctor to directly inspect the entire inner lining of the colon.

Colonoscopy: the examination of the colon using a flexible, lighted instrument called a colonoscope.

Colorectal surgeon: a doctor trained in general surgery who also has advanced training in the treatment of colon and rectal problems.

Colostomy: an operation sometimes used when a portion of the large intestine (usually the rectum; less often, the colon) is removed or bypassed. The end of the remaining portion of the functioning colon is brought through the abdominal wall, creating a stoma. This results in a change of normal body function to allow the body's wastes (feces and gas) to be eliminated into a special pouch.

Complementary therapies: treatments used in addition to standard medical treatment to reduce symptoms and improve quality of life.

Computed tomography (CT) scan: a computerized diagnostic test using a highly specialized X-ray that produces cross-sectional images of the body. Also called a CAT scan.

Constipation: hard, dry stools that are difficult to pass in a bowel movement.

Crohn's disease: a disorder of the small and large intestine that is characterized by diarrhea, cramping, and loss of appetite and weight. Also called granulomatous enterocolitis.

Cryosurgery: a type of ablative surgery using freezing to destroy a tumor.

CT colonography: *see virtual colonoscopy.*

CT scan: *see computed tomography scan.*

Curative-intent therapy: a term used when the proposed treatment is intended to cure the cancer.

Cure: the term often used when a patient has had cancer, receives treatment, and all signs of the cancer disappear. However, most doctors avoid the word "cure" because it suggests cancer will never return. However, since the disappearance of the signs and symptoms of cancer in response to treatment does not necessarily mean all cancer is gone (microscopic traces may remain at the site of the primary cancer or elsewhere in the body), "remission" is generally a more useful term. *See remission.*

Cystoscope: a tube with a small camera used to examine the urinary bladder, remove biopsy samples, and perform some kinds of bladder operations. *See endoscope.*

D

DCBE: *see double-contrast barium enema.*

Deliberate model: a decision-making model in which the final choice of treatment is made by the patient.

Deoxyribonucleic acid (DNA): DNA molecules carry the genetic information necessary for the organization and functioning of most living cells and control the inheritance of characteristics.

Depression: a feeling of extreme sadness and loss of enjoyment in normally rewarding activities.

Descending colon: the portion of the colon that goes down to the left lower abdomen and connects to the sigmoid colon.

Diarrhea: an abnormal increase in the frequency and liquidity of your stools. Sometimes accompanied by abdominal pain or cramping, sweating, or nausea.

Dietary supplement: vitamins, minerals, herbs, animal products, and synthetic versions of chemicals naturally found in the body.

Dietitian: a specially trained health care professional who can help you make diet choices before, during, and after cancer treatment. A

registered dietitian (RD) has at least a bachelor's degree and has passed a national competency exam.

Digestive system: a series of organs responsible for both the digestion of food and the absorption of nutrients that extends from mouth to anus. Also called the digestive tract or gastrointestinal system.

Digital rectal examination (DRE): digital rectal examination. A test in which a doctor inserts a gloved finger into the patient's rectum to detect abnormalities.

Disparity: the unequal burden of cancer on certain racial and ethnic groups, the poor, and medically underserved populations.

DNA: *see deoxyribonucleic acid.*

Dosimetrist: a health care professional who helps plan and calculate the dosage, number, and length of radiation treatments.

Double-barrel stoma: brings both ends of a separated bowel onto the surface of the skin. The top one is functioning, and the bottom one is for mucus drainage.

Double-contrast barium enema (DCBE): a procedure that studies the colon using barium sulfate, a thick, chalky substance that allows X-ray viewing of the lining of the bowel. Also called barium enema with air contrast because air is introduced into the rectum to outline the barium and colon interface.

Down-staging: a reassessment of the cancer's stage when it shrinks due to treatment.

DPOA: *see durable power of attorney for finances* or *durable power of attorney for health care.*

DRE: *see digital rectal exam.*

Dukes staging system: a standardized classification scheme used to describe the extent of a cancer, the Dukes system uses the letters A, B, and C. Developed in the 1930s, it was the most widely used classification until recent years.

Duodenum: the first part of the small intestine, where digestive juices from the pancreas and bile from the liver and gall bladder are added to the intestinal contents.

Durable power of attorney (DPOA) for finances: a legal document that allows you to name a person to handle your finances if you are unable to handle them for yourself.

Durable power of attorney (DPOA) for health care: a legal document that allows you to name a person who will make decisions about your health care if you are unable to make them yourself. Also called a medical DPOA.

Dysplasia: abnormal changes in cells and tissues that can lead to cancer

E

Edrecolomab: a cancer vaccine under investigation.

EGF: *see epidermal growth factor.*

EGFR antagonist: epidermal growth factor receptor antagonist. An antagonist interferes with the attachment of the EGFR stimulus (growth factor), thereby interfering with its actions.

EGFR: epidermal growth factor receptor. A receptor is an "address" on the surface of a cell to which a protein (which is a stimulus to growth control) can attach.

Electrocautery: a surgical technique that uses electrical current to cauterize (burn) the tissues while it cuts to seal the blood vessels.

Electrosurgery: a type of ablative surgery using electrocautery to burn and destroy a tumor. Also called fulguration.

End stoma: brings the end of the bowel out onto the skin surface. This is usually a permanent stoma, and the rest of the bowel has either been removed or has been sewn shut inside the abdomen.

Endocavitary radiation therapy: a special technique that delivers radiation directly to a rectal cancer by using a radiation source that is passed through a special proctoscope inserted into the rectum through the anus.

Endorectal ultrasound: the use of sound waves to evaluate the extent that a rectal cancer has grown into the wall of the rectum. Also called transrectal ultrasound or TRUS.

Endoscope: a narrow, flexible fiber optic instrument that conducts light used to examine the interior of a body cavity or hollow organ such as the colon.

Endoscopy: a method of examining the interior of a body cavity or hollow organ such as the colon using an endoscope.

Epidermal growth factor (EGF): a growth factor that, if found on the surface of colorectal cells, may indicate a mechanism by which these cells can multiply. Twenty-five to 75 percent of colorectal cancer cells have abnormally high numbers of EGF receptors.

Epithelium: the layer of cells that lines the inner surface of the colon and rectum, part of the mucosa.

Excision: surgical removal of a tumor.

Excisional biopsy: the process in which an entire abnormal growth (rather than just a small tissue sample) is surgically removed so it can be tested by the pathologist.

Exploratory laparotomy: an operation to examine (explore) the organs and other parts of the body within the abdominal cavity.

Extended radical left colectomy: a type of surgery that may be used for cancers in the left transverse colon. This procedure extends the left colectomy to the right side of the transverse colon by dividing the right branch of the middle colic artery. The anastomosis connects the right transverse colon with the descending or sigmoid colon.

Extended radical right hemicolectomy: a type of surgery to treat cancers in the hepatic flexure or right transverse colon. It is similar to the radical right hemicolectomy, but it is considered extended because it reaches to the left side of the transverse colon by dividing the left branch of the middle colic artery and resecting the associated additional mesentery. The anastomosis connects the ileum and the left transverse colon.

External beam radiation: the most common type of radiation therapy, external beam radiation involves delivering radiation from a source outside of the body to a precise location inside the body.

F

False negative: a test result that says there is no cancer when there really is.

False positive: a test result that says cancer is present when it really isn't.

Familial adenomatous polyposis (FAP): a relatively rare genetic syndrome that accounts for approximately 1 percent of all colorectal cancers. Also called familial polyposis coli or adenomatous polyposis of the colon

FAP: *see familial adenomatous polyposis.*

Fatigue: a feeling of being overwhelmingly tired or drained of energy.

Fecal DNA test: an exam designed to evaluate the DNA in a stool sample.

Fecal immunochemical test: a newer, less widely used form of fecal occult blood testing that appears to be more accurate than the older method, which was based on detection of a color change.

Fecal occult blood test (FOBT): a screening test for colorectal cancer that involves examining a small sample of stool to determine if any occult (hidden) blood is present in the feces.

FOBT: *see fecal occult blood test.*

Frozen section: a slide made of frozen tissue from the biopsy, used by the pathologist to diagnose cancer. Unlike a permanent section, a frozen section can be done less than 15 minutes, and is used to help the surgeon make an immediate decision during the surgical procedure about the extent of the operation before the procedure is completed.

Fulguration: a type of ablative surgery using a controlled electric current to burn and destroy a tumor. Also called electrosurgery.

G

Gastroenterologist: a doctor who specialize in diseases of the digestive tract.

Gastrointestinal (GI) system: *see digestive system.*

Gene therapy: gene therapy involves inserting a specific gene into cells to restore a missing function or to give the cells a new function. Because missing or damaged genes cause certain diseases such as cancer, it makes sense to try to treat these diseases by adding the missing gene or fixing the damaged one.

General surgeon: a doctor trained to operate on all parts of the body, including the digestive tract.

Genetic counselor: a health professional trained to guide people through the process of obtaining accurate family history, assembly of a detailed pedigree, and helping to decide whether genetic testing should be performed.

Genetic testing: laboratory tests that are conducted to see if a person has certain inherited gene mutations known to increase the risk for a specific disease.

Grade: a measure of the aggressiveness of cancer based on how like normal cells the cancer cells appear under the microscope. Grade 1 (well differentiated) cancers are the least aggressive while grade 3 or 4 (poorly differentiated or undifferentiated) cancers are the most aggressive. Also called histologic grade.

Growth factors: hormone-like substances that activate cell growth. These often work through receptors on cell surfaces.

H

Hereditary nonpolyposis colorectal cancer (HNPCC): the most common form of hereditary colorectal cancer, accounting for approximately 3-5 percent of all colorectal cancers. Also known as Lynch syndrome.

Heredity: the transmission of characteristics from parents to children through genes.

Histology: the study of microscopic structures of tissue.

HNPCC: *see hereditary nonpolyposis colorectal cancer.*

Home equity: the difference between a home's fair market value and the unpaid balance of the mortgage.

Hyperplastic polyps: these polyps are generally not precancerous, although those that grow in the right side of the colon or are detected in multiple family members have a greater tendency to be precancerous.

Hypnosis: the induction of a deeply relaxed state followed by the use of suggestion.

I

IBD: *see inflammatory bowel disease.*

Ileostomy: an operation that brings the ileum (last part of the small intestine) through a hole in the abdominal muscles and sews an open end of the ileum to the abdominal skin so the body's wastes (feces and gas) can be eliminated into a special pouch.

Ileum: the part of the small intestine that attaches to the colon.

Immune system: defends the body against disease, infection, and foreign substances.

Immunotherapy: treatment to help a person's own immune system recognize and fight cancer.

In situ: latin for "in the original place," it refers to a noninvasive cancer

Inflammatory bowel disease (IBD): chronic diseases that cause irritation in the intestinal tract. Crohn's disease and ulcerative colitis are the most common chronic inflammatory bowel diseases.

Inflammatory polyps: nonprecancerous polyps.

Informative or consumer model: a decision-making model in which the doctor presents the information and works together with the patient to make the decision.

Informed consent: a process formalized by the signing of a document by prospective volunteers for a clinical trial that indicates their understanding of why the research is being done, what researchers want to accomplish, what will be done during the trial and for how long, what risks are involved, what, if any, benefits can be expected from the trial, what other interventions are available, and the participant's right to leave the trial at any time.

Infusion: a prolonged intravenous injection given over several hours or days.

Integrative medicine: an approach that combines conventional medical treatments with complementary therapies.

Intraoperative radiation therapy: external beam radiation or brachytherapy delivered during surgery.

Intraoperative ultrasound: ultrasound using a special probe designed for use during an operation.

Intravenous (IV): insertion through your skin into a blood vessel.

J

Juvenile polyposis: a rare syndrome characterized by growth of a particular type of polyps in the gastrointestinal tract; this condition is associated with an increased risk of developing colorectal cancer.

L

Laparoscope: a tube containing a tiny camera that allows the surgeon to see inside the abdominal cavity and perform certain operations

Laparoscopic surgery: surgery performed through multiple small incisions using specially designed surgical instruments and viewed through a laparoscope.

Large intestine: the part of the digestive system where liquid is absorbed and stool is formed and expelled from the body. The large intestine includes both the colon and the rectum.

Late effects: side effects that may emerge many months or years after cancer treatment has been given. If they arise, they tend to be permanent.

Living will: a document that gives instructions about the use of medical treatments at the end of life.

Local excision: a procedure in which superficial cancers and a small amount of nearby tissue are removed without making a major abdominal incision.

Loop stoma: brings out a loop of bowel; a plastic rod is placed beneath it and the skin is stitched shut between the two ends. An opening is made in the top of the bowel to allow drainage from both loops. This is usually a temporary ostomy.

Lymph nodes: small bean-shaped organs that make and store infection-fighting white blood cells.

Lymphocytes: white blood cells that produce antibodies and kill cells infected by viruses and other abnormal cells such as cancer cells.

Lynch Syndrome: *see hereditary nonpolyposis colorectal cancer.*

M

Magnetic resonance imaging (MRI): a type of imaging that uses a combination of radio waves and a strong magnet instead of X-rays.

Malignant: cancerous.

Margin: the edge of the tissue removed during surgery. A clear or negative surgical margin is a sign that no cancer was left behind. A positive surgical margin means that cancer cells were found at the edge of the tissue removed, suggesting some cancer remains in the body.

Massage: the manipulation of the soft tissue of whole or partial body areas to induce general improvements in health or specific physical benefits.

Median survival time: the length of time half the patients in a group will live. This is the statistic most commonly meant when you hear someone has an expected survival expressed in terms of a number of months or years. Because half the individuals will survive less than this time and half will live longer, the predicted number of months is rarely correct for the individual patient.

Medical oncologist: a doctor who is specially trained to diagnose and treat cancer with chemotherapy and other drugs.

Meditation: conscious attempts to calm the mind and body.

Mesentery: tissue that contains the blood vessels that nourish that segment of intestine as well as the lymph glands that drain the area.

Metachronous cancer: a second cancer that develops after initial cancer treatment.

Metastasis: the spread of cancer to other body sites.

Molecularly targeted therapy: treatment that targets the abnormal mechanism responsible for cancer growth. Compare to chemotherapy, which targets all rapidly dividing cells, both normal and cancerous.

Monoclonal antibody: a special infection-fighting protein cloned in a laboratory. These immune system proteins are also used to diagnose and treat some forms of cancer.

MRI: *see magnetic resonance imaging.*

Mucosa: the innermost tissue layer that forms a continuous lining of the gastrointestinal tract from the mouth to the anus.

Mucositis: the presence of inflammation and/ or ulceration of the mouth or other parts of gastrointestinal tract. In the mouth, this is also called stomatitis.

Multimodal treatment: a combination of different therapies (such as surgery and chemotherapy), each having a specific purpose in the treatment of cancer.

Muscularis mucosa: the thin muscle layer of the mucosa.

Muscularis propria: includes two thick layers of muscle fibers that line the digestive tract: one that runs lengthwise and one that encircles the bowel. These muscles control bowel motility and propulsion of waste products through the intestine.

Music therapy: the controlled use of music for clinical benefit.

N

Nausea: upset stomach or feeling of queasiness.

Neoadjuvant therapy: adjuvant therapy given before the primary treatment (for example, radiation therapy or chemotherapy to shrink a tumor before surgery).

Neutropenia: low counts of a particular type of white blood cell known as neutrophils. This condition is often a side effect of chemotherapy and can lower a person's resistance to infections.

Nurse practitioner (NP): a registered nurse who also has a master's or doctoral degree. Nurse practitioners are licensed to diagnose conditions, prescribe medications, and order diagnostic tests.

Nurse: a health professional who can monitor your condition, administer treatment, provide information, and help you adjust physically and emotionally to your cancer diagnosis.

O

Occult: invisible or hidden. *See fecal occult blood test.*

Oncology: the field of medicine concerned with the diagnosis, treatment, and study of cancer.

Oncology-certified nurse (OCN): a registered nurse who has demonstrated an in-depth knowledge of cancer care. They have passed a certification exam and can be found in all areas of oncology (cancer) practice. AOCNs, AOCNSs, and AOCNPs have achieved advanced-level oncology certification.

Osteoporosis: a decrease in bone mass and density that makes bones brittle and liable to break.

Ostomate: person with an ostomy

Ostomy nurse: *see wound, ostomy, and continence nurse.*

Ostomy: a type of surgery required when a person does not have the normal function of the bladder or bowel because of birth defects, disease, injury, or other disorders. The ostomy surgery allows for normal bodily wastes to be expelled through a stoma. Types of ostomies include colostomies, ileostomies, and urostomies. Generally, the term "ostomy" can be used to refer to the site at which the internal organ (such as the colon, in the case of a colostomy) is connected to the skin or to the operation by which that connection is made.

P

Pain specialists: doctors, nurses, and pharmacists who are experts in managing pain.

Pain: a symptom of some physical or emotional hurt or disorder. Pain can be described as acute (sharp or intense with rapid onset), chronic (persistent), breakthrough (a sudden spike in lower-level pain), visceral (pain in the organs), somatic (pain experienced in the skin and soft tissues), or neuropathic (pain caused by nerve pressure or injury).

Palliative care: the goal of palliative care is to ensure the best possible quality of life for people with cancer and their families throughout the course of disease, with a particular emphasis on pain relief and comfort care in the final stages of life.

Palliative chemotherapy: chemotherapy given if surgery is not a treatment option, which may also temporarily shrink or stabilize a tumor, thus reducing symptoms.

Pancolitis: inflammation of the entire colon as a result of inflammatory bowel disease

Papillon technique: a treatment that delivers radiation through a specially designed instrument called a proctoscope that is inserted into the rectum.

Paternalistic model: a decision-making model in which the oncologist is the primary decision maker.

Pathologic stage: determination of the cancer's stage based on tissue collected during surgery. Sometimes the pretreatment clinical stage is different from the final pathologic stage.

Pathologist: a doctor whose area of expertise is the study of diseases' effects on human tissues and the examination of cells and tissues to diagnose diseases.

Pathology report: a report from the pathologist containing the results of his or her analysis of tissue samples to the doctors who are directly caring for the patient.

Pedunculated polyps: polyps that grow on stems or stalks (called pedicles), causing them to look like mushrooms.

Pelvic exenteration: a radical surgical treatment for rectal cancer that is invading nearby organs such as the bladder, nearby pelvic bones, or the female reproductive organs.

Perforate: to puncture or produce a hole; in this case, in the bowel.

Peripheral neuropathy: lack of feeling accompanied by tingling or shooting pains caused by damage to the nerves.

Peritonitis: inflammation of the lining of the abdomen.

Permanent section: a slide made of tissue from the biopsy, used by the pathologist to diagnose cancer.

PET scan: *see positron emission tomography scan.*

Peutz-Jeghers syndrome: disease involving polyps in the gastrointestinal tract associated with dark freckled pigmentation that occurs in and around the mouth and lips and an increased risk of colorectal cancer.

Physician assistant: a health care professional licensed to practice medicine under physician supervision.

Piece-meal polypectomy: a technique that involves repeatedly using a snare to cut into and remove a polyp on the inner lining of the colon in small pieces.

Placebo: an inactive substance or treatment often used in clinical trials

Platelets: small cell fragments essential for blood clotting or coagulation.

Polyp: a growth that develops, in this case, on the lining of the colon or rectum. There are many types of polyps, some of which are precancerous.

Polypectomy: surgical removal of polyps.

Positron emission tomography (PET) scan: a scanning device that uses low-dose radioactive tracers to detect cancer in the body.

Posterior approach: a surgical approach in which the surgeon makes a skin incision in the low back area to gain access to the anal canal or lower rectum.

Presenting symptom: a symptom at the time of diagnosis

Primary care physician: the doctor who takes care of your general health needs. He or she may be a family doctor, internist, general practitioner, or gynecologist.

Proctectomy: an operation to remove the rectum.

Prognosis: the probable outcome of the course of a disease; a prediction of or a patient's chance of recovery and/or survival.

Proxy: the person you designate in a durable power of attorney to execute your decisions. Also called an agent.

Psychiatrist: a medical doctor who specializes in mental health and behavioral disorders. They can counsel you during your cancer care and also prescribe medication, if necessary, for depression or anxiety.

Psychologist: a health care professional with a doctoral degree in mental health and behavior disorders. Psychologists can counsel you during your cancer care but cannot prescribe medication.

R

Radiation oncologist: a medical doctor who specializes in treating cancer with radiation therapy.

Radiation physicist: a health care professional trained to ensure that you receive the right dose of radiation treatment as prescribed by the radiation oncologist.

Radiation therapist: *see radiation oncologist.*

Radiation therapy: the medical use of this energy to treat diseases.

Radical left colectomy: a type of surgery to treat cancers of the splenic flexure and descending colon that involves removal of the left half of the transverse colon and the descending colon. In this case, the anastomosis is between the middle portion of the transverse colon and the sigmoid colon, and is called a colocolostomy or a colocolic anastomosis.

Radical resection: an operation to remove a cancer with margins of normal intestine on either side of the cancer and to remove the adjacent mesentery that contains the blood vessels that nourish the intestine and the lymph nodes that drain the intestine in an attempt to cure the cancer.

Radical right hemicolectomy: a type of surgery to treat cancers in the cecum or ascending colon (parts of the colon in the right half of the abdomen) that removes the right half of the colon. After the colectomy, an anastomosis is done between the last part of the small intestine (ileum) and the mid-transverse colon. Also called an ileocolostomy or ileocolic anastomosis.

Radical sigmoid colectomy: a type of segmental resection surgery to treat cancers in the sigmoid. Depending on the location of the tumor, the resection may include a portion of the descending colon or a portion of the upper rectum. The anastomosis is between the descending colon and the rectum, and is also called a colocolostomy or colorectal anastomosis.

Radical subtotal colectomy: a type of surgery that involves removal of the right, transverse, and descending colon segments with the adjacent mesentery. This may be done if more than one cancer is present in different parts of the colon or if there are multiple polyps in other parts of the colon in addition to the colon cancer. The anastomosis is between the ileum and the sigmoid colon, called an ileosigmoidostomy or ileosigmoid anastomosis.

Radical total colectomy: surgical removal of the entire colon. This procedure is similar to the subtotal colectomy but also removes the sigmoid and its mesentery. The anastomosis between the ileum and the rectum is called an ileorectal anastomosis.

Radiologist: a doctor who use imaging techniques (such as X-rays or ultrasound) to see inside the body.

Radiosensitization: the use of chemotherapy medications to make cancer cells more vulnerable to radiation. Also called radiation sensitization.

Rectum: the final part of the large intestine where stool is stored until it is evacuated.

Recurrence: cancer that re-emerges after treatment because of incomplete removal of the primary cancer or from cells that spread from the original (primary) cancer to another place in the body. Recurrences are classified as local if they develop in the tissues at the site where the primary cancer was originally found, regional if they develop in the nearby lymph nodes, or distant or metastatic if they develop at sites far away from the original tumor.

Reflexology: a special type of massage given to the feet.

Registered nurse (RN): a nurse with an associate's or bachelor's degree in nursing or a diploma from a hospital-based program. He or she has also passed a state licensing exam.

Reiki: a form of massage that uses light touch.

Remission: the complete or partial disappearance of the signs and symptoms of a disease such as cancer in response to treatment. A remission does not necessarily mean that there has been a cure or a permanent disappearance of cancer.

Reporting bias: errors in the reporting of results by study participants to researchers. Blind studies, in which participants do not know whether they have received an actual treatment intervention or a placebo, tend to prevent reporting bias.

Resection: a general type of surgery in which diseased tissue is removed along with a margin of surrounding healthy tissue. For resection of a colorectal cancer, a length of normal bowel tissue on either side of the cancer, as well as the nearby lymph nodes, is usually removed (resected). Then the remaining sections of the colon are attached back together (anastomosed). A resection can be partial, limited, or radical. Also called a colectomy.

Reverse mortgage: a loan against the equity in your home that doesn't have to be repaid for as long as you live there.

Risk factor: a factor (such as age, gender, or a lifestyle choice, such as alcohol or tobacco use) that increases your chance of getting a disease such as cancer.

Risk pool: state-run guaranteed-access programs that serve people who have pre-existing health conditions and are often denied or have difficulty finding affordable coverage in the private market.

S

Sacrectomy: an operation to remove the lower sacral vertebrae, the bones around the spinal cord at the base of the spine. May be used to gain surgical access to tumors in the lower rectum.

Screening: the term doctors use when they perform tests to diagnose or rule out diseases before the patient experiences any symptoms.

Selection bias: errors in the selection and placement of study participants into groups that result in differences between groups that could affect the results of a clinical trial. Randomization tends to prevents selection bias.

Serosa: a thin membrane that produces fluid to lubricate the outer surface of the bowel so that it can slide against the organs and structures that surround it.

Sessile polyps: polyps that grow directly onto the inner wall of the colon.

Sigmoid colon: the portion of the colon that typically has an "S"-shaped turn.

Sigmoidoscope: a thin, flexible, lighted tube that is inserted through the rectum into the lower part of the colon that can be hooked up to video camera and display monitor to allow a doctor to directly view the lower third of the colon.

Sigmoidoscopy: the examination of the sigmoid colon (the lower transverse part of the colon) using a flexible, lighted instrument. Also called flexible sigmoidoscopy.

Simulation: the process of planning radiation treatment using computer technology.

Small intestine: the section of the digestive tract between the stomach and the colon where food is broken down into nutrients that the body can absorb and use.

Snare polypectomy: a process in which the doctor passes a wire through a chamber in the colonoscope and loops or snares the polyp. The polyp is removed using electrocautery.

Social worker: a trained specialist in the social, emotional, and financial needs of individuals and families. Medical social workers are health specialists with master's degrees in social work and, in most cases, are licensed or certified by the state in which they work.

Sphincter: the ring of muscle that contracts to close the anus and relaxes to allow feces to be eliminated from the body.

Spiral CT: a new generation of computed tomography that is used in virtual colonoscopy. Also called helical CT.

Stage: a measure of how widespread a cancer may be.

Staging system: a standardized classification scheme explaining the extent of a cancer that allows physicians to quickly and accurately describe a patient's cancer using a universal language that all specialists can understand.

Standard of care: the recommended treatment

Stent: a device implanted in a body part to support its structure and help keep it open

Stoma: the name for the opening that is created during surgery between the skin's surface and an organ. Can refer to the opening created from a colostomy or an ileostomy.

Stool: fecal matter.

Submucosa: the second layer of tissue that lines the gastrointestinal tract from the mouth to the anus, the submucosa contains blood vessels, lymph vessels, nerves.

Subserosa: a thin layer of connective tissue.

Surgeon: *see general surgeon.*

Surgical oncologist: a surgeon who has had advanced training in the surgical treatment of people with cancer.

Survival rate: a general measure of the percentage of patients alive after a certain interval of time.

> **Disease-free survival rate:** the percentage of patients who live a certain number of years after their initial diagnosis and don't have any evidence of cancer.

> **Five-year relative survival rate:** the percentage of patients diagnosed with cancer who live at least five years after cancer is diagnosed, excluding anyone who has died of causes unrelated to colon cancer. Relative survival rates are considered to be a more accurate measure of prognosis than five-year survival rates.

Five-year survival rate: the percentage of patients diagnosed with cancer who live at least five years after their cancer is diagnosed. *See five-year relative survival rate.*

Ten-year survival rate: the percentage of patients diagnosed with cancer who live at least 10 years after their cancer is diagnosed. Sometimes used to estimate "cure" rates.

Survivor: a word adopted by cancer advocates to refer to anyone who has been diagnosed with cancer, someone living with cancer, someone who has completed cancer treatment, or someone who has lived several years past a cancer diagnosis. The American Cancer Society considers a survivor to be anyone who defines himself or herself this way, from the time of diagnosis through the balance of his or her life.

Survivorship: the process of adjusting to life after cancer.

Synchronous cancer: a cancer found at the same time you were found to have the first such cancer but in a different place.

T

T'ai Chi: an ancient Chinese practice in which sequences of movements are performed slowly, softly, and gracefully. Sometimes described as "moving meditation."

TEM: *see transanal endoscopic microsurgery.*

Temporary colostomy: to prevent stool from reaching a part of the colon that has been surgically resected, a temporary colostomy diverts stool so it can be eliminated through the stoma, allowing the colon time to heal after surgery. Temporary colostomies are reversible and normal bowel elimination can be restored.

Temporary proximal diversion: a surgical process that temporarily diverts feces into a pouch to prevent stool from going through

the newly resected colon. Once the anastomosis is totally healed, a second operation is done six to twelve weeks later to reverse the temporary colostomy or ileostomy.

Tenesmus: spasms or cramping of the anal sphincter muscle.

TNM staging system: currently the standard staging system for colorectal cancer, the TNM system uses three elements to describe how widespread a cancer is. T stands for the extent of the primary (main) colorectal tumor, N for the extent of lymph node involvement, and M for distant metastasis (spread) to other organs or tissues. Each of these letters is followed by a number that provides more details about that element. The higher the number, the more serious the state of each element in the system.

Transanal approach: a surgical approach in which the surgeon works through the anus without a skin incision.

Transanal endoscopic microsurgery (TEM): a specialized technique used in the local treatment of sessile polyps and favorable T1 cancers of the middle to upper third of the rectum. It requires special instruments and its availability is limited to a few cancer centers.

Transverse colectomy: a type of surgery occasionally used to treat a cancer growing in the middle portion of the transverse colon. After removal of the cancer and the adjacent mesentery, the surgeon must free up both the hepatic and splenic flexures (the two "corners" of the colon) to bring the two ends of the colon together for an anastomosis.

Transverse colon: the portion of the colon that crosses the upper abdomen from right to left.

Tubular adenomas: one of two major types of adenomatous polyps found in the colon and rectum, tubular adenomas get their name from the round or tubular appearance of the glands in the polyp.

Tubulovillous adenomas: adenomas that contain both tubular and villous features. Although less common than tubular adenomas, villous and tubulovillous adenomas are more likely to give rise to cancer.

Tumor markers: proteins or other substances that can signify the presence of cancer somewhere in the body. *See carcinoembryonic antigen.*

Type 2 diabetes: a condition characterized by high blood glucose levels caused either by a lack of insulin or the body's inability to use insulin efficiently. Formerly called "adult-onset" diabetes; however, this term is no longer used because the condition may develop earlier in life.

U

Ulcerative colitis: a disease that causes ulcers and chronic inflammation of the lining of the colon that is linked to an increased risk for colon cancer.

Ultrasound: uses sound waves rather than X-rays to create images of the body.

Urgency: a feeling like you have to go to the bathroom "right now" and are unable to hold back stool. This sensation can be a symptom of colorectal cancer.

Urologist: a doctor that specializes in treating problems of the urinary tract in men and women and of the genital area in men.

Urostomy: a surgical procedure that diverts urine away from a diseased or defective bladder.

V

Vascular endothelial growth factor (VEGF): a growth factor that helps tumors develop new blood vessels and has been linked to colorectal cancer. VEGF inhibitors are used in treatment combinations.

Viatical: the sale of a life insurance policy for cash.

Villi: tiny fingerlike projections that are normally found on the surface of the mucous membrane of the small intestine (singular is villus)

Villous adenomas: less common than tubular adenomas, this type of adenomatous polyps found in the colon and rectum are so named because their glands have a villous, or frond-like, appearance under the microscope. This type is more likely than tubular adenomas to lead to cancer.

Virtual colonoscopy: an imaging procedure that uses a CT scan to create two- or three-dimensional images of the lining of the colon. Also called CT colonography.

Visualization and imagery: techniques that involve the use of visual images such as a mountain or peaceful beach scene to enhance relaxation.

Vomiting: regurgitation or "throwing up."

W

WOCN: *see wound, ostomy, and continence nurse.*

Wound, ostomy, and continence nurse (WOCN): a nurse who is specially trained to teach people how to care for an ostomy, a temporary or permanent opening that is sometimes created in the abdomen during colorectal cancer surgery. Also called an enterostomal therapist, or ET nurse.

X

X-rays: very short wavelengths of high-energy electromagnetic radiation that are used to provide images of the body.

Y

Yoga: a philosophy and exercise system that combines movement and simple poses with deep breathing and meditation to promote relaxation and to reduce fatigue.

About the Editors

Lead Editor

Bernard Levin, MD, is Vice President for Cancer Prevention and Population Sciences at The University of Texas M. D. Anderson Cancer Center in Houston. Dr. Levin was the first recipient of the Betty B. Marcus Chair in Cancer Prevention. He was chair of the ASCO Committee on Cancer Prevention from 2002-2004 and is chair of the American Cancer Society National Advisory Committee on Colorectal Cancer (1993-present) and chair of the National Colorectal Cancer Roundtable (1998-present). Dr. Levin's research interests include seeking molecular markers for detection of colorectal cancer, chemoprevention of colorectal adenomas, and better methods for enhancing public awareness of colorectal cancer prevention.

Editorial Panel

Terri Ades, MS, APRN-BC, AOCN, is Director of Cancer Information at the American Cancer Society. Before joining the American Cancer Society, Ades worked with adults and children with cancer at the Medical College of Georgia, Indiana University Medical Center in Indianapolis, the Medical University of South Carolina in Charleston, and the University of Alabama in Birmingham.

Durado Brooks, MD, MPH, is Director of Prostate and Colorectal Cancer at the American Cancer Society's national home office. A specialist in internal medicine, Dr. Brooks has spent much of his career working to improve the plight of medically underserved populations. In addition to his work in cancer control, Dr. Brooks has written and spoken extensively on disease prevention and health promotion, disparities in healthcare and health outcomes, and cultural competency of health care providers and systems.

Christopher H. Crane, MD, is Associate Professor and Program Director of gastrointestinal radiation oncology at The University of Texas M.D. Anderson Cancer Center. His research focuses on the multidisciplinary care of patients with gastrointestinal malignancies.

Paulo M. Hoff, MD, FACP, is Associate Professor of Medicine and Deputy Chairman of Clinical Research in the Department of Gastrointestinal Medical Oncology at The University of Texas M. D. Anderson Cancer Center.

Paul J. Limburg, MD, MPH, is Director of the Gastrointestinal Neoplasia Clinic at the Mayo Clinic in Rochester, Minnesota. Dr. Limburg is the Principal Investigator for the NCI-sponsored Cancer Prevention Network, a multicenter consortium that conducts clinical trials of new cancer prevention agents. He is a practicing gastroenterologist and has research interests in cancer epidemiology and cancer chemoprevention.

David A. Rothenberger, MD, is Professor of Surgery and Chief of the Division of Colon and Rectal Surgery, Department of Surgery, at the University of Minnesota. He is the Associate Director for Clinical Research and Outreach at the University's Comprehensive Cancer Center and the John P. Delaney Chair in Clinical Surgical Oncology. His clinical practice is heavily focused on rectal cancer, inflammatory bowel disease, and complex reconstructive pelvic surgery.

LIST OF CONTRIBUTORS

Lead Editor

Bernard Levin, MD, *Vice President for Cancer Prevention and Population Sciences,* The University of Texas M. D. Anderson Cancer Center, Houston, TX

Editorial Board

Terri Ades, MS, APRN, AOCN, *Director of Cancer Information,* American Cancer Society, Atlanta, GA

Durado Brooks, MD, MPH, *Director,* Prostate and Colorectal Cancer, American Cancer Society, Atlanta, GA

Christopher H. Crane, MD, *Associate Professor,* Radiation Oncology, The University of Texas M. D. Anderson Cancer Center, Houston, TX

Paulo M. Hoff, MD, FACP, *Associate Professor,* GI Medical Oncology, The University of Texas M. D. Anderson Cancer Center, Houston, TX

Paul J. Limburg, MD, MPH, *Director of Gastrointestinal Neoplasia Clinic,* Mayo Clinic, Rochester, MN

David A. Rothenberger, MD, *Professor of Surgery,* Department of Surgery, and *Chief,* Division of Colon and Rectal Surgery, University of Minnesota, and *Associate Director for Clinical Research and Outreach,* University of Minnesota Cancer Center, Minneapolis, MN

Contributing Authors

Dennis J. Ahnen, MD, *Staff Physician and Head,* Section of Gastroenterology and Hepatology, Denver VA Medical Center, and *Professor of Medicine,* University of Colorado School of Medicine, Denver, CO

Robert P. Akbari, MD, *Student Clerkship Director,* Division of Colorectal Surgery, The Western Pennsylvania Hospital, Clinical Campus of Temple University School of Medicine, Pittsburgh, PA

Aaron C. Baltz, MD, *Gastroenterology Fellow,* University of Colorado Health Sciences Center, Denver, CO

Barrie R. Cassileth, MS, PhD, *Chief,* Integrative Medicine Service, and *Laurance S. Rockefeller Chair in Integrative Medicine,* Memorial Sloan-Kettering Cancer Center, New York, NY

Maureen E. Coyle, MSW, LCSW-C, *Clinical Social Worker,* Department of Medicine/Surgery Social Work, Johns Hopkins Hospital, Baltimore, MD

Christopher Crane, MD, *Associate Professor,* Radiation Oncology, The University of Texas M. D. Anderson Cancer Center, Houston, TX

Cathy Eng, MD, *Assistant Professor,* Gastrointestinal Medical Oncology, The University of Texas M. D. Anderson Cancer Center, Houston, TX

Edward Giovannucci, MD, ScD, *Professor,* Departments of Nutrition and Epidemiology, Harvard School of Public Health, and *Associate Professor,* Channing Laboratory, Brigham and Women's Hospital and Harvard Medical School, Boston, MA

Richard M. Goldberg, MD, *Chief,* Division of Hematology and Oncology, and *Professor,* Department of Medicine, University of North Carolina at Chapel Hill, Chapel Hill, NC

Edward W. Greeno, MD, *Assistant Professor,* Department of Medicine, Division of Hematology,

Oncology, and Transplantation, and *Medical Director,* Masonic Cancer Clinic, University of Minnesota, Minneapolis, MN

Hanna Kelly, MD, *Fellow,* Department of Medicine, Division of Hematology and Oncology, University of North Carolina at Chapel Hill, Chapel Hill, NC

Amy E. Kelly, *Co-founder* and *Director,* Colon Cancer Alliance, New York, NY

Kandice L. Knigge, MD, *Assistant Professor of Medicine,* Division of Gastroenterology, Oregon Health and Science University, Portland, OR

Simon Kung, MD, *Instructor of Psychiatry,* Department of Psychiatry and Psychology, Mayo Clinic College of Medicine, Rochester, MN

Paul J. Limburg, MD, MPH, *Assistant Professor of Medicine,* Division of Gastroenterology and Hepatology, Mayo Clinic College of Medicine, Rochester, MN

Marilyn Mulay, RN, MS, OCN, *Director,* Clinical Research Unit, Premiere Oncology, Santa Monica, CA

Pamela J. Netzel, MD, *Instructor of Psychiatry,* Department of Psychiatry and Psychology, Mayo Clinic College of Medicine, Rochester, MN

Amy S. Oxentenko, MD, *Assistant Professor of Medicine,* Division of Gastroenterology and Hepatology, Mayo Clinic College of Medicine, Rochester, MN

Michelle Rhiner RN, MSN, NP, CHPN, *Patient Coordinator* and *Manager,* Supportive Care, Pain and Palliative Medicine, City of Hope National Medical Center, Duarte, CA

Rocco Ricciardi, MD, *Instructor of Surgery,* Department of Surgery, Division of Colon and Rectal Surgery, University of Minnesota, Minneapolis, MN

David A. Rothenberger, MD, *Professor of Surgery,* Department of Surgery, and *Chief,* Division of Colon and Rectal Surgery, University of Minnesota, and *Associate Director for Clinical Research and Programs,* University of Minnesota Cancer Center, Minneapolis, MN

Teresa A. Rummans, MD, *Professor of Psychiatry,* and *Consultant,* Department of Psychiatry and Psychology, Mayo Clinic College of Medicine, Rochester, MN

Catherine Tomeo Ryan, MPH, *Project Coordinator,* Harvard Center for Cancer Prevention, Boston, MA

Brenda K. Shelton MS, RN, CCRN, AOCN, *Clinical Nurse Specialist,* The Sidney Kimmel Comprehensive Cancer Center at Johns Hopkins, Baltimore, MD

Neal E. Slatkin, MD, DABPM, *Director,* Supportive Care, Pain and Palliative Medicine, City of Hope National Medical Center, Duarte, CA

Eden Stotsky, *Health Educator,* Johns Hopkins Colon Cancer Center, Baltimore, MD

Alan G. Thorson, MD, *Clinical Associate Professor of Surgery* and *Program Director,* Section of Colon and Rectal Surgery, Creighton University School of Medicine, and *Clinical Associate Professor of Surgery,* University of Nebraska College of Medicine, Omaha, NE

Andrew Vickers, PhD, *Biostatistician* and *Research Methodologist,* Integrative Medicine Service, Memorial Sloan-Kettering Cancer Center, New York, NY

Esther K. Wei, ScD, *Instructor in Medicine,* Channing Laboratory, Brigham and Women's Hospital and Harvard Medical School, Boston, MA

K. Simon Yeung, MBA, MS, RPh, LAc, *Research Pharmacist,* Integrative Medicine Service, Memorial Sloan-Kettering Cancer Center, New York, NY

INDEX

travel after, 286

types of, 274–276

what is, 272–274

Comfrey, 227

Communication

with employer and coworkers, 289, 291

getting information, 124–125

giving information, 124

with health care professionals, 342

with loved ones, 340–342

with others about ostomies, 281–282

resolving problems with, 126

taking enough time for, 125–126, 340–342

Community resources, 131–132

becoming involved with, 334

Complementary treatments, 124, 134, 221–222.
See also Alternative treatments

acupuncture and acupressure, 222, 245, 248

for anxiety and depression, 225

difference between alternative and, 222

herbs and supplements used in, 225–230

mind-body, 223

movement therapies, 224

music therapy, 224

for nausea and vomiting, 225

for pain, 224–225, 245

questions to ask about, 235

for symptoms and side effects, 224–225

therapeutic massage, 224

what are, 222–224

Complete blood count, 64

Computed tomography (CT), 64, 66–67, 197, 322

Conscious sedation, 43, 45, 46

Consolidated Omnibus Budget Reconciliation Act (COBRA), 297

Constipation, 28, 58, 244, 249

after colostomy, 283

managing, 252

Consumer Credit Counseling Service, 304

Coping with a colostomy, 280–282

Coping with diagnosis of colorectal cancer

building support networks in, 108–110

consider the whole self in, 99–101

with emotions, 101–104

after initial cancer is treated, 323

by looking ahead, 110

taking action and, 104–106

talking about cancer and, 106–108

Corticosteroids, 246, 248

CPT-11, 198, 199, 260t

Crohn's disease, 17, 52t

CT colonography, 38, 48–49

CT-guided needle biopsy, 67

D

Decision making

about enrolling in clinical trials, 212–213

patients' role in, 137–139

about treatment choices, 133–137, 206

Deep breathing, 224, 246

Denial, 37, 101

Department of Labor, U.S., 293

Depression

complementary treatments for, 225

managing, 100, 103, 245–246

Descending colostomy, 274, 276

Detection of colorectal cancer. *See* screening and early detection

Diabetes, type 2, 17

Diagnosis. *See also* screening and early detection

and grading of cancer, 73, 75

initial, 72–73

pathology reports and, 83–86

role of pathologist in, 72–75

second opinions and, 86, 128

and staging of cancer, 75–81

Diarrhea, 58, 190, 193, 203, 256–257

after colostomy, 283

managing, 251–252

NOTES

NOTES

NOTES

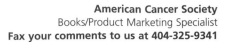
No Matter Who You Are, We Can Help.

Your feedback can help the American Cancer Society help others. Please complete this very brief "reader survey" and drop it in the mail or fax it to us today. Thank you!

The American Cancer Society respects your privacy. *Your contact information will not be distributed.*
PLEASE PRINT CLEARLY.

First Name _____   Last name _____

Street _____

City _____   State _____   Zip _____

E-mail _____

Please choose one answer for each question.

❏ Yes, I would like more information about other books published by the American Cancer Society.
I prefer to be contacted via: ❏ e-mail   ❏ US mail

I am   ❏ a patient   ❏ a caregiver   ❏ a friend or family member

I am   ❏ female   ❏ male   Age: ❏ 60+   ❏ 40–59   ❏ 20–39

I have bought or read _____ health books in the past 12 months.

American Cancer Society's Complete Guide to Colorectal Cancer

This book is for   ❏ me   ❏ someone else

How I found out about this book (please choose one):
❏ American Cancer Society—Hope Lodge _____ (location)
❏ American Cancer Society—Local Division _____ (location)
❏ 1.800.ACS.2345   ❏ www.cancer.org/bookstore   ❏ Online retailer_____   ❏ Recommendation
❏ Store display   ❏ Catalog/Mailing   ❏ Advertisement_____   ❏ TV/Radio

The most helpful parts of this book are:
❏ the organization of the book
❏ the tips shared by other patients and caregivers
❏ the resources provided at the back of the book
❏ the information about coping
❏ the information about cancer and its treatment
❏ the information about medical care and talking to my doctor
❏ the information about insurance, finances, and/or legal issues
❏ other (please specify _____)

I think that the next edition should include this topic: _____
_____

Thank you for sharing your thoughts!